Transferring Nanotechnology Concept Towards Business Perspectives

About The Centre

The Centre for Science and Technology of the Non-Aligned and Other Developing Countries (NAM S&T Centre) is an inter-governmental organisation with a membership of 47 countries spread over Asia, Africa, Middle East and Latin America. Besides this, 12 S&T agencies and academic/research institutions of Bolivia, Botswana, Brazil, India, Nigeria and Turkey are the members of the S&T-Industry Network of the Centre. The Centre was set up in 1989 to promote South-South cooperation through mutually beneficial partnerships among scientists and technologists and scientific organisations in developing countries. It implements a variety of programmes including international workshops, meetings, roundtables, training courses and collaborative projects and brings out scientific publications, including a quarterly Newsletter. It is also implementing 6 Fellowship schemes, namely, NAM S&T Centre Research Fellowship, South Africa Mineral Processing Training Fellowship, Joint NAM S&T Centre – ICCBS Karachi Fellowship, Joint CSIR/CFTRI (Diamond Jubilee) - NAM S&T Centre Fellowship, Joint NAM S&T Centre – ZMT Bremen Fellowship and Research Training Fellowship for Developing Country Scientists (RTF-DCS) in Indian institutions. These activities provide, among others, the opportunity for scientist-to-scientist contact and interaction, training and expert assistance, familiarising the scientific community on the latest developments and techniques in the subject areas, and identification of technologies for transfer between member countries. The Centre has so far brought out 64 publications and has organised 95 international workshops and training programmes.

For further details, please visit www.namstct.org or write to the Director General, NAM S&T Centre, Core 6A, 2nd Floor, India Habitat Centre, Lodhi Road, New Delhi-110003, India (Phone: +91-11-24645134/24644974; Fax: +91-11-24644973; E-mail: namstcentre@gmail.com; namstct@bol.net.in).

Transferring Nanotechnology Concept Towards Business Perspectives

— Editors —

Prof. Dr. Shogo Shimazu
and
Prof. Dr. Silvester Tursiloadi

CENTRE FOR SCIENCE & TECHNOLOGY OF THE
NON-ALIGNED AND OTHER DEVELOPING COUNTRIES
(NAM S&T CENTRE)

2016
DAYA PUBLISHING HOUSE®
A Division of
ASTRAL INTERNATIONAL PVT. LTD.
New Delhi – 110 002

Cataloging in Publication Data--DK
Courtesy: D.K. Agencies (P) Ltd. <docinfo@dkagencies.com>

International Workshop on 'Nanotechnology: Transferring Nanotechnology Concept towards Business Perspectives' (2013 : Serpong, Indonesia)
Transferring nanotechnology concept towards business perspectives / editors, Prof. Dr. Shogo Shimazu and Prof. Dr. Silvester Tursiloadi.
pages cm
Papers presented at the International Workshop on 'Nanotechnology: Transferring Nanotechnology Concept Towards Business Perspectives' organised by Centre for Science and Technology of the Non-Aligned and Other Developing Countries at Serpong during 2-4 October 2013.

ISBN 978-93-5130-877-5 (International Edition)
1. Nanotechnology--Industrial applications--Developing countries--Congresses.   I. Shimazu, Shogo, editor. II. Tursiloadi, Silvester, editor. III. Centre for Science and Technology of the Non-Aligned and Other Developing Countries.organizer. IV. Title.
T174.7.I58 2013 DDC 620.5091724   23

Centre for Science and Technology of the Non-Aligned and Other Developing Countries (NAM S&T Centre)
Core-6A, 2nd Floor, India Habitat Centre, Lodhi Road,
New Delhi-110 003 (India)
Phone: +91-11-24644974, 24645134, Fax: +91-11-24644973
E-mail: namstct@gmail.com
Website: www.namstct.org

Published by	:	**Daya Publishing House®**
		A Division of
		Astral International Pvt. Ltd.
		4760-61/23,. Ansari Road, Darya Ganj,
		New Delhi - 110 002
		Phone: 011-4354 9197, 2327 8134
		E-mail: info@astralint.com
		Website: www.astralint.com
Laser Typesetting	:	**Classic Computer Services,** Delhi - 110 035
Printed at	:	**Replica Press**

Foreword

Following the ground-breaking successes of Biotechnology and Information Technology in the 21st Century, Nanotechnology has now emerged as a new field with vast potential for applications in all perceivable areas varying from engineering to medicine and other frontiers of science and technology. The beginning of applications is evident in commercial products, although most applications are limited to the bulk use of passive nanomaterials. Globally, availability of innovation based technology and consequent products has become an indicator of prosperity of any nation. Nanotechnology has tremendous applications in the widespread industrial growth by development of new products, value additions and cost reduction. Many nanotechnology based industries have already made substantial progress, e.g., in opto-electronics with products like flat plate displays using carbon nanotubes electron field emission; devices using antimicrobial activity of nano-silver for water purification; crease free and anti-stain textile materials; nano sensors and nano probes, etc. The near future nanotechnology based products being envisaged include fuel cell, hydrogen storage devices, solar cell, super capacitors, lithium battery, microwave absorption, bullet proof jackets, drug delivery and diagnostic devices.

While many of the more developed nations have had an early lead in nanotechnology and its applications, the developing countries have also made substantial contributions despite serious limitations on their research base and budgetary support.

The present book is highly informative and brings out the efforts of developing nations with focus on growth and profitability balanced with social concerns. I am sure this effort will lead to enhanced global cooperation.

I compliment the NAM S&T Centre, particularly its Director General, Prof. Arun Kulshreshtha and his team, for this initiative in bringing out a very important publication for wider dissemination of the knowledge generated on Nanoscience and Nanotechnology with a view to enhanced South-South cooperation.

Prof. Ashutosh Sharma

Secretary to the Government of India,
Department of Science & Technology,
Ministry of Science and Technology
New Delhi - 110 016

Preface

In 21st century there have been several paradigm changes in the technology, where properties and performance of materials could be modified in many different ways more effectively and efficiently. In fact, in nanometer scale (10^{-9} m) the materials have properties and performance with unique phenomena more superior compared to micrometer scale (10^{-6} m). By rearranging or modifying material's structure in nanometer level, a certain excellent material can be obtained. That is why, nanotechnology has become center of attention in the world concerning with its applications in industrial world. For developing countries, nanotechnology can open up new avenues for research for rapid progress in priority areas.

However, it is important to note that nation's capacity to benefit from such revolutionary technology would depend on the prevailing institutional and human capacities and the embedded social culture of innovation and entrepreneurship. Successful research and technology transfer activities will depend on cooperative endeavors between developed and developing countries and between public and private institutions. In conjunction with other technologies like information technology and biotechnology, nanotechnology will usher in social and economic transformations.

Therefore, the NAM S&T Center with the Ministry of Research and Technology of the Republic Indonesia (RISTEK), Indonesian Institute of Science (LIPI), Indonesia Chemistry Society (HKI) and Indonesian Society for Nanotechnology (MNI) initiated to hold an International Workshop on Nanotechnology (IWON) with the theme "Transferring Nanotechnology Concept Toward Business Prespective". Over 150 participants including representative delegates from 31 countries participated in this event. The workhsop was conducted for three days on 2-4 October 2013 in Puspiptek, Serpong. Each delegate presented his or her report regarding the progress of nanotechnology development in his/her country.

On the last day of conference, all participants discussed and formulated a manuscript of "Serpong Declaration" to show their commitment toward the mutual development of nanotechnology in the future.

This book is a compilation of all qualified papers from participants of workshop. There are two types of papers published in this book, i.e. technical work and country report. Both were peer reviewed carefully by editors with relevant backgrounds. The subject of study varied from nanotechnology material synthesis and preparation, technology process selection and formulation, production initiative and development, till product application and market opportunity. The reviewing process was conducted by considering the similarity in case studies, research novelty, complexity of challenges and solutions, wide scope of applications and collaborative opportunities. As a result, 20 papers representing broad topic areas of workshop were selected for this publication.

We are delivering thank you very much for all stakeholders who were involved in the success of the workshop and this follow up publication- especially for our NAMs country partners.

Shogo Shimazu
Silvester Tursiloadi

Introduction

It is estimated that by ~2050 the world population may rise to around 9-10 billion, which will not only require an increased consumption of resources, but the demand pattern will also severely alter as compared to the existing scenario. To cope up with the situation, the changing society will be in need of radically new technologies. In this context, nanoscience, which began ~30 years ago as a research theme on the manipulation of materials at nano scale, presents itself as a saviour as it has undergone a revolution in these few decades and has emerged as an innovation-driven high-tech field of science penetrating to almost all spheres of lives, especially in the context of pressing global challenges such as those related to energy, healthcare, clean water and climate change. Broader societal implications indicate that globally a plethora of opportunities and windows exists and around 2 million nanotechnology workers will be needed and $1- $2.5 trillion products incorporating nanotechnology will be achieved worldwide within 2015.

Although nanotechnology is in its infancy, the governments around the world have invested almost $67 billion in last decade with the developed countries being a level ahead and possessing large number of nanotechnology companies and skilled nano-researchers, including professors and students. However, for the developing countries too this is the right time to invest in this new arena and explore cooperative ventures between developed and developing countries and between public and private institutions. Individual developing countries may take their own policy decisions to identify the facets of advancements in nanotechnology which can address their unique economic, social and environmental needs. And then these countries will benefit through South-South and North-South cooperation to make them prosperous.

In order to explore the wider prospects and share the best practices on Nanotechnology, the Centre for Science and Technology of the Non-aligned and Other Developing Countries (NAM S&T Centre) jointly with the Ministry of Research and Technology (RISTEK), Government of Indonesia and the Indonesian Institute of Sciences (LIPI), and in collaboration with Indonesian Society for Nanotechnology, organised an international workshop on 'Nanotechnology (IWoN) 2013: Transferring Nanotechnology Concept towards Business Perspectives' in Serpong, Indonesia during 2-5 October 2013. The workshop provided a valuable platform for sharing of knowledge, transfer of technology and capacity building, coordination and networking among the experts and professionals of the developing countries and was attended by 104 experts, professionals, researchers and administrators from 33 countries including Australia, Cambodia, China, Egypt, The Gambia, Hong Kong, India, Indonesia, Iran, Iraq, Japan, Kenya, Republic of Korea, Madagascar, Malawi, Malaysia, Mauritius, Myanmar, Nepal, Nigeria, Pakistan, South Africa, Sri Lanka, Sudan, Taiwan, Tanzania, Thailand, Togo, Uganda, Venezuela, Vietnam, Zambia and Zimbabwe, of which 24 were the member countries of the NAM S&T Centre. Of these, 30 participants were sponsored by the NAM S&T Centre; a resource person was invited from Japan; 31 researchers from 11 countries were from the Asia Nano Forum Society (ANF), Singapore sponsored under Asia Nanotech Camp (ANC); and 35 participants were from Indonesian R&D and academic institutions.

The present publication comprises 20 selected scientific and technical papers including those presented at the above International Workshop and some other papers contributed by eminent experts on the subject.

I gratefully acknowledge the dynamic involvement and untiring efforts of Prof. Dr. Silvester Tursiloadi of the Research Centre for Chemistry, Indonesian Institute of Sciences (LIPI), Indonesia and Prof. Dr. Shogo Shimazu of Chiba University, Japan for learned technical editing of this publication. I also appreciate the valuable services provided by the entire team of the NAM S&T Centre, in particular, Mr. M. Bandyopadhyay for overall supervision, and Ms. Radhika Tandon and Mr. Pankaj Buttan in compiling the papers and giving shape to this volume.

I hope that the information provided and suggestions and recommendations made in the papers included in this book will be a good reference material on Nanotechnology for all.

Prof. Dr. Arun P. Kulshreshtha,
Director General, NAM S&T Centre

Contents

Chapter 1

Formulation and *in vitro* Evaluation of Albumin Nanoparticles Containing Temozolomide

M. Ravikiran[1], V. Murugan[2] and B. Wilson[1]

[1]*Department of Pharmaceutics,*
[2]*Department of Pharmaceutical Chemistry,*
Dayananda Sagar College of Pharmacy, Kumaraswamy Layout,
Bangalore – 560 078, Karnataka, India

ABSTRACT

Cancer is a disease in which cells divide in an abnormal manner without any control. Temozolomide is an alkylating agent with broad spectrum anti tumor activity, mostly used for treating malignant gliomas. It is a white to off white powder with slight water. Elimination half-life is 1.29 h and 1.13 h following per orally and intraperitoneal administration respectively. Temozolomide is less stable at plasma pH and it is associated with many side effects upon oral administration. To deliver temozolomide to targeted tumor site and to avoid side effects after administration, the stability of temozolomide under physiological conditions has to be improved. It is reported that nanoparticles can deliver drugs to cancer cells at a controlled rate. Recently, albumin based nanoparticles are used by researchers for targeting owing to its biodegradability, biocompatibility and its versatility. The objective of the present study was to formulate and evaluate albumin nanoparticles containing temozolomide. The albumin nanoparticles containing the drug temozolomide were prepared by desolvation method. The particles were characterized for size, charge, and drug loading. The in vitro release studies showed a bi-phasic drug release. Drug release from the particles was diffusion controlled and the mechanism was Fickian.

Keywords: Temozolomide, Albumin nanoparticles, Anticancer.

INTRODUCTION

Cancer is a type of disease in which cells divide in an abnormal manner without any control. Moreover, the cancer cells are able to enter into other tissues. Cancers are, generally, named after the organ they affect (Anonymous, 2011a). It is highly difficult to specify the exact cause for cancer. It is known that many factors increase cancer risk. They are usage of tobacco, exposure to radiation, infection, deficient in physical activities, improper diet, obesity, and environmental pollutants. Life style and environment attribute for 90–95 per cent cases, while 5–10 per cent of cases can be due to genetic defects (Anand *et al.*, 2008). In 2008, about 12.7 million people were suffered by cancer worldwide and about 7.6 million people died because of cancer (Jemal *et al.*, 2007). Every year about 440000 people die because of various types of cancers in India and 7 to 9 lakhs of new cases are diagnosed (Anonymous, 2011b). About 70 per cent of all cancer deaths occurred in low- and middle-income countries. It is estimated that in 2030 over 13.1 million people will be suffered by cancer globally (Anonymous, 2011c). All these factors tell about the need for active research in this field.

Nanoparticles, for drug delivery, are generally made of polymers in which the active principle is dissolved, entrapped, or encapsulated, and their size ranges from 1nm to 1000 nm (Sivabalan *et al.*, 2011). Recently, drug targeting especially targeting of drugs by nanoparticles have been getting much attention by the researchers for treating cancer. Nanoparticles have been successfully used to deliver anticancer drugs into tumor cells. The natural leaky vasculature along with enhanced penetration and retention effect of cancerous tissues provide advantages in treating cancer using nanoparticles (Peppas and Blanchette, 2004). Albumin is one of the most commonly used polymers for making nanoparticles (Davaran *et al.*, 2006).

Temozolomide is an anticancer drug belonging to class of alkylating agents. It appears as a white to off white non-hygroscopic powder that is freely soluble in dimethylsulfoxide, slightly soluble in water and acetonitrile and very slightly soluble in methanol (Anonymous, 2011d). Temozolomide has broad spectrum anti-umor activity. It is used for treating brain tumors specifically glioblastoma multiformae, astrocytoma and also useful in the treatment and prevention of brain metastases in melanoma patients (Narayanan, 1992). Unfortunately temozolomide usage is restricted due to side effects such as cardiomyopathy owing to the accumulation of drug. It also produces acute toxicities such as bone marrow depression and oral ulcerations (Du, 2000). Hence, an attempt was made to prepare temozolomide loaded albumin nanoparticles in the present study.

MATERIALS AND METHODS

Temozolomide was a kind gift from Celon Laboratories Ltd., Hyderabad,India. Bovine serum albumin was purchased from Central Drug House, India. All the other chemicals used for the study were analytical grade.

Preparation of Temozolomide Loaded Bovine Serum Albumin Nanoparticles

Temozolomide loaded albumin nanoparticles were prepared by desolvation method. Accurately weighed quantity of temozolomide was added to albumin solution that was made up between pH 5-6 with 0.1N HCl and incubated for 1 h (Das *et al.*, 2005). Ethanol was added to this at a rate of 1 ml/min under continuous magnetic stirring at 500 rpm. The formed nanoparticles were cross linked with 100 µl of 4 per cent glutaraldehyde-ethanol and stirring was continued at room temperature for another 3 h (Vijayarajkumar and Jain, 2007). Dried nanoparticles were obtained by freeze drying the nanosuspension (Das *et al.*, 2005).

Characterization

Particle Size Analysis

Malvern system was used to determine the particle size, with vertically polarized light supplied by an argon-ion laser (Cyonics) operated at 40 mW. Experiments were carried out at a temperature of $25 \pm 0.1°C$. The measuring angle was 90° to the incident beam (Vijayarajkumar and Jain, 2007).

Surface Charge Analysis

Charge of the nanoparticles was determined by a Malvern Zetasizer. Measurements were done at $25 \pm 0.10°C$. For this, particles were dispersed in distilled water and measured (Vijayarajkumar and Jain, 2007).

Determination of Percentage Drug Loading Capacity

Drug loading was determined by extracting the drug completely from known amount of particles in pH 1.2 acidic buffer (Huang *et al.*, 2008). The drug concentration in the solution was determined spectrophotometrically at a wavelength of 329 nm against blank.

In vitro Drug Release Studies

Drug release from nanoparticles was studied by dialysis method. Nanoparticles equivalent to 5 mg drug were transferred into a dialysis bag, and to this 1 ml of dissolution media was added. It was arranged such that the dialysis membrane was completely immersed into the dissolution medium in receptor compartment, which was stirred continuously at 100 rpm maintained at 37°C. At regular time intervals samples were collected and the same were replaced with fresh medium and drug concentration in the samples were determined by UV spectrophotometer at a wavelength 329 nm against blank.

Release Kinetics

The *in vitro* release study data was fitted to kinetic models such as zero order, first order, Higuchi model and Kosmeyer-Peppas model to find out mechanism of drug release (Costa and Lobo, 2001).

RESULTS AND DISCUSSION

Albumin nanoparticles containing temozolomide were prepared by desolvation method. Ethanol was added to facilitate the formation of nanoparticles. Glutaraldehyde-ethanol solution was added as cross linking agent and also to harden the coacervates. The particle size was determined by Zetasizer (Malvern system). The mean particle size was found to be 160.42 nm (Figure 1.1). Nanoparticles have the ability to change the biodistribution and pharmacokinetics of drugs. This is important and plays a central role for therapeutic applications. Moreover, the size and charge play an important role in the interaction between the particles and tissue surface followed by their uptake by cells. Nanoparticles made of hydrophilic polymers have longer circulation in blood which inturn enhance the targeting efficiency.

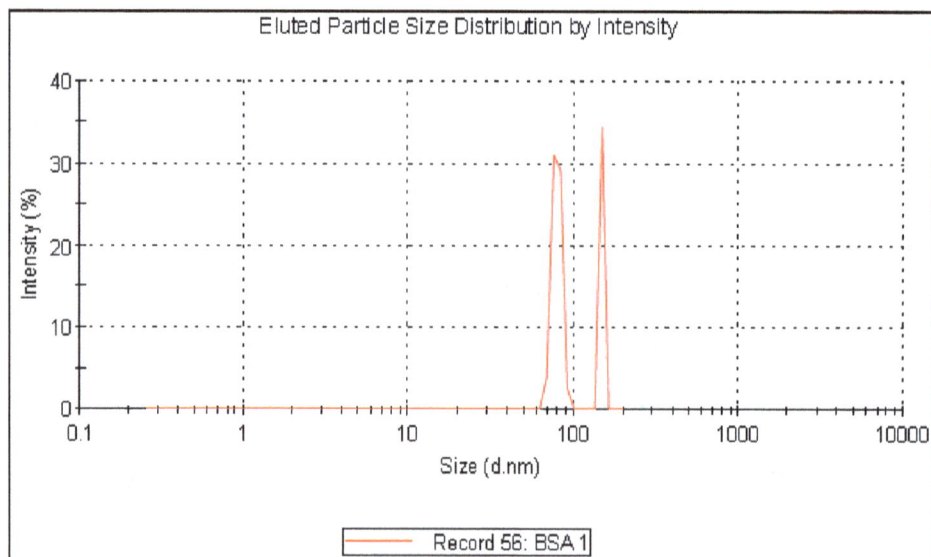

Figure 1.1: Particle Size Distribution of Temozolomide Loaded Bovine Serum Albumin Nanoparticles

Nanoparticles' surface charge was determined in distilled water by Zetasizer (Malvern systems). Zeta potential of drug loaded particles was found to be -33.6 mV. (Figure 1.2). The zeta potential tells about the particles' charge which is important for products stability. Larger the value then more repulsive interactions between particles and more stable the product.

The prepared nanoparticles showed a high drug loading capacity of 29.10 w/v per cent. More percent of drug loading is one of the desired criteria to minimize the solid content per ml during injection. The *in vitro* drug release of drug temozolomide from the nanoparticle formulation was carried out by using dialysis method in 1.2 pH acidic buffer for 24 h. The temozolomide release from the nanoparticles was 92.75 per cent which indicates the ability of particles to release the drug in a sustained manner.

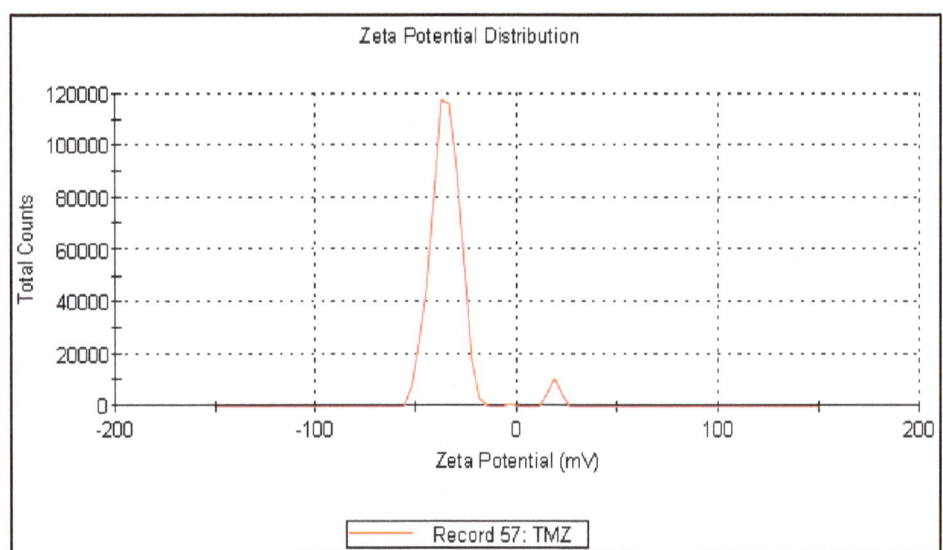

**Figure 1.2: Zeta Potential Distribution of Temozolomide Loaded
Bovine Serum Albumin Nanoparticles**

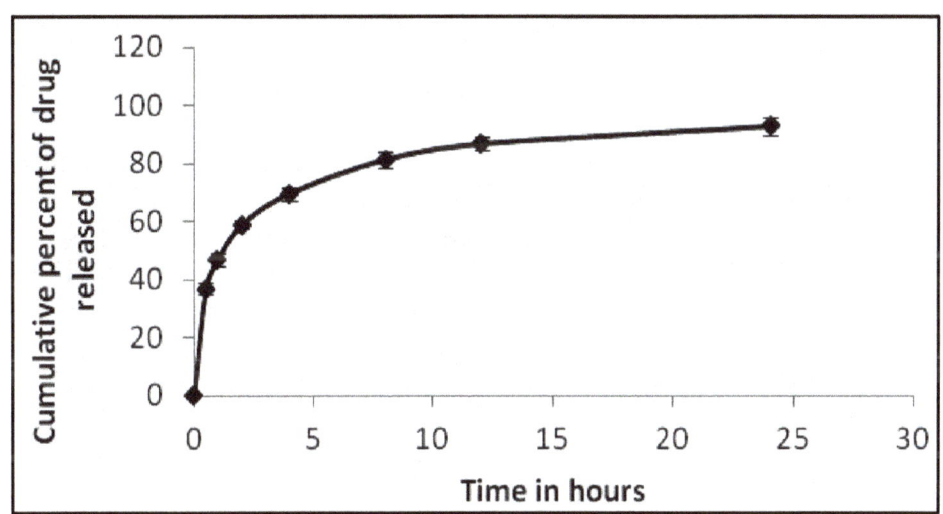

**Figure 1.3: *In vitro* Release of Temozolomide from
Bovine Serum Albumin Nanoparticles**

Release kinetics study revealed that temozolomide release was diffusion controlled as indicated with higher r^2 values in Higuchi model. Korsmeyer-Peppas model showed an n value of 0.45 indicating the release mechanism was Fickian.

CONCLUSIONS

Present study deals with the development of nanoparticulate delivery system for slightly water soluble drug temozolomide. Bovine serum albumin nanoparticles of drug temozolomide were prepared by desolvation method. The method produced small and uniform sized nanoparticles with good drug loading efficiency. Nanoparticles were able to sustain the drug release for a period of 24 h. The temozolomide release from the particles was diffusion controlled and the mechanism was Fickian. Hence, it can be concluded that the formulated nanoparticulate delivery system of slightly water soluble drug temozolomide using albumin was capable of exhibiting sustained release properties for a period of 24 h. This may reduce dose needed for the therapy and minimize dose relared side effects. But, it requires further studies to consider as a drug delivery system.

REFERENCES

1. Anand, P., Kunnumakkara, A.B., Sundaram, C., Harikumar, K.B., Tharakan, S.T., Lai, O.S., Sung, B., Aggarwal, B.B., 2008. Cancer is a preventable disease that requires major lifestyle hanges. *Pharm Res*, 25 (9): 2097–116.

2. Anonymous, 2011a. Htpp://www.cancer.gov/cancertopics/cancerlibrary/what-is-cancer. Accessed on 11/11/2011.

3. Anonymous, 2011b. http://www.globalcancer.org/WhatIsCancer.aspx. Accessed on 11/11/2011.

4. Anonymous, 2011c. http://www.who.int/mediacentre/factsheets/fs297/en/ Accessed on 11/11/2011.

5. Anonymous, 2011d. European medical agency. Temozolomide SUN. CHMP assessment report.

6. Costa, P., Lobo, J.M.S., 2001. Modeling and comparison of dissolution profiles. *Eur J Pharm Sci*, 13, 123-133.

7. Das, S., Banerjee, R., Bellare, J., 2005. Aspirin loaded albumin nanoparticles by coacervation: Implications in drug delivery. *Trends Biomater*, 18(2):203-212.

8. Davaran, S., Rashidi, M.R., Pourabbas, B., Dadashzadeh, M., Haghshenas, N.M., 2006. Adriamycin release from poly(lactide-co-glycolide)-polyethylene glycol nanoparticles: synthesis and *in vitro* characterization. *Int J Nanomed*, 1(4):535-539.

9. Du, X.L., 2000. Temozolomide: a new drug for the treatment of intractable and polymorphism glioma. *Chin Pharm J*, 35:135.

10. Huang, G., Zhang, N., Bi, X., Dou, M., 2008. Solid lipid nanoparticles of temozolomide: Potential reduction of cardial and nephric toxicity. *Int J Pharm*, 355: 314–320.

11. Jemal, A., Bray, F., Center, M.M., Ferlay, J., Ward, E., Forman, D., 2011. Global cancer statistics. *CA Cancer J Clin*, 61(2): 69–90.

12. Narayanan, S.R., 1992. Immobilized proteins as chromatographic supports for chiral resolution. *J Pharm Biomed Anal*,10(4): 251-262.

13. Peppas, L.B., Blanchette, J.O., 2004. Nanoparticle and targeted systems for cancer therapy. *Adv Drug Deliv Rev*, 56:1649-1659.

14. Sivabalan, M., Anto, S., Phaneendhar, R., Vasudevaiah., Anup, J., Nigila, G., 2011. Formulation and evaluation of 5-fluorouracil loaded chitosan and Eudragit® nanoparticles for cancer therapy. *Pharmacie Globale (IJCP)*, 1 (07): 1-4.

15. Vijayarajkumar, P., Jain, N.K., 2007. Suppression of agglomeration of ciprofloxacin-loaded human serum albumin nanoparticles. *AAPS Pharm Sci. Tech.*, 8(1): E1-E6.

Chapter 2

Transferring Nanotechnology Concept for Industrial Use: Applications of Nanotechnology for Agriculture, Food and Medicine

Parul Sehgal

Research Assistant,
Centre for Science and Technology of the Non-Aligned and
Other Developing Countries (NAM S&T Centre), New Delhi, India
E-mail: parulsehgal1989@gmail.com

ABSTRACT

Nanoscale science, engineering, and technology, more widely known using the novel term 'nanotechnology', is an emerging interdisciplinary area of research dealing with the processes that occur at molecular level and of nanolength scale size that can have enormous potential impact on all areas of the society. Since the US National Nanotechnology Initiative was announced in the year 2000, almost every developed and developing economy has initiated national nanotechnology programs. According to an estimate, an amount of $10 billion is currently spent per year across the world on nanotechnology research and development, which is projected to grow by 20 per cent over the next three years.[1]

Vast opportunities have opened up for significant applications of nanotechnology for developing industrial products in diverse fields such as agriculture, processed food products, pharmaceuticals, cosmetics, textiles, environmental sciences, chemical engineering, high performance materials, electronics and communications, optics, sensors, energy production, and construction etc. As of March 10, 2011, the Project on Emerging Nanotechnologies estimated that over 1300 manufacturer-identified nanotech products are publicly available, with new ones hitting the market at a pace of 3–4 per week.[2]

Nanotechnology has great potential for application in agriculture for plant disease diagnostics and plant protection, crop improvement, post-harvest management, food technology etc. Nanotechnology-based food products, and food packaging materials have been developed and are already available to consumers in some countries and more products and applications are currently in the research and development stage. Applications of nanotechnology in the food industry can be utilized to detect microorganisms in packaging, or produce stronger flavours and colour quality, and help provide enhanced barrier performance.

Pharmaceutical nanotechnology presents revolutionary opportunities to fight against many diseases including diabetes mellitus, respiratory disorders, neurodegenerative diseases, AIDS etc. and has led to more improved diagnosis and treatment of disease at a molecular level. It helps in detecting the microorganisms and viruses associated with various infections.[3] Drug delivery is one of the areas where this technology has made remarkable progress. It is predicted that nanotechnology will revolutionize the diagnostics, imaging and therapy segments of healthcare and in next ten years market will be flooded with nanotechnology-devised medicine or nanomedicine.

The purpose of this paper is to provide an overview of nanotechnology and its applications, with particular focus on food, agriculture and medicine.

Keywords: Nanotechnology, Pharmaceutical nanotechnology, Nanomedicine, Drug delivery.

INTRODUCTION

The term nanotechnology comes from the combination of two words: the Greek numerical prefix nano referring to a billionth and the word technology. It is a multidisciplinary field of applied science and technology dealing with the processes occurring at molecular level and Nanoscale *i.e.* 10^{-9}. Nanotechnology or Nanoscaled Technology is generally considered to be at a size below 100 nm (a nanometer is one billionth of a meter, 10^{-9} m) and below this level, the resulting materials exhibit physical and chemical properties that are significantly different from the properties of macro scale materials composed of the same substance.

Nanomaterials with unique properties such as: nanoparticles carbon nanotubes, fullerenes, quantum dots, quantum wires, nanofibers, and nanocomposites allow completely new applications to be found. Products containing engineered nano-materials are already in the market. The range of commercial products available today is very broad, including metals, ceramics, polymers, smart textiles, cosmetics, sunscreens, electronics, paints and varnishes. However new methodologies and instrumentation have to be developed in order to increase our knowledge and information on their properties.[4]

What's so Special about the Nanoscale?

Nanotechnology is not simply working at ever smaller dimensions; rather, working at the nanoscale enables scientists to utilize the unique physical, chemical, mechanical, and optical properties of materials that naturally occur at that scale.

When particle size is made to be nanoscale, properties such as melting point, fluorescence, electrical conductivity, magnetic permeability, and chemical reactivity change as a function of the size of the particle.[5]

A fascinating and powerful result of the quantum effects of the nanoscale is the concept of "tunability" of properties. That is, by changing the size of the particle, a scientist can literally fine-tune a material property of interest (*e.g.*, changing fluorescence color; in turn, the fluorescence color of a particle can be used to identify the particle, and various materials can be "labeled" with fluorescent markers for various purposes). Over millennia, nature has perfected the art of biology at the nanoscale. Many of the inner workings of cells naturally occur at the nanoscale. For example, hemoglobin, the protein that carries oxygen through the body, is 5.5 nanometers in diameter. A strand of DNA, one of the building blocks of human life, is only about 2 nanometers in diameter.[5]

Many medical researchers are working on designing tools, treatments, and therapies that are more precise and personalized than conventional ones—and that can be applied earlier in the course of a disease and lead to fewer adverse side-effects.

Nanoscale materials have far larger surface areas than similar masses of larger-scale materials. As surface area per mass of a material increases, a greater amount of the material can come into contact with surrounding materials, thus affecting reactivity. This makes them better catalysts and also makes nanostructured membranes and materials ideal for water treatment and desalination.

Scientists have recognized potential uses of nanotechnology in a wide range of applications such as pharmaceutics, cosmetics, processed food, chemical engineering, high-performance materials, electronics, precision mechanics, optics, energy production, and environmental sciences. This paper attempts to review nanotechnology applications in a few important sectors such as food, agriculture and medicine.

The current picture of Pharmaceutical Nanotechnology includes development of nanomedicine, tissue engineering, biosensors, diagnostic tools, new drugs and drug delivery, biomarkers etc.

Thus in the coming years advancements in this field will lead to improvement in drug delivery as well as in other areas of medicine.

APPLICATIONS OF NANOTECHNOLOGY IN THE FOOD SECTOR

The term "nanofood" describes the food which has been cultivated, produced, processed or packaged using nanotechnology techniques or tools, or to which manufactured nanomaterials have been added.[6] Nanofood has, in fact, been part of food processing for centuries, since many food structures naturally exist at the nanoscale.[7] The applications of nanotechnology for the food sector fall into the following main categories[8]:

☆ Where nano-sized, nano-encapsulated or engineered nanoparticle additives have been used

☆ Where food ingredients have been processed or formulated to form nanostructures

☆ Where nanomaterials have been incorporated to develop improved, active, or intelligent materials for food packaging or in food contact materials or surfaces

☆ Where nanotechnology-based devices and materials have been used, *e.g.* for nanofiltration, water treatment

☆ Where nanosensors have been used for food safety and traceability and contaminant detection.

Biologists and nanotechnologists have recognized potential uses of nanotechnology in almost every sphere of the food industry (Figure 2.1). Examples in agriculture (pesticide and vaccine delivery; detection of pathogens; and targeted genetic engineering, etc.) in food processing (nanoencapsulation of avor or odour enhancers; food textural or quality improvement; viscosifying agents, etc.) in nutrient supplements (*e.g.*, nutraceuticals with higher stability and absorption) and in food packaging (*e.g.*, sensing and signalling of information; UV-protection; improvement of plastic materials barriers) which is the most identified and flourishing area of food nanotechnology.

The main areas of application include food packaging and food products that contain nanosized or nanoencapsulated ingredients and additives. The potential for food nanotechnology applications seems unlimited. All facets of the food industry from ingredients to packaging to food analysis methods are already looking into nanotech applications. These are resulting in numerous promising applications for

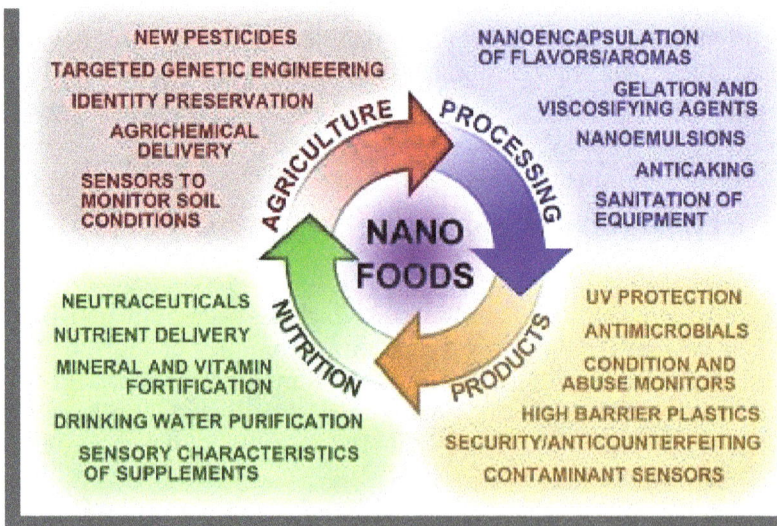

Figure 2.1: Applications of Nanotechnology in the Food Industry
Source: Duncan, 2011

improved food production, processing, packaging, and storage. Bacteria identification and food quality monitoring using biosensors; intelligent, active, and smart food packaging systems; nanoencapsulation of bioactive food compounds are a few examples of emerging applications of nanotechnology for the food industry.

The main areas of application include food packaging and food products that contain nanosized or nano-encapsulated ingredients and additives. The main principle behind the development of nanosized ingredients and additives appears to be directed towards enhanced uptake and bioavailability of nanosized substances in the body, although other beneûts, such as improvement in taste, consistency, stability and texture, etc., have also been claimed.[9]

Bacteria identification and food quality monitoring using biosensors; intelligent, active, and smart food packaging systems; nanoencapsulation of bioactive food compounds are a few examples of emerging applications of nanotechnology for the food industry.

Carbon nanotubes can be used in food packaging to improve its mechanical properties. It has been recently discovered that carbon nanotubes exhibited powerful antimicrobial effects and *Escherichia coli* bacteria died on immediate direct contact with aggregates of carbon nanotubes. In fact, the long, thin nanotubes puncture *E. coli* cells, causing cellular damage.

Processed Nanostructures in Food

Another area of application of nanotechnology in food processing includes nanostructures/nanotextures in foods.

This gives new tastes, improved textures, consistency and stability compared with other conventional products. Another area of application involves the use of nanosized or nano-encapsulated food additives.

Nanoencapsulation

Nanoencapsulation is defined as a technology to pack substances in miniature making use of techniques such as nanocomposite, nanoemulsification, and nanoestructuration and provides final product functionality that includes controlled release of the core. The protection of bioactive compounds, such as vitamins, antioxidants, proteins, and lipids as well as carbohydrates may be achieved using this technique for the production of functional foods with enhanced functionality and stability.

Nano-encapsulation offers benets that are similar to, but better than, those of microencapsulation, in terms of preserving the ingredients and additives during processing and storage, masking unpleasant tastes and avours, controlling the release of additives, better dispersion of water-insoluble food ingredients and additives, as well as improved uptake of the encapsulated nutrients and supplements. After food packaging, nano- encapsulation is currently the largest area of nanotechnology application in the food sectors, and a growing number of products based on nanocarrier technology are already available on the market.[10]

Lipid-based nanoencapsulation systems enhance the performance of antioxidants by improving their solubility and bioavailability, *in vitro* and *in vivo* stability, and preventing their unwanted interactions with other food components.

Nanoliposome technology is used for encapsulation and controlled release of food materials, as well as the enhanced bioavailability, stability and shelf-life. Nanoencapsulation can also be used to design de novo vaccines.

Nano-Packaging

When food will not be consumed immediately after production, it must be contained in a package that serves numerous functions. In addition to protecting the food from dirt or dust, oxygen, light, pathogenic microorganisms, moisture, the packaging must also be safe under its intended conditions of use, inert, cheap to produce, light-weight, easy to dispose of or reuse, able to withstand extreme conditions during processing or lling, impervious to a host of environmental storage and transport conditions, and resistant to physical abuse.

The main areas of application include the following:

☆ Improved packaging properties (flexibility, gas barrier properties, temperature/moisture stability, light and flame resistance, transparency, mechanical stability)

☆ Nanoparticles with antimicrobial or oxygen scavenging properties

☆ "Intelligent" or "smart" food packaging: Nanosensors for sensing and signalling of microbial and biochemical changes, release of antimicrobials, antioxidants, enzymes, flavours and nutraceuticals to extend shelf-life

☆ Biodegradable polymer–nanomaterial composites by introduction of inorganic particles, such as clay, into the biopolymeric matrix and can also be controlled with surfactants that are used for the modification of layered silicate (Sozer and Kokini, 2009; Chaudhry *et al.*, 2008; Miller and Sejnon, 2008; Joseph and Morrison, 2006; Doyle, 2006; Lopez- Rubio *et al.*, 2006; Brody, 2007)

NANOTECHNOLOGY IN THE AGRICULTURE SECTOR

Agriculture is an integral part of the wider biological industry. Given that the world of biology is at the scale of microns and below region where the sphere of nanotechnology resides, the convergence of biotechnology, bioengineering and nanobiology to solve practical problems facing agricultural is logical.

1. Nanosensors to monitor the health of crops and farm animals and magnetic nonoparticles to remove soil contaminants. Dispersed throughout fields, a network of nano-sensors would relay detailed data about crops and soils. The sensors will be able to monitor plant conditions, such as the presence of plant viruses or the level of soil nutrient.

2. Livestock may be identified and tracked using implanted **nanochips** (Holden and Ortiz, 2003).

3. **Animal feed**: Researchers have developed a nanoparticle that adheres to E. coli consisting of a polystyrene (PS) base, polyethylene glycol (PEG) linker, and mannose targeting biomolecule. These nanoparticles are designed to be administered through feed to remove food-borne pathogens in the GI tracts of livestock, and their potential risks, benefûts and societal issues have been explored (Kuzma *et al.*, 2008).

4. **Agrochemicals:** Nanoparticles or nanocapsules could provide a more efficient means to distribute pesticide and fertilizers reducing the quantitites of chemicals released into the environment.

5. **Crop Improvement:** The genetic constitution of the crop plants can be modified using Nanotechnology leading to crop improvement.

6. **Therapeutics**: A wide range of applications of nanobiotechnology are found in the areas like disease prevention, diagnosis, and treatment including gene therapy.

   (*a*) **Nanovaccines:** Nanobeads (10-500 nm) are used as adjuvants in injected formulations of microparticles (1-100μm) of DNA vaccines are effective in stimulation of both B and T cell immunity.

   (*b*) **Disease diagnosis and drug delivery:**

   (*i*) **Dendrimers** are synthetic polymers, a thousand times smaller than cells which can be used in the diagnosis, treatment and eradication of malignant tumors in animals.

   (*ii*) **Buckyballs,** another category of nanomaterials, are a novel form of carbon and are only a nanometer long, smooth and round. They are inert and nontoxic and because of their size they can easily interact with cells, proteins and viruses. Because of them being hollow inside, pharmacological agents can be put inside them.

   (*iii*) Diseases are one of the major factors limiting crop productivity. The problem with the disease management lies with the detection of the exact stage of prevention. Nano-based viral diagnostics and biomarkers have taken momentum in order to detect the exact strain of virus and stage of application of some therapeutic to stop the disease. These nano-based diagnostic kits not only increase the speed of detection but also increase the power of the detection.

   (*iv*) Nanoparticles have been effectively used in drug delivery with drugs or antigens encapsulated in **biodegradable nanoparticles**.

   (*v*) Monomeric polypeptides are used as a **nanotube** with the encapsulated drug molecule.

   (*vi*) Quantum dots may also be injected into the bloodstream of animals and they may detect cells that are malfunctioning. Because quantum dots respond to light it may be possible to illuminate the body with light and stimulate the quantum dot to heat up enough to kill the cancerous cell.

(c) **Gene Therapy:** Nanotechnology based gene therapy has minimal side effects on normal cells. In-vivo gene transfer with DNA- nanoparticle suspension is effective for targeted drug delivery for wound healing.

APPLICATIONS OF NANOTECHNOLOGY IN PHARMA-CEUTICALS INDUSTRY AND MEDICINE

Nanomedicine involves utilization of nanotechnology for the benefit of human health and well being. Nanoparticles are used for diagnostics, therapeutics and as biomedical tools for research. A greater degree of cell specificity improves efficacy and minimizes adverse effects. Diagnostic methods with greater degree of sensitivity aid in early detection of the disease and provide better prognosis. Various nano materials like fullerenes, nanotubes, quantum dots, nanopores, dendrimers, liposomes, magnetic nanoprobes and radio controlled nanoparticles are being developed.[11] Table 2.1 shows various nanosystems along with their characteristics and applications. Some of them are described below:

1. Carbon Nanotubes

Carbon nanotubes are hexagonal networks of carbon atoms, 1 nm in diameter and 1–100 nm in length, as a layer of graphite rolled up into a cylinder. There are two types of nanotubes: single-walled nanotubes (SWNTs) and multi-walled nanotubes (MWNTs), which differ in the arrangement of their graphene cylinders (Figure 2.2).

These are characterized by greater strength and stability hence can be used as stable drug carriers. Cell specificity can be achieved by conjugating antibodies to carbon nanotubes with fluorescent or radiolabelling. Entry of nanotubes into the cell may be mediated by endocytosis or by insertion through the cell membrane.

It was observed that carbon nanotubes, when bonded with a peptide produce a higher immunological response compared to free peptides. This property can be used in vaccine production to enhance the efficacy of vaccines.

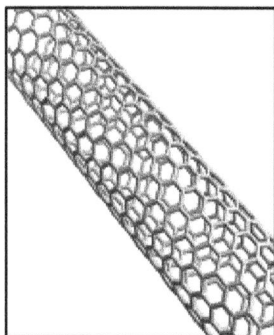

(a) Single Walled (SWNTs)   (b) Multi Walled (MWNTs)

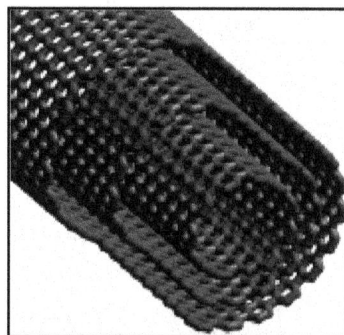

Figure 2.2: Structure of Carbon Nanotubes

Source: (a) www.3dchem.com/ images of molecules/Buckytubes2.jpg
(b) www.msm.cam.ac.uk/./msps100/cutMWNT.jpg

2. Quantum Dots

Quantum dots are nanocrystals measuring around 2-10 nm which can be made to fluorescence when stimulated by light. Their structure consists of an inorganic core, the size of which determines the colour emitted; an inorganic shell and an aqueous organic coating to which biomolecules are conjugated. The biomolecule conjugation of the quantum dots can be modulated to target various biomarkers. Quantum dots can be used for biomedical purposes as a diagnostic as well as therapeutic tool. These can be tagged with biomolecules and used as highly sensitive probes.

3. Dendrimers

Cavities within the dendrimer molecule can be used for drug transport. The ends of the dendrimer molecule can be attached with other molecules for transport. Dendrimers can be used for gene therapy.

4. Liposomes

They are spherical nanoparticles used as effective drug delivery systems made up of lipid bilayer membranes with an aqueous interior but can be unilamellar with a single lamella of membrane or multilamellar with multiple membranes (Figure 2.3). These can be loaded with drugs either in the aqueous compartment (water soluble drugs) or in the lipid membrane (lipid soluble drugs). The major limitation is their rapid degradation and clearance by the liver macrophages.

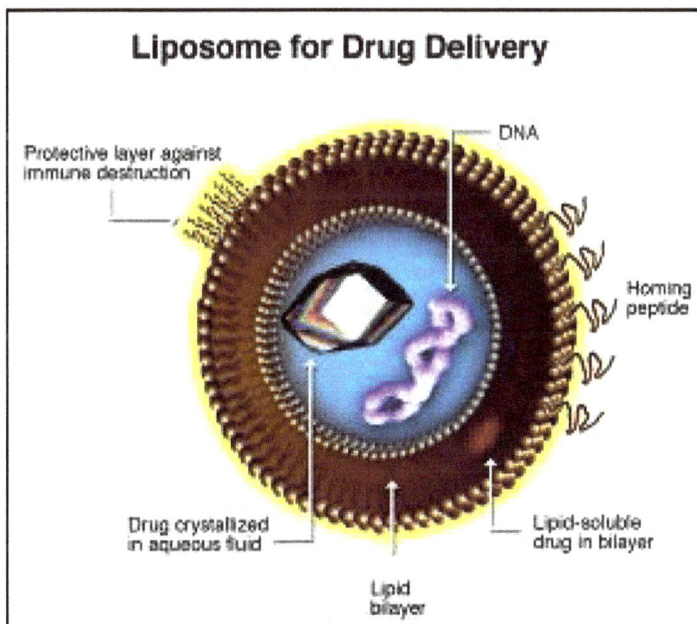

Figure 2.3: Liposome Structure
Source: Torchilin, V (2006). "Multifunctional nanocarriers". *Advanced Drug Delivery Reviews* 58 (14): 1532 55. doi:10.1016/j.addr.2006.09.009.PMID 17092599

Table 2.1: Brief Descriptions of Nanosystems (Nahar et al., 2006)

Types of Nanosystems	Size	Characteristics	Applications
Polymeric nanoparticles	10-1000 nm	Biocompatible, biodegradable, offer complete drug protection	Excellent carrier for controlled and sustained delivery of drugs.
Nanocrystals Quantum dots	2–9.5 nm	Semi conducting material; Size between 10-100 Å; Bright fluorescence, narrow emission, Broad UV excitation and high photostability	Long term multiple color imaging of liver cell; DNA **hybridization**, **immunoassay**; receptor mediated **endocytosis**; labeling of breast cancer marker HeR2 surface of cancer cells
Carbon nanotubes	0.5–3 nm diameter and 20–1000 nm length	Third allotropic crystalline form of carbon sheets either single layer (single walled nanotube, SWNT) or multiple layers (multi-walled nanotube, MWNT). These crystals have remarkable strength and unique electrical properties (conducting, semiconducting, or insulating)	Functionalization enhanced solubility, penetration to cell cytoplasm and to nucleus, as carrier for gene delivery, peptide delivery
Dendrimer	<10 nm	Highly branched, nearly monodisperse polymer system produced by controlled polymerization; three main parts core, branch and surface	Long circulatory, controlled delivery of bioactives, targeted delivery of bioactives to **macrophages**, liver targeting
Metallic nanoparticles	<100 nm	Gold and silver colloids, very small size resulting in high surface area available for functionalization, stable	Drug and gene delivery, highly sensitive diagnostic assays, thermal ablation and radiotherapy enhancement
Polymeric micelles	10-100nm	Block **amphiphilic** copolymer micelles, high drug entrapment, payload, biostability	Long circulatory, target specific active and passive drug delivery, diagnostic value
Liposome	50-100 nm	Phospholipid vesicles, biocompatible, versatile, good entrapment efficiency, offer easy face functionalization	Long circulatory, offer passive and active delivery of gene, protein, peptide and various other bioactives
Iron oxiden anocrystal	4–5 nm	Superparamagnetism	Magnetic resonance imaging (disease detection such as cancer, arthritis, and atherosclerosis); intracellular monitoring
Silica Nanoparticles	10 nm–50 μm	Silanised and coated with **oligonucleotide**. Observable by fluorescence method.	Efficient nucleic acid hybridization. Detection of DNA Nanobiosensor for trace analysis

CHALLENGES ASSOCIATED WITH NANOTECHNOLOGICAL APPLICATION IN INDIA AND INDIA'S PREPAREDNESS TO FACE THEM

Nanotechnology has still not caught on in India in a big way, though several Indian and multinational companies such as Reliance Industries, the Tata Group, Mahindra and Mahindra, Intel, General Electric and General Motors are investing in it.

Dabur Pharma, which was recently acquired by the Singapore based Fresenius Kabi, is using nanotechnology for a novel cancer drug delivery system. It has used nanotechnology to increase patients' tolerance to the anti-cancer drug Paclitaxel.

Bharat Biotech, is conducting nanotechnology research on products (like oestrogen therapy) using herbal bases.

The following companies are engaged in nanotechnology R&D, though final consumer-oriented products are still some way off:

- ☆ **Dabur Pharma:** Launched anti-cancer drug Nanoxel and Docetaxel using nanotech drug delivery

- ☆ **Tata Group:** Experimenting with nanotech to make fertilisers more efficacious and its vehicles lighter and stronger

- ☆ **Eureka Forbes:** Uses a technology for its water filter, developed by IIT Madras, to remove pesticides from water with the help of silver nano particles

RECENT INITIATIVES

- ☆ Indian Universities and R&D Centres have taken Nanotechnological research very aggressively

- ☆ The Government of India launched a Mission on Nano Science and Technology (Nano Mission) in May 2007. An allocation of Rs. 10 billion for 5 years was made to build, ground up, the nanotech industry in India. Nanotech Mission that will fund R&D by industry and also give grants to leading educational and research institutes engaged in nanotech research. The plan envisages developing cutting-edge products and services in drug delivery, cosmetics, consumer durables and engineering[12, 13]

- ☆ India is trying to rapidly close the gap with Europe, the US and East Asia in finding commercial applications for basic research in Nanosciences

- ☆ Government is shifting funding priority from scientific research to more application-oriented ventures

- ☆ Between early 2002 and March 2009, the Nano Science and Technology Initiative and the Nano Mission have funded 193 different research projects with another 100 currently being evaluated for funding[12, 13]

- ☆ Between 1990 and 2008, Indian scientists contributed to a total of 11,000 publications

☆ Indians held 167 patents on nanotechnology in 2007

☆ The most dominant sectors by far are health care and textiles. There are numerous nanotech applications that are either currently on the market in India or are planned to be marketed over the coming years

☆ Bangalore-based Velbionanotech, a Bio- Nanotechnology Product Development Company has developed nano-based treatments for Atherosclerosis, Nephrolithiasis and Diabetes

☆ IIT Bombay has developed I-sens, a cardiac diagnostic device that uses Nanotechnology for blood analysis and a drug for lung cancer that is inhaled in the form of nano particles

☆ Some of the Indian and Multinational Companies investing in Nanotechnology are: Reliance Industries, TATA Group, Mahindra and Mahindra, INTEL, General Electric and General Motors.

CHALLENGES

☆ With the emerging focus on nanotechnology, an increasing demand for qualified manpower will arise in the next few years in industrial fields such as production, quality assurance etc.

☆ In Academia and R&D labs, still there is emphasis on presenting research papers in the conferences/seminars in India and abroad. Publications provide only an analytical overview. Product development is lacking

☆ Private Sector R&D is minimal and is mostly in Pharmaceuticals, Consumer goods (Water Filters)

☆ Nano-foodtechnology R&D is in its infancy

☆ Nanomaterial risk assessment in India is so far mostly limited to a few individual toxicity programmes and studies

☆ Currently there is no regulatory framework, no clear policy/guidelines on regulation. The Department of Science and Technology, Govt. Of India has constituted a working group on regulation of Nanotechnology.

CONCLUSIONS

☆ Nanotechnology has immense potential for on-farm and off-farm agricultural applications

☆ ~ 44 countries including India are pursuing R&D for Nanotechnology application in agriculture for alleviating malnutrition and to ensure food security

☆ Pharmaceutical Nanotechnology is now well-established for drug delivery, diagnostics, prognostic and treatment of diseases through nanoengineered tools. Few Nanotechnology based products and delivery systems are already in the market

☆ Research must be carried out towards understanding public health and safety of all nanotechnology products

- ☆ Institutions for education and training, centres of excellence exclusively in the area of nanotechnology should be more strongly promoted by the Government

- ☆ Suitable mechanisms for translating nanotechnology R&D results to commercially viable technologies should be developed and adopted

- ☆ NT Parks and NT Transfer Centres should be set up in R&D Institutions and research-industry linkages should be encouraged to ensure smooth transfer of technology

- ☆ Nanotechnology needs due attention and importance in policy formulation and proper government intervention in funding

- ☆ India is trying to rapidly close the gap with Europe, the US and East Asia in finding commercial applications for basic research in Nanosciences. The DST is currently shifting its funding priority from purely scientific research to more application-oriented ventures

- ☆ Risk assessment activities have only just begun and are few and far between. The pharmaceutical sector is an exception and is, in terms of regulatory policy, ahead of other sectors

- ☆ If more nano-enabled products are on the market, civil society interest will grow, as also the industry involvement in the policy-making process.

Given the right impetus, India can emerge as a huge nanotech hub, as in the case of information technology. Given this potential, it's just a matter of time before this trickle turns into a deluge.

REFERENCES

1. Harper, Tim. (2011). Global Funding of Nanotechnologies and Its Impact, July 2011, Global-Nanotechnology-Funding-Report-2011. Available from: http://cientifica.com/wp-content/uploads/downloads/2011/07/Global-Nanotechnology-Funding-Report-2011.pdf

2. The Project on Emerging Nanotechnologies. 2008. Retrieved 13 May 2011

3. Varshney, H.M. and Shailender, M. (2012). "Nanotechnology" Current Status in Pharmaceutical Science: A Review". *International Journal of Therapeutic Applications*, Volume 6, 2012, 14 - 24.

4. S. Logothetidis (ed.), *Nanostructured Materials and Their Applications*, NanoScience and Technology, DOI 10.1007/978-3-642-22227-6_1, © Springer-Verlag Berlin Heidelberg, 2012, p. 3

5. National Nanotechnology Initiative. Available from: http://www.nano.gov/nanotech-101/special

6. Morris, V. 2007. Nanotechnology and food. Available from: http://www.iufost.org/reports_resources/bulletins/documents/IUF.SIB.Nanotechnology.pdf

7. T.V. Duncan, J. Colloid Interface Sci. (2011), Applications of nanotechnology in food packaging and food safety: Barrier materials, antimicrobials and sensors.

8. Šimon, P., Chaudhry, Q. and Bakoš, D. 2008. Migration of engineered nanoparticles from polymer packaging to food – a physiochemical view. *J. Food Nutr. Res.*, 47(3): 105–113.

9. Jafarali K. Momin, Chitra Jayakumar and Jashbhai B. Prajapati. Potential of nanotechnology in functional foods. *Emir. J. Food Agric*. 2013. 25 (1): 10-19

10. World Health Organization, Expert meeting on the application of nanotechnologies in the food and agriculture sectors: potential food safety implications (2010).

11. A. Surendiran, S. Sandhiya, S.C. Pradhan and C. Adithan. Novel Applications of Nanotechnology in Medicine. *Indian J Med Res 130*, December 2009, pp 689-701

12. Annual Report 2012-13, Department of Science and Technology, Government of India.

13. Nanotechnology developments in India – a status report, The Energy and Resources Institute, April 2010.

Chapter 3

Synthesis of Hydroxyapatite Nanofiber from Tutut Shells by Use of Hydrothermal Method for Biomaterial Application

Lenita Herawaty[1] and Wisnu Ari Adi[2]

[1]*Graduate Students of Department of Chemistry,*
Faculty of Mathematics and Natural Science,
Bogor Agricultural University, Indonesia
[2]*Center for Science and Technology of Advance Materials,*
National Nuclear Energy Agency, South Tangerang 15314, Indonesia
[1]*E-mail: land_nn@yahoo.com*

ABSTRACT

The synthesis of hydroxyapatite (HAp) nanofiber by hydrothermal method has been performed. Cetryltrimethylammonium bromide (CTAB) was dissolved in a mixture of $Ca(OH)2$, $H3PO4$, $NaOH$ and water, and then put in autoclave at temperature 150 °C for 18 hours. The resulting suspension was heated in a furnace at temperature of 1000 ° C for 3 hours. Base on the result of element analysis showed that the Ca/P ratio of HAp sample is 2.03. The refinement results of x-ray diffraction patterns showed that the sample consist of two phase, namely, hydroxyapatite $Ca_{10}(PO_4)_6(OH)_2$ phase and lime CaO phase. The $Ca_{10}(PO_4)_6(OH)_2$ phase had a hexagonal structure (P63/m) with lattice parameters a = b = 9.4163(5) Å, c = 6.8791(4) Å, $\alpha = \beta = 90°$, dan dakua = 120°, V = 528.23(7) Å^3, dan ρ = 3.142 gr.cm^{-3}. And CaO phase had a cubic structure (Fm-3m) with lattice parameters a = b = c = 4.807(1) Å, $\alpha = \beta$ = dakua = 90°, V = 111.1(1) Å^3, dan ρ = 3.353 gr.cm^{-3}. The HAp had crystallite and particle sizes are 53.4265 and 147.95 nm, respectively. Base on data of TEM showed that the hydroxyapatite particles shaped rod with diameter and length rod are around 15-20 and

40-60 nm, respectively. It was concluded that the synthesis of hydroxyapatite nanorod from tutut shells by using hydrothermal method has been successfully carried out and expected to be used for biomaterial application.

Keywords: Tutut shells, Hydroxyapatite, Hydrothermal, Crystal structure, Nanofiber.

INTRODUCTION

The case of broken bones and tooth decay increased very high, so the material needs of biomaterials is also increasing. Efforts to find alternative materials that can replace biomaterials in bone tissue structure or teeth without causing side effects draw attention at the present. One of the biomaterials that are being developed is hydroxyapatite (HAp). Hydroxyapatite (HAp) is a bioceramic the most widely studied and used in various biomedical applications, especially in the fields of orthopedics and dentistry (Nayak, 2010). HAp is very similar to the inorganic mineral component of bone and teeth. This material has excellent biocompatibility and bioactivity of unique (Chen Q.Z., 2004). Natural HAp has a hexagonal structure with the chemical formula of $Ca_{10}(PO_4)_6(OH)_2$ (Zhang, 2003). The mechanical properties of HAp is affected by a form of powder, pores, grain size, particle size and fabrication methods. HAp powder with the proper stoichiometry molar ratio of Ca/P = 1.67 can produce superior mechanical properties (Chow, 2009).

Previous study, HAp nanoparticles were successfully prepared by chemical precipitation method using calcium nitrate tetrahydrate and diammonium phosphate as a precursor. Particle measurements used AFM (atomic force microscopy) produces spherical particles 30-50 nm in diameter and aggregate (Dedourkova, 2012). It is known that hydroxyapatite crystals in bone are generally needle shaped nanometer-size range of 5-20 nm in wide and 60 nm in length. And development of other methods that serves as a HAp nanoparticles were sol-gel, hydrothermal, multiple emulsion, and electrode position methods (Vijayalakshmi, 2006). At this study will be carried out synthesis HAp nanoparticle by hydrothermal method. And the aim of this study is to synthesize HAp nanoparticles from Tutut Shells material by hydrothermal method. The study will be focussed on understanding the process of synthesis of HAp nanoparticle from tutut shells material, and understand the characterization of HAp the terms of crystal structure, microstructure, functional groups, and particle size, so that will be obtained HAp nanofiber are expected able to be used as materials for biomaterial application.

MATERIALS AND METHODS

The main source of raw material for synthesis of HAp is calcium hydroxide $(Ca(OH)_2)$ from tutut shells as shown in Figure 3.1. While the source of tutut shells retrieved from conch paddy, Sumatra, Indonesia. Tutut shells are waste of tutut meat consumption. This waste is rich in various minerals including calcium. Calcium contained in the shells of mollusks are generally in the form of calcium carbonate $(CaCO_3)$ which is incorporated in the shell structure as calcite and aragonite crystals associated to the organic matrix of conchiolin (Soido, 2009).

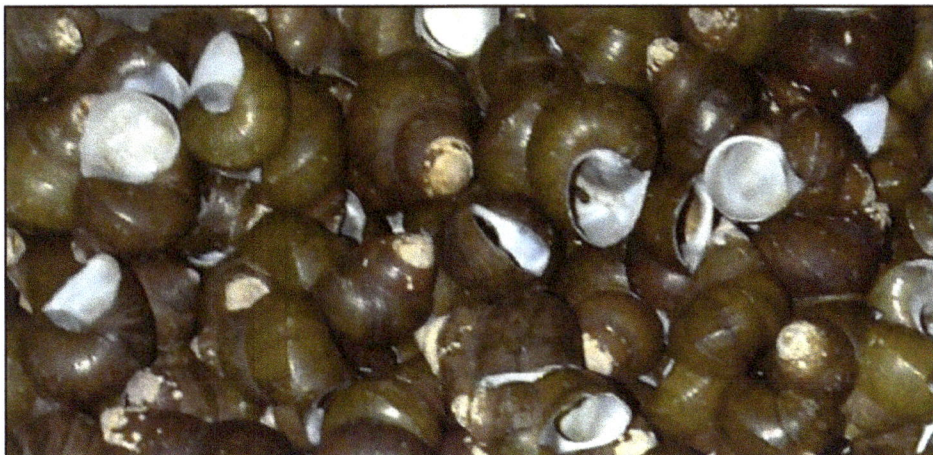

Figure 3.1: Conch Paddy, Sumatra, Indonesia

2 grams cetryltrimethylammonium bromide (CTAB) was dissolved in a mixture 100 ml of $Ca(OH)_2$ from tutut shells and H_3PO_4, then stirred for 30 minutes. Add 2 ml of 1M NaOH and 10 ml of water and stirred again for 30 minutes. Since H_3PO_4 solution is acidic, it requires monitoring and adjustment of the pH in order to produce HAp. When the pH drops below 9 or 7 would lead to the formation of calcium monophosphate and calcium dehydrated (Afshar A, 2003). Therefore it is used pH meter to monitor pH and 1 M NH_4OH solution as pH adjustment. In this study, the final pH is kept around 10. After that the solution is put in autoclave and heated at 150 °C for 18 hours. The resulting suspension was cooled at room temperature and washed several times by deionized water. The deposition is dried in the oven at 90 °C for 20 hours and heated in a furnace at 1000 °C for 3 hours.

The surface morphology and element identification of the sample were analyzed by using the JEOL scanning electron microscope (SEM) and energy dispersive spectroscopy (EDS), respectively. Analysis of functional groups used Fourier transformation infra red (FTIR). The phase qualitative and quantitative of analysis were carried out using the PW1710 Philips diffractometer equipped (XRD). The Rietveld analysis was performed applying GSAS program (Toby B.H., 2001). Particle size of the sample is analyzed by using the particle size analyzer (PSA) and transmission electron microscope (TEM).

Results and Discussion

The element identification was analyzed by using energy dispersive spectroscopy (EDS) of samples was shown in Figure 3.2. The elements content of the sample is shown in Table 2.1.

HAp powder with the stoichiometry molar ratio of C/P about 1.67 can result in superior mechanical properties of HAp (Chow, 2009). And the results of measurement by using energy dispersive spectroscopy showed that the molar ratio of Ca/P in the

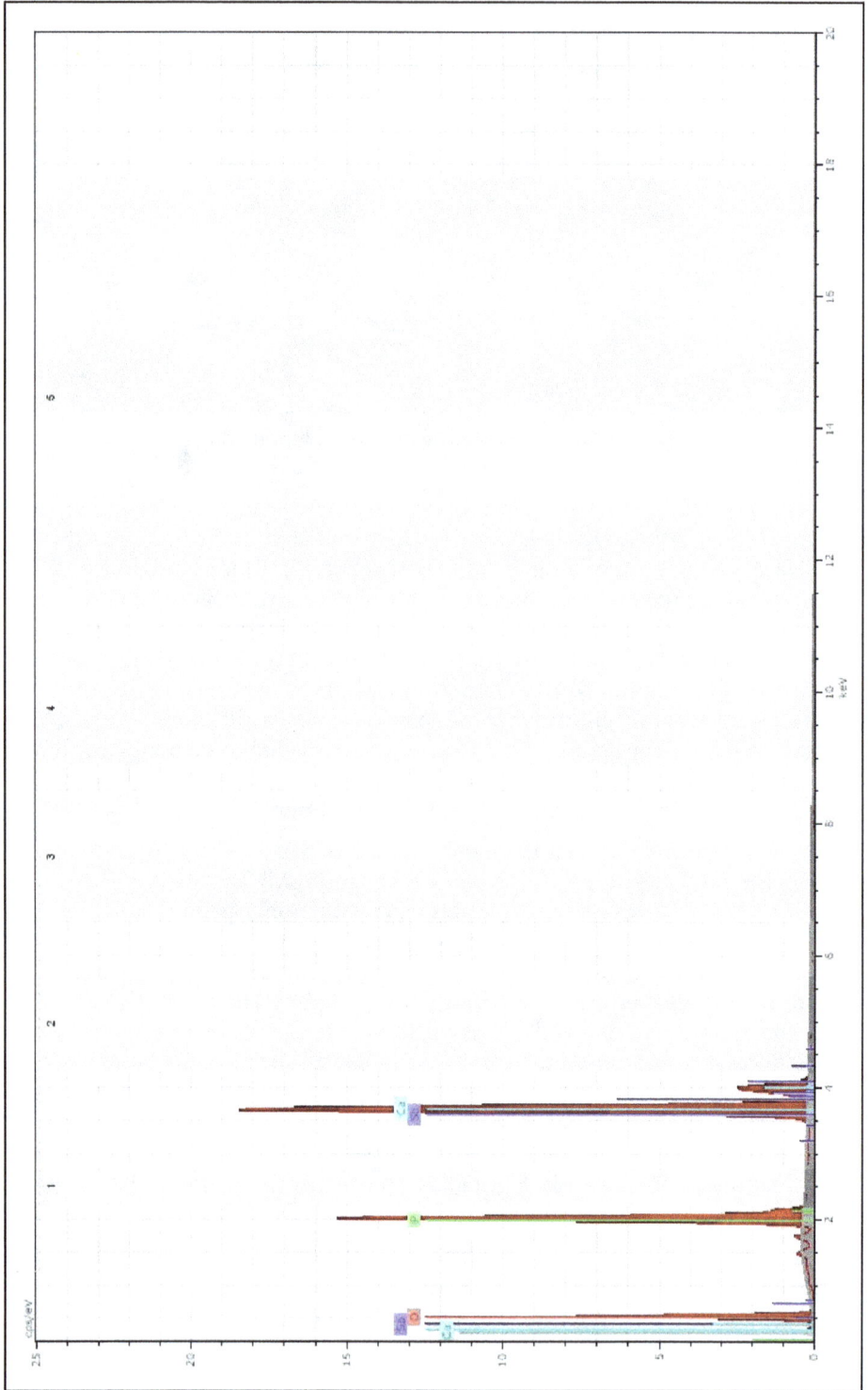

Figure 3.2: The Element Analysis Result of the Sample

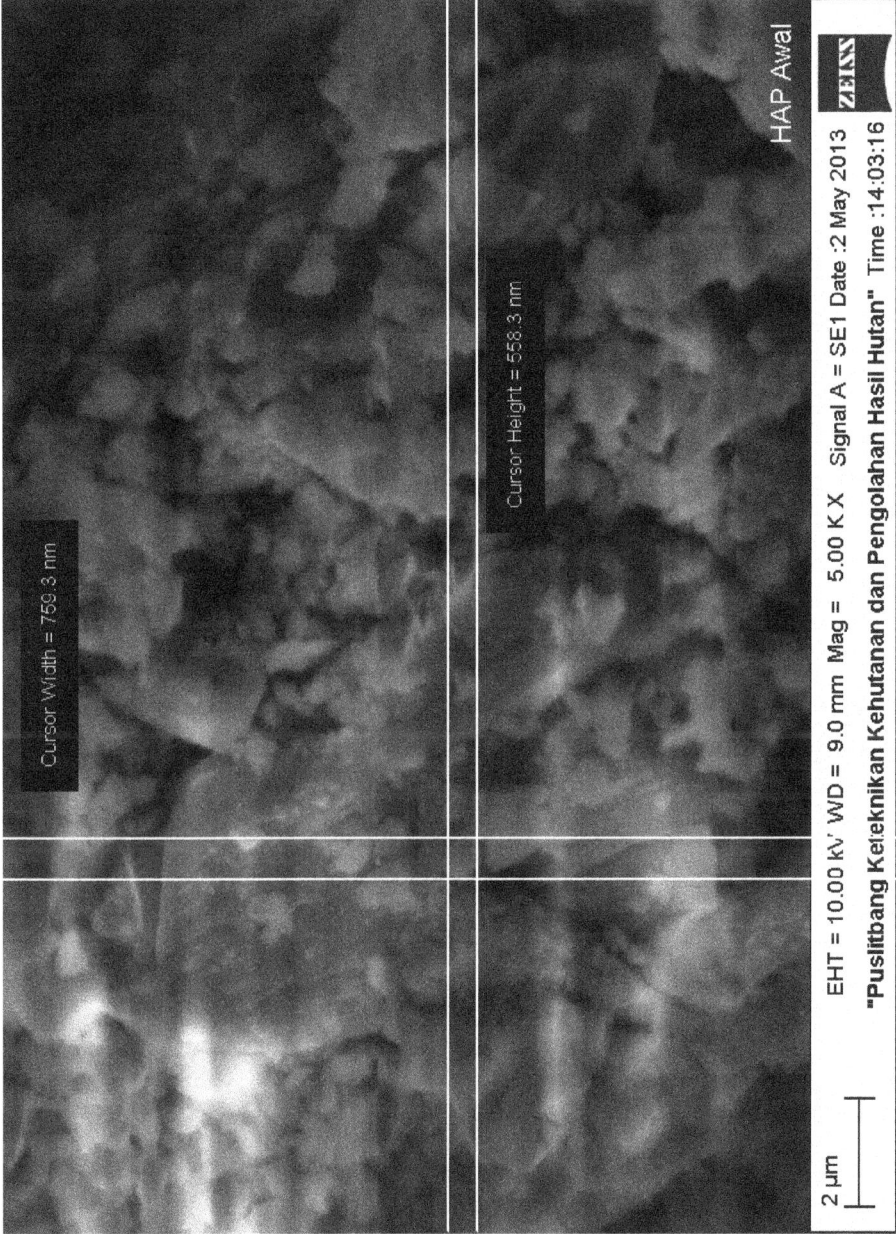

Figure 3.3: Surface Morphology Photo of the Sample

samples synthesized using hydrothermal method is equal to 2.03. This indicates that the samples contain elements the excess calcium which possible form multiphase.

Tabel 3.1: The Results of Element Analysis by Using Energy Dispersive Spectroscopy

Sl.No.	Font Appearance	
	Unsure	Mass Fraction (wt per cent)
1.	Kalsium (Ca)	38.15 ± 1.4
2.	Phsopor (P)	18.76 ± 0.9
3.	Oksigen (O)	39.26 ± 8.2
4.	Antimony (Sb)	3.83 ± 0.2

The surface morphology results of observations by scanning electron microscope on the samples showed that the sample has been well established as shown in Figure 3.3.

Based on morphological observations appears that the sample HAp of hydrothermal product has two particles form a relatively distinct and evenly distributed throughout the sample surface. Thus it is also suspected that HAp of hydrothermal product had multiphase compositions. Further confirmation observed functional groups of sample by using FTIR as shown in Figure 3.4.

In Figure 3.4 are shown the results of the analysis of functional groups HAp samples synthesized by hydrothermal method using fourier transform infrared spectroscopy (FTIR) of wave numbers 4000-400 cm^{-1}.

Absorbance peaks of the FTIR spectra indicate the presence of vibration of the hydroxyl functional groups (OH$^-$), phosphate (PO$_4^{3-}$), carbonate (CO$_3^{2-}$), hydrogen phosphate (HPO$_4^{2-}$), and water (H$_2$O). Hydroxyl group (OH$^-$) has absorption bands at wave numbers around 3572-3570 cm^{-1} and 634-632 cm^{-1} (Destainville A., 2003). Absorbance peaks of the samples appeared at wave numbers around 3572.17 and 632.65 cm^{-1} that indicated the presence of O–H vibrations of the hydroxyl group (–OH). And adsorption peaks at 1658.78 cm^{-1} indicates O–H bond in the form of water absorption (Meejoo S., 2006). Whereas phosphate group (PO$_4^{3-}$) has absorption bands at wave numbers around 473, 550-640, 963, and 1120 to 1000 cm^{-1} (Destainville A., 2003). Absorbance peaks in this sample appeared at 470.63, 570.93, 601.79, 964.41, 1053.13, and 1091.71 cm^{-1} that indicates P–O vibrations of the –PO$_4$ groups. Then carbonate group (CO$_3^{2-}$) has absorption bands at wave numbers around 875, 1418, 1456, 1466, 1636 cm^{-1} (Meejoo S., 2006). Absorbance peaks of this sample appeared at wave numbers 1442.75 cm^{-1} that indicated the presence of C–O vibration of the –CO$_3$ groups. Thus based on the above analysis, it can be assumed that the presence of the –OH, –PO$_4$ and –CO$_3$ indicate hydroxyapatite phase have formed properly. And also appears the bond Ca-O and Ca-OH bonding overlap indicating that the phase is built from Ca-O bond group. Absorbance peaks of this sample appeared at wave numbers 3641.60, and 405.05 cm^{-1} that indicated the presence of Ca–O groups (Ji G., 2009). Further confirmation is measuring the x-ray diffraction pattern on the samples of hydrothermal product to determine the phase of hydroxyapatite formed.

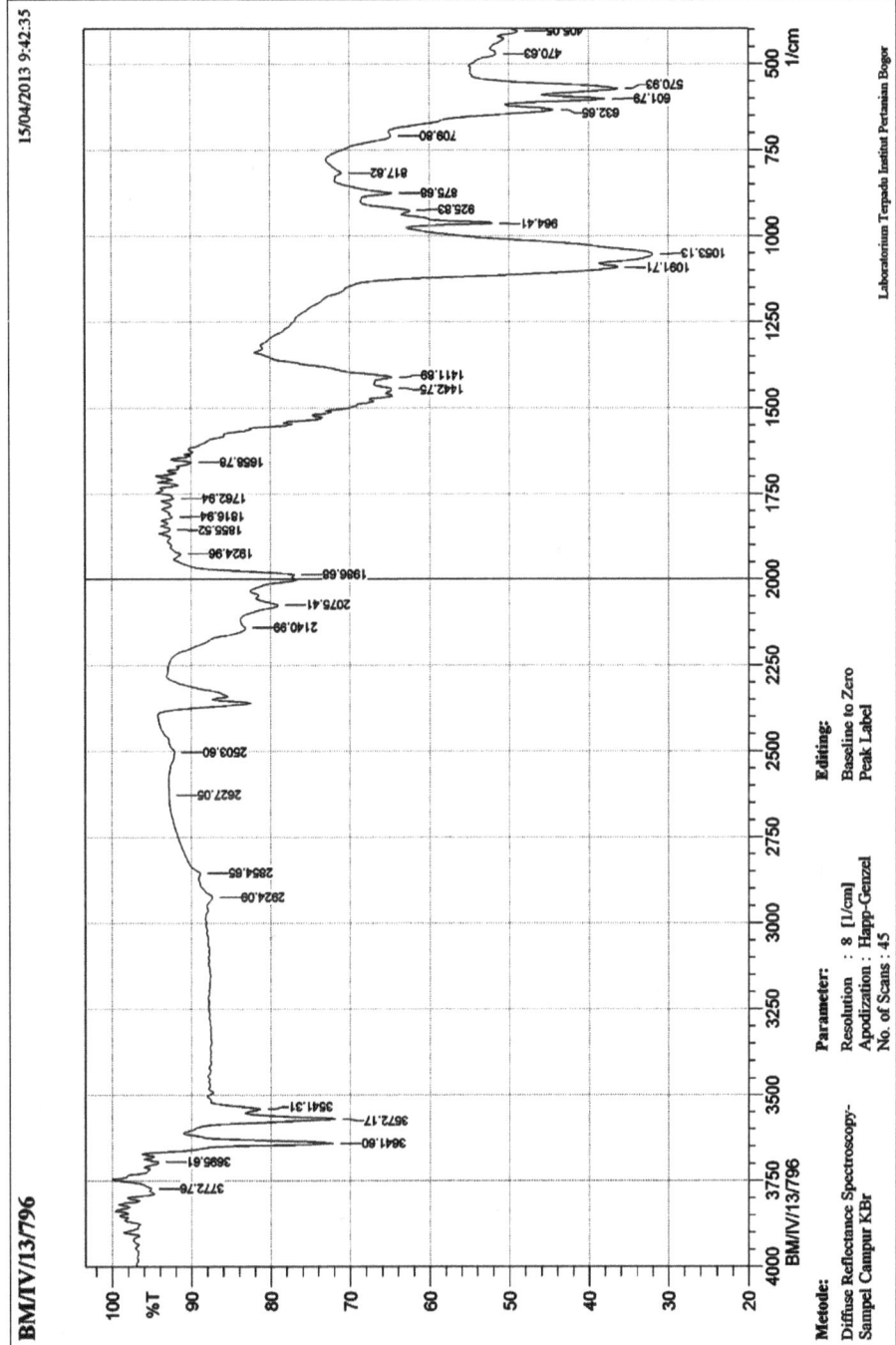

Figure 3.4: The FTIR Absorbance Spectral of the Sample

The phase identification referred to Lee Y, *et al.* (Lee Y. J., 2009) and Wyckoff, *et al.* (Wyckoff R. W. G., 1963) for $Ca_{10}(PO_4)_6(OH)_2$ and CaO phases, respectively. Therefore, it was necessary for the analysis of phase content in the samples using the GSAS software as shown in Figure 3.5. The analysis results of X-ray diffraction patterns showed that the sample consist of two phases. The $Ca_{10}(PO_4)_6(OH)_2$ phase has a hexagonal structure (P63/m) with lattice parameters a = b = 9.418(3) Å, c = 6.885(2) Å, $\alpha = \beta = 90°$, dakua = 120°, V = 528.9(4) Å^3, and ρ = 3.084 gr.cm^{-3}. And CaO phase has a cubic structure (Fm-3m) with lattice parameters a = b = c = 4.807(1) Å, $\alpha = \beta$ = dakua = 90°, V = 111.1(1) Å^3, and ρ = 3.353 gr.cm^{-3}.

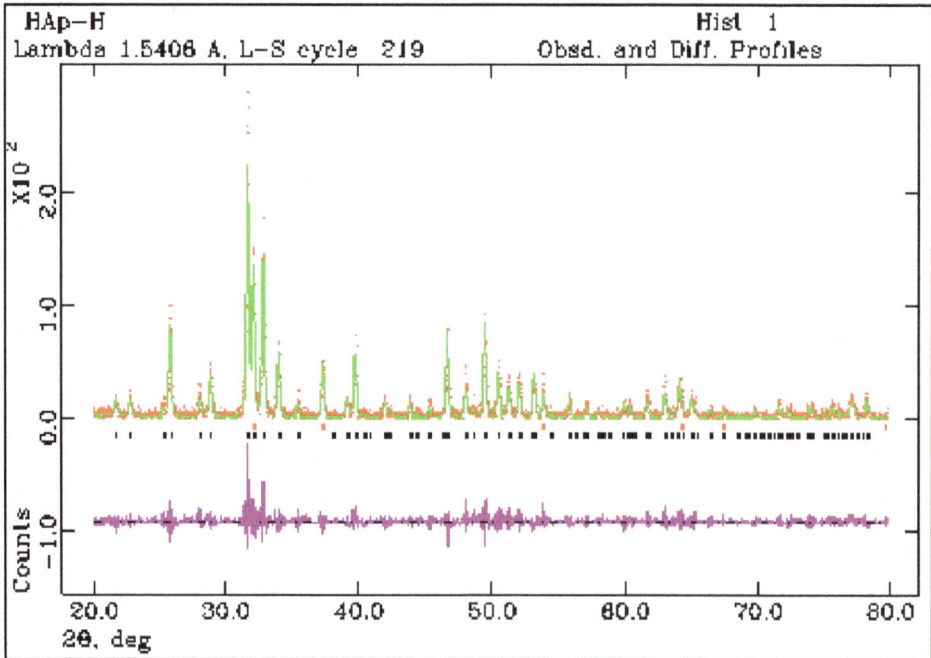

Figure 3.5: The Analysis of XRD Pattern of the Sample

The refinement result has produced very good quality of fitting with R factor is very small. And goodness of fit value 2 (chi-squared) according to rietveld agreement (Izumi, 1994).

This result is evidenced by the calculation results of the mass fraction as shown in Table 3.2.

Table 3.2: Mass Fraction of the Sample

Sl.No.	Phase	Mass Fraction (per cent)
1.	HAp – $Ca_{10}(PO_4)_6(OH)_2$	94.55
2.	Lime – CaO	5.45

And crystallite size of HAp hydrothermal product after calcination can be calculated by Scherrer formula using X-ray diffraction data is 53.42 nm. However, these results need further confirmation by measurement of particle size using a particle size analyzer as shown in Figure 3.6.

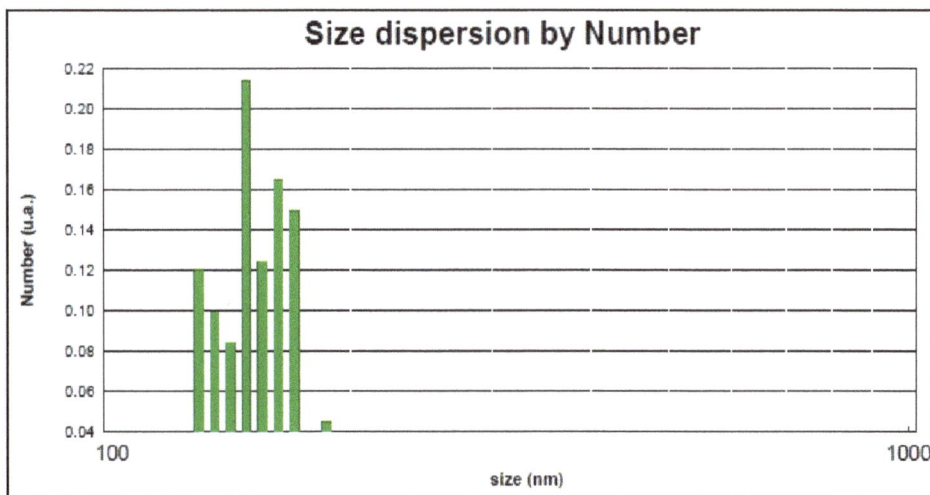

Figure 3.6: Particle Size Distribution of HAp Hydrothermal Product by Using Statistical Methods

The results of particle size measurements using a particle size analyzer by statistical methods obtained that the majority of the particles size of HAp precipitation product was 147.95 nm reached 21 per cent. Visually, particles size of the sample can be observed by using a transmission electron microscope as shown in Figure 3.7.

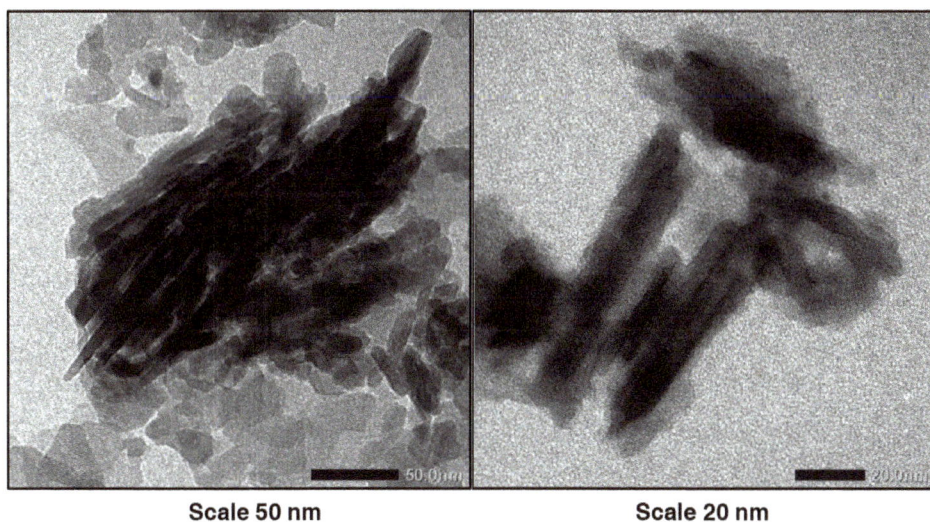

Scale 50 nm   Scale 20 nm

Figure 3.7: Photo of Transmission Electron Microscope on the HAp Sample of Hydrothermal Product

The observation by transmission electron microscopy indicated that HAp hydrothermal product has a particle size of diameter and length rod are around 15-20 and 40-60 nm, respectively.

CONCLUSIONS

Synthesis of hydroxyapatite from tutut shells by using hydrothermal method has been successfully carried out. The elementary analysis showed that the ratio of Ca/P on HAp sample was 2.03. The results of analysis of x-ray diffraction patterns showed that the sample consist of two phases, namely $Ca_{10}(PO_4)_6(OH)_2$ and CaO phases. The $Ca_{10}(PO_4)_6(OH)_2$ phase has a hexagonal structure (P63/m) with lattice parameters a = b = 9.418(3) Å, c = 6.885(2) Å, $\alpha = \beta = 90°$, dakua = 120°, V = 528.9(4) Å^3, and ρ = 3.084 gr.cm^{-3}. And CaO phase has a cubic structure (Fm-3m) with lattice parameters a = b = c = 4.807(1) Å, $\alpha = \beta$ = dakua = 90°, V = 111.1(1) Å^3, and ρ = 3.353 gr.cm^{-3}. The HAp had crystallite and particle sizes are 53.42 nm and 147.95 nm, respectively. Base on data of TEM showed that the hydroxyapatite particles shaped spherical-polygonal with an average size of diameter and length rod are around 15-20 and 40-60 nm, respectively. Synthesis of hydroxyapatite nanoparticles from tutut shells by using a hydrothermal method has been successfully made and expected able to be used as materials for biomaterial application.

REFERENCES

1. Afshar A, Ghorbani M, Ehsani N, Saeri MR, Sorrell CC. 2003. Some important factors in the wet precipitation process of hydroxyapatite. *Materials and Design*. 24:197–202.

2. Chen QZ, Wong CT, Lu WW, Cheung KMC, Leong JCY, Luk KDK. 2004. Strengthening mechanisms of bone-bonding to crystalline hydroxyapatite *in vivo*. *Biomaterials*. 25: 4243-4254.

3. Chow LC. 2009. Next generation calcium phosphate-based biomaterials. *Dent Mater. J Nat Institute of Health*. USA. 28(1):1–10.

4. Dedourkova T, Zelenka J, Zelenkova M, Bene L, Svoboda L. 2012. Synthesis of sphere-like nanoparticles of hydroxyapatite. Prague. Czech Republic. *J Procedia Engineering*. 42:1816–1821.

5. Destainville A., Champion E., Bernache-Assollante D., 2003. Synthesis, characterization and thermal behaviour of apatite tricalcium phosphate/ Materials Chemistry and Physics, No. 80, pp. 269 – 277.

6. Izumi F., 1994. "A Rietveld-Refinement Program RIETAN-94 for Angle-Dispersive X-Ray and Neutron Powder Diffraction", National Institute for Research in Inorganic Materials 1-1 Namiki, Tsukuba, Ibaraki 305, Japan.

7. Ji G., Zhu H., Jiang X., 2009. Mechanical Strenght of Epoxy Resin Composites Reinforced by Calcined Pearl Shell Powders. *J. Appl. Polym. Sci.*, Vol.114, pp. 3168.-3176.

8. Lee Y. J., Stephens P. W., Tang Y., Li W., Phillips B. L., Parise J. B., Reeder R. J., 2009. "Arsenate substitution in hydroxylapatite: Structural characterization of

the Ca5(PxAs1-xO4)3OH solid solution Sample: As0 Locality: synthetic", American Mineralogist 94, 666-675.

9. Meejoo S., Maneeprakorn W., Winotai P. 2006. Phase and thermal stability of nanocrystalline hydroxyapatite prepared via microwave heating. *Thermochimica Acta*, No. 447, pp. 115–120.

10. Nayak AK. 2010. Hydroxyapatite synthesis methodologies: an overview. Int J *Chem Tech Res* 2(2): 903-907.

11. Soído C, Vasconcellos MC, Diniz AG, Pinheiro J. 2009. An improvement of calcium determination technique in the shell of molluscs. *Brazilian archives of Bio Tech* 52(1): 93-98.

12. Toby B.H., 2001. EXPGUI, A Graphical User Interface for GSAS, *J. Appl. Cryst*. 34 210-213.

13. Vijayalakshmi U, Rajeswari S. 2006. Preparation and characterization of microcrystalline hydroxyapatite using sol gel method. Trends *Biomaterial Artificial Organs*. 19(2):57-62.

14. Wyckoff R. W. G., 1963. "Second edition. Interscience Publishers, New York, New York rocksalt structure", *Crystal Structures* 1, 85-237.

15. Zhang H., Yao X., Wu M., Zhang L., 2003. Complex Permittivity and Pearmibility of Zn-Co Substituted Z-type Hexaferrite Prepared by Citrate Sol-gel Process, *British Cer. Transc.*, Vol. 102, pp. 01-10.

Chapter 4

Isolation and Characterization of Cellulose Nanofibers from Sludge of Pulp and Paper Industry

Lisman Suryanegara[1], Dian Susanthy[2]*,
Muhamad Alif Hamimdal[2] and Purwantiningsih Sugita[2]

[1]*Research and Development Unit for Biomaterials,*
Indonesian Institute of Sciences, Cibinong Science Center,
Cibinong-Bogor 16911, Indonesia
[2]*Department of Chemistry, Bogor Agricultural University,*
Dramaga, Bogor 16680, Indonesia
*E-mail: diansusanthy@yahoo.co.id

ABSTRACT

This paper describes the isolation of cellulose nanofibers from sludge of pulp and paper industry. The sludge was first repulped in distillated water and then pretreated with commercial surfactant to remove the pollutant particle. After pre-treatment, the fibers bleached with hydrogen peroxyde for several times until the brightness reach constant. This bleached fibers were then converted into cellulose nanofibers by mechanical treatment using high-performance dispersing instrument (ultra turrax) for 120 minutes at speed of 5000 rpm. The dispersed fibers processed in ultrasonic equipment for 120 minutes at 40 per cent amplitude. The morphology of isolated cellulose nanofibers was then characterized by light microscope and SEM. The starting sludge contains many pollutant particles. After pre-treatment and bleaching process, cellulose fibers became cleaner and brighter. However, the pollutant particles still can not be completely removed and they became interference on the fiber characterization. The fibers that isolated after dispersion and sonication process had diameter about 300-700 nm. These fibers still have not become nanofibers, but cellulose microfibers. More mechanical treatment was suggested to convert this microfibers to cellulose nanofibers.

Keywords: *Cellulose microfibers, Cellulose nanofibers, Dispersion, Sludge of pulp and paper industry, Sonication.*

INTRODUCTION

Recently, nanotechnology has been a common way to develop the utilization of materials. One of the novel nanostructured material during recent years is cellulose nanofibers. Because cellulose is the most abundant biomass source on earth, cellulose nanofibers becomes a promising material to develop. With a size range of 5-100 nm, cellulose nanofibers have the potential to be a low cost renewable material that has many applications, such as reinforcing polylactic acid (Iwatake *et al.*, 2008), polyvinyl alcohol (Bhatnagar and Sain, 2005), polyethylene (Wang and Sain, 2007), polyurethane (Jonoobi *et al.*, 2010), chitosan films (Azeredo *et al.*, 2010), etc. Nanocellulose-based biomaterials have the potential to be truly green nanomaterials because they are carbon-neutral, sustainable, recyclable, and non-toxic (Dufrense., 2013). Cellulose nanofibers surfaces has abundant hydroxyl groups, allowing potential hydrogen bonding and surface modification. Although the morphology and dimensions of cellulose nanofibers can vary substantially, depends in the fibrillation degree and any pre-treatment that involved, generally cellulose nanofibers has long flexible fiber networks form (Xi *et al.*, 2013). Cellulose nanofibers can be obtained from many sources, such as wood pulp (Abe *et al.*, 2007;Siddiqui *et al.*, 2013), kenaf fiber (Jonoobi *et al.*, 2010), sugarcane bagasse (Li *et al.*, 2012), pineapple leaf fibres (Cherian *et al.*, 2010), soybean (Wang and Sain, 2007), and many other sources that contain cellulose.

Nowadays, people become more concern about the sustainability of their areas of activity, which is usually called humanosphere. Realizing that natural resources is soon to exhaust available ones in this earth, people need more prudent ways to utilize them. One of many ways to do it is by recycling waste. In 2010, Japan paper industry discharged around 5 million tons of paper sludge as their solid waste (Prasetyo *et al.*, 2011). Some of paper sludge's apllication are sludge-cement composites (Balwaik and Raut, 2012), sludge concrete brick (Wattimena *et al.*, 2011), bioethanol production (Pezsa and Ailer, 2011), as filler in composites (Edalatmanesh *et al.*, 2011), as fertilizer (Lesmono, 2005), and as fiber additive for asphalt road pavement (Mari *et al.*, 2009). The composition of pulp and paper industry sludge is different, depends on the paper production process in the factory. The most paper sludge has average composition of cellulose about 50 per cent (Edalatmanesh *et al.*, 2011). This high cellulose composition is a potential point, so it can be developped to explore the utilization of paper sludge. Because sludge contain many cellulose, cellulose nanofibers could be isolated from it. Converting this sludge to cellulose nanofibers can improve the economy of pulp and paper industry, besides it can reduces the industry waste which will become environmental pollution.

There are many methods to obtain cellulose nanofibers, but generally there are two types of cellulose nanofibers isolation processes: simple mechanical methods or a combination of both mechanical and chemical methods. Although chemo-mechanical method can result smaller nanofibers (Wang and Sain, 2007), but their waste can be hazardous for the environment because they using medium concentrate sulphuric acid. So that mechanical methods was choosen to convert sludge to cellulose nanofibers without producing more hazardous waste. There are several mechanical methods to convert cellulose fibers to cellulose nanofibers, they are high-pressure homogenizer, sonication, high-speed blender, cryocrushing, and grinder/refiner (Moon *et al.*, 2011). But high-pressure homogenizer, grinder, and cryocrushing were too expensive to use in waste management. So the most possible method to converts sludge fiber become cellulose nanofibers is by sonication. Beside that, Zhao *et al.* (2007) showed that ultrasonication can be a cost-effective technique for fabricating bionanofibers from nature.

In this study, the cellulose nanofibers was isolated from paper sludge by mechanical treatment. The sludge was gained from PT Indah Kiat Pulp and Paper. The sludge was first pretreated with commercial deterjent to remove impurities from the sludge, such as ink, sand, plastic, etc. Pretreated sludge was then bleached to increase the optical properties of the fiber. After that, the sludge was processed through several mechanical treatments, such as dispersion and sonication, to make the fiber fibrillated become thinner fibers or cellulose nanofibers. The morphology of isolated cellulose nanofibers was then characterized using light microscope and SEM.

RESEARCH METHODS

Materials

Paper sludge was obtained from PT. Indah Kiat Paper and Pulp, in the dark grey solid (Figure 4.1). The sludge contains many impurities, like ink, sand, paint, and plastic pieces.

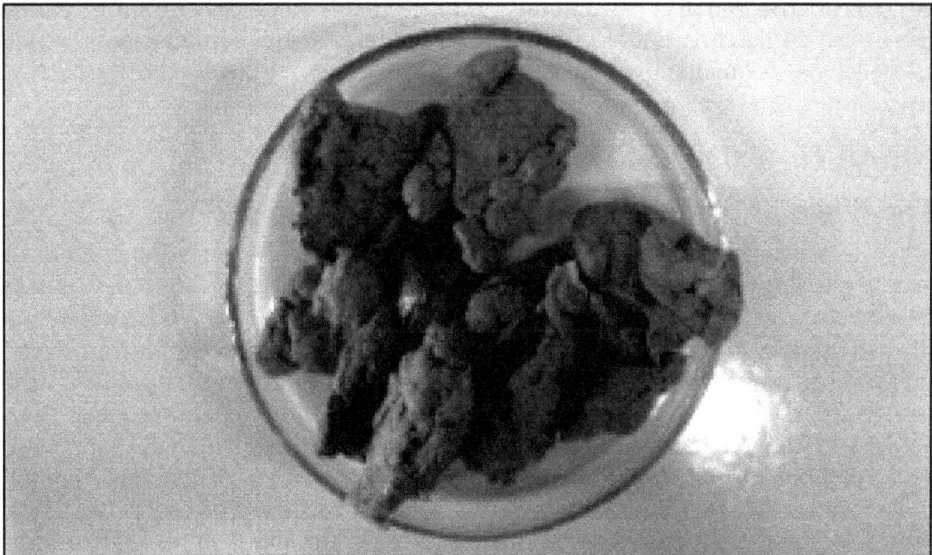

Figure 4.1: Sludge from PT Indah Kiat Pulp and Paper

Sludge Pre-treatment

The sludge was first pretreated with modified Masruchin *et al.* (2010) method. In this method, 100 g of sludge was repulped in 500 ml of aquadest in blender for 30 minutes and poured into 2L beaker glass. Approximately, 500 ml of aquadest was then added again into beaker glass. Detergent was then added into the mixture for about 2 per cent according to the sludge weight. This mixture then stirred with overhead stirrer for 30 minutes. The mixture was then filtered with a fabric filter and the solid part was collected. This process was repeated three times with the same proportion of sludge, water, and the detergent.

Sludge Bleaching

The sludge was bleached with modified Fuadi and Sulistya (2008) method. About 6 gram (dried weight) deinked sludge was put into 250 ml Erlenmeyer flask and then added with aquadest until its volume reached 180 ml. Then, 4.5 ml of H_2O_2 50 per cent was then added into the mixture. This mixture then sealed with plastic cover and then heated at 80 °C for 1 hour while shaked periodically. This procedure was repeated 4 times and then the mixture was filtered with vacuum pump filter.

Mechanical Treatment

The sludge was treated mechanically with modified Syamani *et al.* (2010) method. About 100 ml fiber suspension with concentration of 1 per cent weight was processed in high-performance dispersing instrument (ultra turrax) for 120 minutes at speed of 5000 rpm. After the dispersion, the suspension was further processed in ultrasonic equipment for 120 min at 30 per cent amplitude.

Morphological Characterization

Morphological characterization of fiber was done by low vacuum type scanning electron microscope (EVO50). For the sample preparation for SEM, glimmer plates were fixed with a carbon tape on a specimen holder. A drop of diluted fiber/water suspension was put on the glimmer plate. The samples were air-dried using oven at temperature 60°C for 3-4 days.

RESULTS AND DISCUSSION

The Effect of Sludge Pre-treatment

The effect of sludge pre-treatment was the color change of sludge, from dark brown into light brown (Figure 4.2). The fibers before and after filtration was also observed using light microscope. This obseration results that after pre-treatment the fiber sludge became so much cleaner than before (Figure 4.3). The filtrate from every pre-treatment process was also collected and observed. The filtrate of first pre-treatment was very dark and it became lighter after the second and third repetition (Figure 4.4). This result showed that in pre-treatment process, there is an ink removal happened. This ink should be removed from the sludge because the metal component from the ink will reduce the performance of peroxyde acid in bleaching process (Li *et al.*, 2011). However, the rendemen of pre-treatment process is just about 30 per cent because there were many small fibers that fall down in the filtration process, together with the

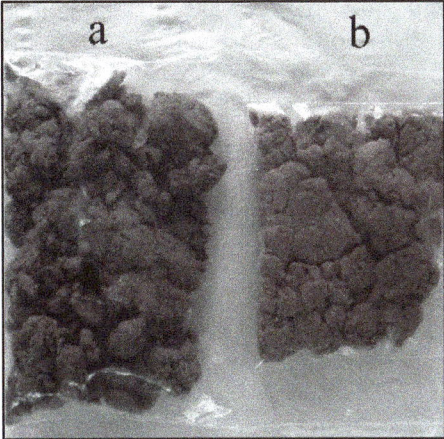

Figure 4.2: Sludge Before (a) and After (b) Pre-treatment

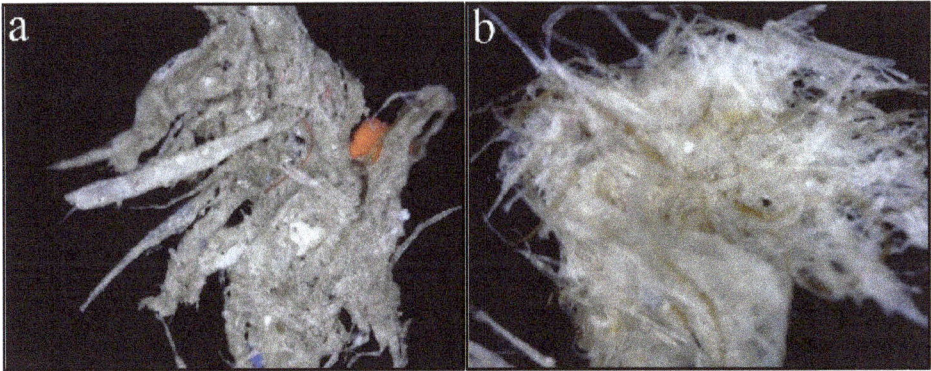

Figure 4.3: Light Microscopic Images of Sludge Fiber Before Pre-treatment (a, in magnificient of 225x) and After Pre-treatment (b, in magnificient of 215x)

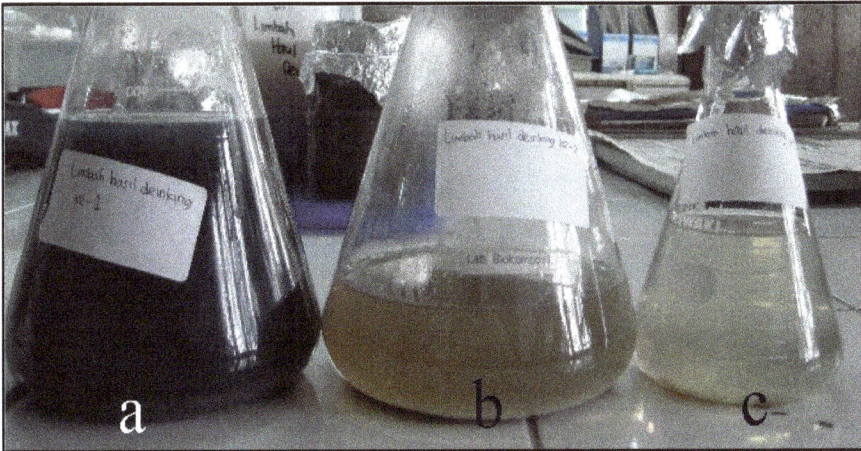

Figure 4.4: Filtrate of First (a), Second (b), and Third (c) Pre-treatment Process

impurities. Beside that, the pollutant particles still can not be completely removed and they became interference on the fiber characterization. Further research was needed to develop the pre-treatment process to get higher rendemen and completely removed impurities.

The Effect of Bleaching Process

In the bleaching process, hydrogen peroxide works in the perhydroxyl ion, OOH^-, that will destroy the chromophore. These reaction will make the fiber became brighter (Li *et al.*, 2011). In this research, after bleaching process the fiber color changed from light brown into white (Figure 4.4). The bleached fiber was also observed using light microscope and it showed a white fiber (Figure 4.5). These results show that the bleaching process was succesfull.

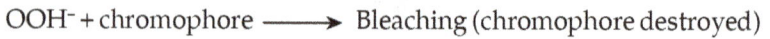

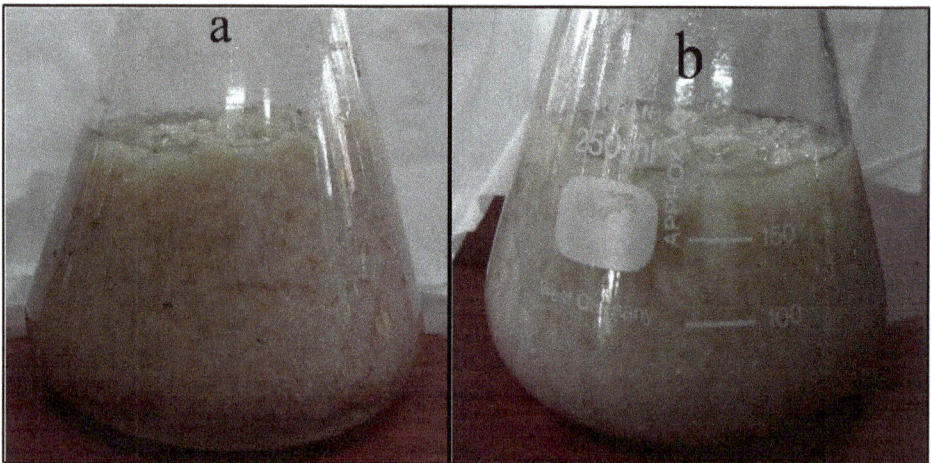

$$OOH^- + chromophore \longrightarrow Bleaching (chromophore destroyed)$$

Figure 4.5: Sludge Before (a) and After (b) Bleaching

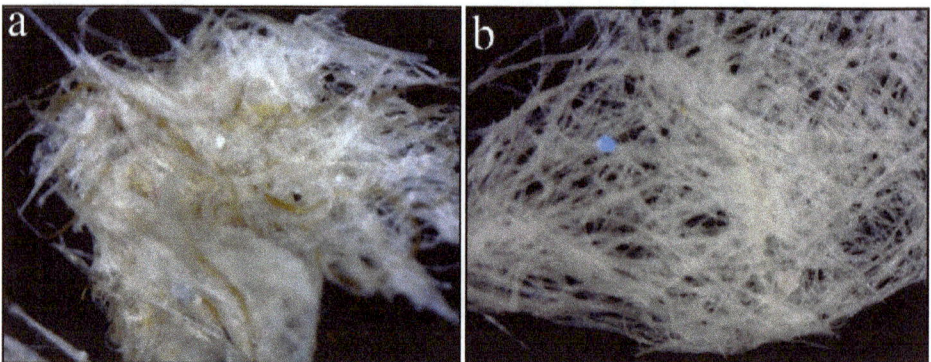

Figure 4.6: Light Microscopic Images of Sludge Fiber Before Bleaching (a) in magnificient of 215x) and After Bleaching (b) in magnificient of 225x)

The Effect of Mechanical Treatment

The effect of mechanical treatment was on the fiber size. Figure 4.7 shows that before mechanical treatment, the sludge fiber was precipitated in water. It fell down to the ground and separated from water. After processed using high performance dispersion instrument (ultratrurrax), it became suspension that stable in water for several days. And after sonication, this suspension became more stable, even for several weeks.

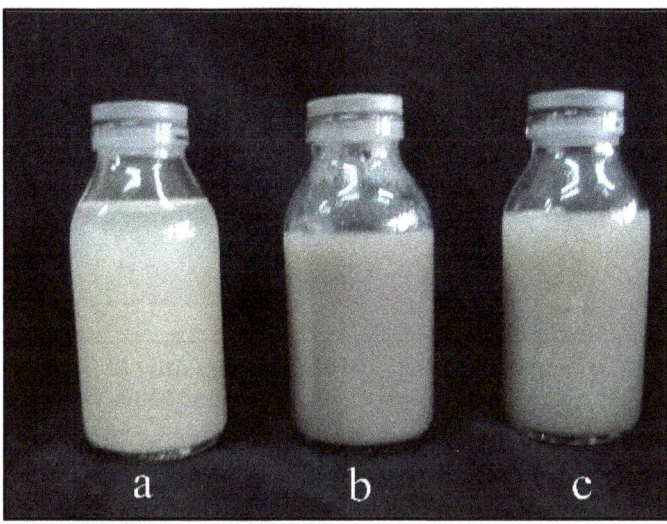

Figure 4.7: Sludge Fiber Suspension before Mechanical Treatment (a), After Processed in Ultraturrax (b), and After Processed in Ultraturrax and Ultrasonic (c)

The morphology of the fiber was observed using light microscope and scanning electron microscope to know the effect of mechanical treatment on the fiber size and its fibrillation. Figure 4.8 shows that before mechanical treatment sludge fiber has

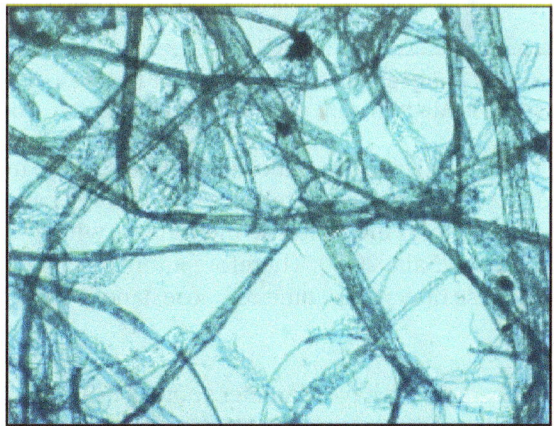

Figure 4.8: Microscopy Images of Sludge Before Mechanical Treatment at Magnificient of 100x

diameter about 800µm. After processed in ultraturrax (Figure 4.9), the diameter of the fiber became about 500-700 nm and the figure also shows that the fibrillation happened but the fibril has not separated completely. Finally, after processed in ultraturrax and ultrasonic (Figure 4.10), the diameter of fiber became 300-500nm and the fibrillation happened better. These results show that mechanical treatment can reduce the diameter of the fiber and make the fibrillation happen.

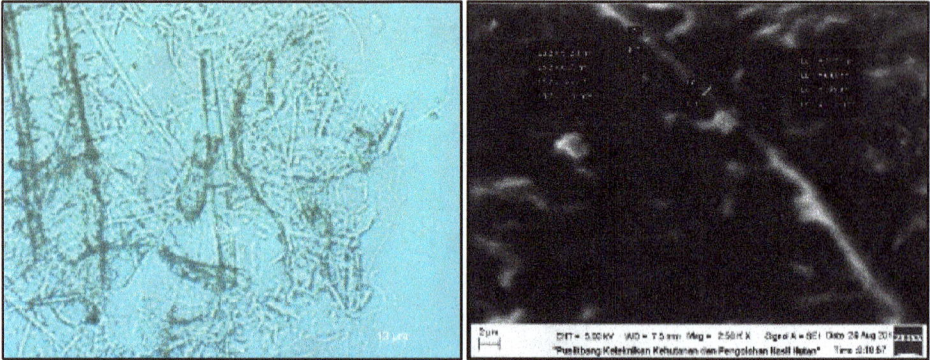

Figure 4.9: Microscopy Images of Sludge Fiber After Processed in Ultraturrax at Magnificient of 500x (Left) and 2500x (Right)

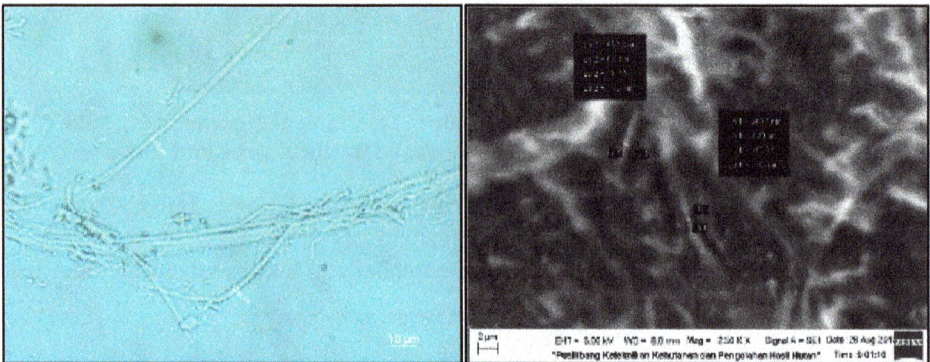

Figure 4.10: Microscopy Images of Sludge Fiber After Processed in Ultraturrax and Ultrasonic at Magnificient of 500x (Left) and 2500x (Right)

According to the general size of cellulose nanofibers, 5-100 nm (Siddiqui *et al.*, 2011), the resulted fibers has not been cellulose nanofibers because the size was about 300-500 nm. These fibers are cellulose microfibers which still have diameter about 0.1-1 µm (Wang and Sain, 2007). Therefore, more mechanical treatment was suggested to convert these fibers to become cellulose nanofibers.

CONCLUSIONS

Cellulose microfibers which have diameter about 300-500 nm was isolated from sludge of pulp and paper industry using high-performance dispersion instrument and sonication. After pre-treatment and bleaching process, cellulose fiber became cleaner and brighter. However, the rendemen was poor and the pollutant particles still can not be fully removed and they became interference on the fiber characterization. More mechanical treatment was suggested to convert these microfibers to cellulose nanofibers.

ACKNOWLEDGMENTS

This research was funded by Competitive Program of Indonesian Institutes of Science (LIPI). The authors also thank to PT Indah Kiat Pulp and Paper for the sludge which be used as the main material of this research.

REFERENCES

1. Abe K, S Iwamoto, H Yano. 2007. Obtaining Cellulose Nanofibers with a Uniform Width of 15 nm from Wood. *Biomacromolecules*, 8 : 3276-3278. DOI:10.1021/bm700624p.

2. Azeredo HMC, LHC Mattoso, RJ Avena-Bustillos, GC Filho, ML Munford, D Wood, TH McHugh. 2010. Nanocellulose Reinforced Chitosan Composite Films as Affected by Nanofiller Loading and Plasticizer Content. *Journal of Food Science*, 75 (1) : N1-N7. DOI: 10.1111/j.1750-3841.2009.01386.x.

3. Balwaik SA and SP Raut, Utilization of Waste Paper Pulp by Partial Replacement of Cement in Concrete. *International Journal of Engineering Research and Applications*, 1(2): 300-309, (2012).

4. Bhatnagar A, Sain M. 2005. Processing of Cellulose Nanofiber-reinforced Composites. *Journal of Reinforced Plastics and Composites*, 24 (12) : 1259-1268. DOI:10.1177/0731684405049864

5. Cherian BM, AL Leao, SF de Souza, S Thomas, LA Pothan, M Kottaisamy. 2010. Isolation of Nanocellulose from Pineapple Leaf Fibres by Steam Explosion. *Carbohydrate Polymers*, 81: 720-725. DOI: 10.1016/j.carbpol.2010.03.046

6. Dufrense A. 2013. Nanocellulose: A New Ageless Bionanomaterial. *Materials Today*, 16 (6): 220-227. DOI: 10.1016/j.mattod.2013.06.004.

7. Edalatmanesh M, M Sain, and Liss SN, Utilization of Secondary Sludge as Filler in Composites: Surface Energy and Final Mechanical Properties, *Journal of Reinforced Plastics and Composites*, 30(10): 864-874, (2011).

8. Fuadi AM and Sulistya H. Pemutihan Pulp dengan Hidrogen Peroksida. *Jurnal Reaktor*, 2008;12(2):123-128.

9. Iwatake A, Nogi M, Yano H. 2008. Cellulose Nanofiber-reinforced Polylactic Acid. *Composites Science and Technology*, 68(2008) 2103-2106. DOI: 10.1016/j.compscitech.2008.03.006

10. Jonoobi M, J Harun, AP Mathew, MZB Hussein, K Oksman. 2010. Preparation of Cellulose Nanofibers with Hydrophobic Surface Characteristics. *Cellulose*, 17 :299-307. DOI 10.1007/s10570-009-9387-9.

11. Lesmono T, *Kajian Pemanfaatan Limbah Sludge IPAL Industri Pulp dan Kertas Sebagai Pupuk*. [Thesis] Sekolah Pascasarjana Institut Pertanian Bogor, (2005).

12. Li J, X Wei, Q Wang, J Chen, G Chang, L Kong, J su, Y Liu. 2012. Homogeneous Isolation of Nanocellulose from Sugarcane Bagasse by High Pressure Homogenization. *Carbohydrate Polymers,* 90 : 1609-1613. DOI: 10.1016/j.carbpol.2012.07.038

13. Li L, S Lee, HK Lee, HJ Youn. 2011. Hydrogen Peroxide Bleaching of Hardwood Kraft Pulp with Asdorbed Birch Xylan and Its Effect on Paper Properties. *BioResources,* 6(1) : 721-736.

14. Mari EL, Moran MSR, Austria CO. Paper Mill Sludge as Fiber Additive for Asphalt Road Pavement. *Philippine Journal of Science*, 138(1): 29-36, (2009).

15. Masruchin N, Kusumaningrum WB, Ismadi, Subyakto. Characteristics of Sugarcane Bagasse Fiber (*Saccharum officinale*) Reinforced Polypropylene Composites. *Journal of Tropical Wood Science and Technology*, 2010;8(1):55-67. ISSN 1693-3834.

16. Moon RJ, A Martini, J Nairn, J Simonsen, J Youngblood. 2011. Cellulose Nanomaterials Review: Structure, Properties, and Nanocomposites. *Chemical Social Review*, 40: 3941-3994. DOI: 10.1039/c0cs00108b.

17. Pezsa N and P Ailer. Bioethanol Production from Paper Sludge Pretreated by Subcritical Water. *Hungarian Journal of Industrial Chemistry Veszprem* 2011;39(2):321-324.

18. Prasetyo J, Naruse K, Kato T, Boonchird C, Harashima S, Park EY. 2011. Bioconversion of Paper Sludge to Biofuel by Simultaneous Saccharification and Fermentation Using A Cellulase of Paper Sludge Origin and Thermotolerant *Saccharomyces cerevisiae* TJ14. *Biotechnology for Biofuels*, 4:35. DOI: 10.1186/1754-6834-4-35.

19. Siddiqui N, Mills RH, Gardner DJ, Bousfiel D. 2011. Production and Characterization of Cellulose Nanofibers from Wood Pulp. *Journal of Adhesion Science and Technology*, 25 (2011) 709-721 DOI:19.1163/016942410X525975

20. Syamani FA, L Astari, Subyakto. 2010. Technology of Producing Cellulose Nanofibers from *Acacia mangium* Pulp. *Proceeding of International Symposium of Indonesian Wood Research Society*, 2010.

21. Wang B, Sain M. 2007. Dispersion of Soybean Stock-based Nanofiber in Plastic Matrix. *Polymer International*, 56:538-546. DOI: 10.1002/pi.2167

22. Wattimena RBI, A Surachman, and W Aziz. Potensi Penerapan Self-locking Wall pada Pemanfaatan Limbah Sludge Deinking Industri Kertas sebagai Batako Interlok. *Jurnal Selulosa*, 1(1): 42-50, (2011).

23. Xi X, F Liu, L Jiang, JY Zhu, D Haagenson, DP Wiesenborn. 2013. Cellulose Nanocrystals vs. Cellulose Nanofibrils: A Comparative Study on Their Microstructures and Effect as Polymer Reinforcing Agents. *ACS Applied Materials and Interfaces*, 5 (8): 2999-3009. DOI: 10.1021/am302624t.

24. Zhao HP, XQ Feng, H Gao. 2007. Ultrasonic Technique for Extracting Nanofibers from Nature Materials. *Applied Physycs Letters* 90, 073112. DOI: 10.1063/1.2450666

Chapter 5

Nano-structured Manganese Titanate Catalysts Prepared in Molten Salts for the Benzylic Oxidation of Alkyl Aromatics under Mild Reaction Conditions

Indri Badria Adilina[1], Syu Takeuchi[2], Takayoshi Hara[2], Nobuyuki Ichikuni[2], Nobuhiro Kumada[3] and Shogo Shimazu[2]*

[1]*Research Centre for Chemistry, Indonesian Institute of Sciences, Kawasan Puspiptek Serpong, Tangerang 15314, Indonesia*
[2]*Graduate School of Engineering, Chiba University, 1-33 Yayoi-cho, Inage-ku, Chiba 263-8522, Japan*
[3]*Graduate School of Medicine and Engineering, University of Yamanashi, 4-4-37 Takeda, Kofu, Yamanashi 400-8510, Japan*
*E-mail: shimazu@faculty.chiba-u.jp

ABSTRACT

A nano-structured Mn-incorporated titanate catalysts (K/MnTO) was synthesised, followed by tuning of its clearance space via cation exchange of the interlayer potassium with alkaline metals in molten salts or proton exchange in acidic media (A/MnTO, A = Li, Na, H). Layered structures were maintained after the exchange with Li^+ and Na^+ whereas a tunnel structure was partly formed when the catalyst was treated with acid. The exchange ratio, clearance space values, and surface properties of the synthesised catalysts varied depending on the interlayer cation. These layered Mn catalysts were applied for the benzylic oxidation of alkyl aromatics using *tert*-butyl hydroperoxide as an oxidant in mild reaction conditions. Li/MnTO catalyst having a 48 per cent exchange ratio, lower water content, and higher surface area, displayed the best catalytic activity among others, exhibiting 80 per cent selectivity toward the aromatic ketone in the oxidation of diphenylmethane and reusable for additional runs.

Keywords: *Nano-structured catalyst, Layered titanate, Manganese, Molten salts, Ion exchange, Benzylic oxidation*

INTRODUCTION

Benzylic oxidation of alkyl aromatics to the corresponding aromatic ketones is of fundamental importance in the synthesis of fine chemicals (Suresh, 2000). Despite good yields, conventional syntheses through a Friedel-Crafts acylation, or by means of transition metal oxidants such as CrO_3, $KMnO_4$, are harsh, and produces large amounts of toxic wastes (Wiberg, 1960; Cullis, 1965). As the demand of clean technology emerges, environmentally benign oxidation processes using supported transition metal-based catalysts under mild reaction conditions are favourable. Although a number of supported metal catalysts of Cr, Mn, Fe, and Co have shown advances for the benzylic oxidation (Tusar, 2011; Jana, 2007; Selvaraj, 2012), leaching of the metal from the catalyst support or relatively high temperature and pressure requirements remain a challenge that must be diminished for industrial purposes.

Layered compounds such as layered silicates or clay minerals are recognised for their host-guest chemistry, which allows strong electrostatic interaction between the interlayer guest species and host lattice (Pinnavaia, 1983; Yamaguchi 2004; Centi 2008). This phenomenon is beneficial in catalysis, since a suitable reaction space and highly stable active sites can be created by easy tune-up of the nanosize interlayer via ion exchange of the guest species (Adilina, 2012; Hara, 2012). While most of the host lattice of layered compounds expands and swells in aqueous media, some types of layered compounds such as layered titanates show low level of expansion and ion exchange ability in aqueous media compared to layered silicates, limiting their use as catalyst precursors. In order to expand the interlayer space, the guest ion is usually exchanged with alkyl ammonium ions, followed by a stepwise exchange process (Sasaki, 1996). In molten salt conditions, however, these materials have proved to show easy ion exchange and give smooth intercalation via simple cation exchange reactions (Adilina, 2013; Lee, 2000).

Manganese titanates, may have a layered lepidocrocite (dakua-FeOOH) structure, by which Mn(III) and Ti(IV) occupy the Fe site and O in the O and (OH) sites (Xu, 2001). Exchangeable cations of alkali metals are located between the manganese titanate layers, balancing the negative charge formed by the replacement of Ti(IV) with Mn(III). In this perspective, the synthesis of cation exchangeable Mn-incorporated layered titanate catalysts (K/MnTO) and their application for the mild benzylic oxidation of aromatic ketones using tert-butyl hydroperoxide (TBHP) as an oxidant is reported. The Mn species was incorporated into the titanate framework to reduce metal leaching, whereas tune-up of the interlayer was controlled by cation exchange of the interlayer potassium with various alkaline metals in molten salts or proton exchange in acidic media (A/MnTO, A = Li, Na, H). The cation exchange ratio of the A/MnTO catalysts was measured by induction coupled plasma-atomic emission spectroscopy (ICP-AES) and their surface properties were analysed by powder X-ray diffraction (XRD), thermogravimetry-differential thermal analysis (TG-DTA), and Brunauer-Emmett-Teller (BET) surface area analysis.

EXPERIMENTAL

Materials

Diphenylmethane and ethylbenzene used as substrates in the oxidation reactions were purchased from Tokyo Chemical Industry Co., Ltd. and distilled under vacuum before use. Catalyst precursor anatase-type TiO_2 was obtained from ST-01, Ishihara Sangyo Co., Ltd. Potassium carbonate and manganese oxide were purchased from Kanto Chemical Co., Inc. Acetonitrile as the solvent was purified before use as in the literature (Armarego, 2005).

Synthesis of Mn-Incorporated Titanate Catalysts

The K/MnTO catalyst was synthesised by first stirring in an alumina crucible a stochiometric mixture of K_2CO_3, Mn_2O_3, and TiO_2 with a molar ratio of 3 : 3 : 10 at 100 °C for 6 h. After cooling to room temperature, the mixture was calcined at 1150 °C for 6 h and a greyish-black powder was obtained. The chemical formula of the synthesised K/MnTO catalyst was found to be $K_{0.36}Mn_{0.36}Ti_{0.59}O_4$ (Mn/Ti = 0.6). Two other catalysts with lower amounts of Mn were synthesised using the same procedure giving a chemical formula of $K_{0.18}Mn_{0.18}Ti_{1.82}O_4$ (Mn/Ti = 0.1) and $K_{0.46}Mn_{0.46}Ti_{1.54}O_4$ (Mn/Ti = 0.3). The three catalysts were denoted as K/MnTO(0.1), K/MnTO(0.3), and K/MnTO(0.6), representing their Mn/Ti ratios of 0.1, 0.3 and 0.6, respectively.

Cation Exchange in Molten Salts or Acidic Media

The cation exchanged A/MnTO(0.6) (A = Li, Na, H) catalysts were prepared by a molten salts technique or acid treatment. An amount of K/MnTO(0.6) catalyst (1.5 g) was treated with either $NaNO_3$ (8 g, 94 mmol) or $LiNO_3$ (8 g, 116 mmol) at 330 °C for 6 h. Proton exchange was performed by acid treatment using 6 M HCl (200 ml) at room temperature. After the cation exchange reaction, an excess of alkaline metal or HCl was adequately washed with distilled water. The final product was filtered and dried at 50 °C.

Characterisation of the Catalysts

The synthesised K/MnTO and A/MnTO(0.6) (A = Li, Na, H) catalysts were characterised by powder X-ray diffraction (XRD) acquired at room temperature from 2°C to 60°C on a MAC SCIENCE MXP3V system operated at 35 kV and 15.0 mA, utilising Cu Kα radiation. The amount of incorporated Mn and intercalated alkaline metal or proton in the A/MnTO catalysts were determined by measuring the amount of unexchanged potassium in the interlayer using inductively coupled plasma atomic emission spectroscopy (ICP-AES) of a Seiko Instruments Inc. SPS 1700 HVR spectrometer, after dissolving the sample in 0.1 M HNO_3 (35 per cent). The Brunauer-Emmett-Teller (BET) specific surface areas were measured using N_2 at -196 °C with a volumetric adsorption analyser BELSORP-max manufactured by BEL Japan, Inc., and all samples were heated at 110 °C for 2 h prior to the analysis. The amount of adsorbed water in the samples was measured using a Rigaku Thermo plus EVO II TG-DTA TG8120 analyser under N_2 atmosphere.

Catalytic Reaction

Catalytic experiments were carried out in a Schlenk flask fitted with a reflux condenser and be settled on a magnetic stirrer. A mixture of diphenylmethane (0.3 mmol), K/MnTO catalyst (0.05 g), and toluene (3 mL) as the solvent was inserted, and TBHP (2.5 eq. relative to diphenylmethane) was added dropwise. The flask was kept at 35 °C and stirred for 24 h. Products of the reaction were analysed by GC and GC-MS analysis using 1,4-dichlorobenzene as the internal standard. GC analyses were performed on a Shimadzu GC-17A Gas Chromatograph packed with a KOCL-3000T column. The mass spectra analyses were conducted with a Shimadzu GC-MS 2010 equipped with an Rtx-5MS column. Oxidation reactions using the cation exchanged A/MnTO catalysts were performed in the same manner.

After the first catalytic reaction, a catalyst was separated by centrifugation, washed with acetonitrile (3 x 10 mL) and dried *in vacuo* before reuse. The recovered catalyst was then characterised by XRD, and the next cycle of oxidation was performed as previously described above.

RESULTS AND DISCUSSION

Powder X-ray Diffraction and ICP-AES Elemental Studies

The XRD patterns of synthesised K/MnTO catalysts with different Mn/Ti ratios are shown in Figure 5.1. At a lower ratio of Mn/Ti = 0.1, the K/MnTO(0.1) catalyst resembled peaks of a tunnel (holladite) structure (Carter, 2005). This was confirmed from the presence of (110), (200), and (310) planes at 12.3°, 17.4°, and 27.5°, respectively. When the manganese molar ratio was increased to Mn/Ti = 0.3, the catalyst structure partly changed to the layered (lepidocrocite) structure (Xu, 1999). Appearance of additional characteristic diffraction peaks of a layered structure at 11.4° (020), 25.2° (040), and 34.5° (060) shows that both tunnel and layered structure existed in the K/MnTO(0.3) catalyst. However, further increasing the molar ratio up to Mn/Ti = 0.6 generated a K/MnTO(0.6) catalyst with dominantly layered structure. The (020) and (130) peaks of a layered structure at 11.3° and 28.7° were observed more intense for the K/MnTO(0.6) catalyst, meanwhile the (200) peak of a tunnel structure was hardly seen. In a previous report, synthesis of a manganese titanate with a reduced cation exchange capacity could not give a layered compound, but a tunnel (hollandite) structure. Similar to this case, K/MnTO catalyst with a lower Mn/Ti ratio indicated lower Mn content (reduced cation exchange capacity) hence the tunnel structure was formed instead of the layered structure. Since the desirable layered structure was best obtained for the K/MnTO(0.6) catalyst, tune-up of the interlayer via cation exchange using different alkaline metal cations or proton species (Li, Na or H) were performed using K/MnTO(0.6) as the catalyst precursor.

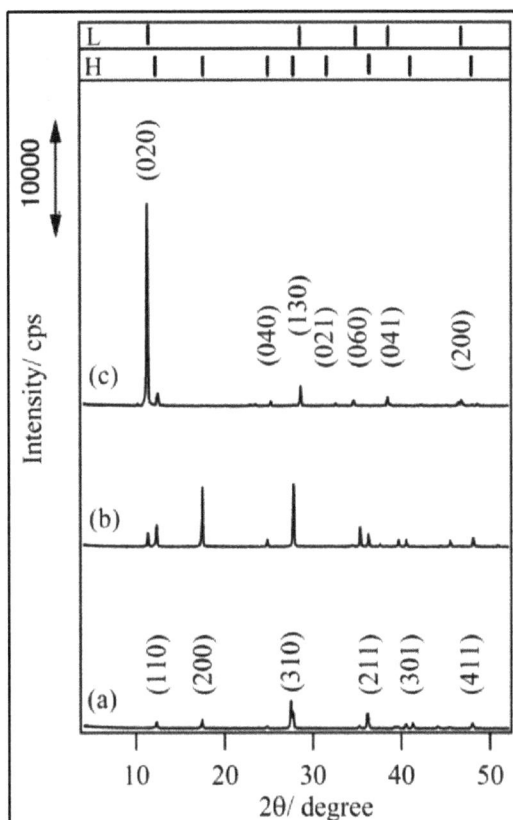

Figure 5.1: Powder X-ray Diffraction Patterns of the Catalyst;
(a) K/MnTO(0.1), (b) K/MnTO(0.3), and (c) K/MnTO(0.6);
L = lepidocrocite phase, H = hollandite phase

Table 5.1: Elemental Analysis Data of K/MnTO(0.6) and
A/MnTO(0.6) (A = Li, Na, H) Catalysts

Entry	Catalyst	Amount[a]/mmol g⁻¹		Exchange Ratio/ Per cent [b]
		Mn	K	
1	K/MnTO (0.6)	2.8	2.8	–
2	Li/MnTO(0.6)	2.8	1.5	48
3	Na/MnTO(0.6)	2.7	0.3	90
4	H/MnTO(0.6)	2.5	0.4	86

[a] Determined by ICP-AES analysis, [b] Calculated based on the amount of K⁺.

Table 5.1 presents the ICP-AES analysis data of K/MnTO(0.6) and cation exchanged A/MnTO(0.6) (A = Li, Na, H) catalysts. The exchange ratio was estimated based on the amount of unexchanged K⁺ and were found as 90 per cent, 86 per cent, and 48 per cent for Na/MnTO(0.6), H/MnTO(0.6), and Li/MnTO(0.6), respectively. The lowest cation exchange ratio was observed for Li/MnTO(0.6) which gave 48 per cent exchange ratio, indicating that the amount of interlayer cations after the exchange reaction was almost an even mixture of K^+ and Li^+. The Mn content in the catalyst framework slightly decreased from 2.8 mmol g^{-1} in the parent K/MnTiO(0.6) catalyst, to 2.7 mmol g^{-1} (Na/MnTO(0.6)) and 2.5 mmol g^{-1} (H/MnTO(0.6)) after the cation exchange. In the case of Li/MnTO(0.6) catalyst, the amount of Mn remained as 2.8 mmol g^{-1}. The preservation of Mn loading showed that the Mn species was not easily removed from the catalysts by cation exchange processes, presumably due to its location is in the titanate framework. Each cation exchanged A/MnTO(0.6) (A = Li, Na, H) catalysts gave different XRD patterns as shown in Figure 5.2 and the calculated clearance space (CS) values of all of the catalysts is summarised in Table 5.2.

Generally, a (020) plane was detected for all catalysts, demonstrating that partly or all of the layered structure was maintained even after the exchange reaction. In the case of H/MnTO(0.6) catalyst, additional phases of tunnel structure were formed. As the previous result of elemental analysis of H/MnTO(0.6) catalyst showed a decrease

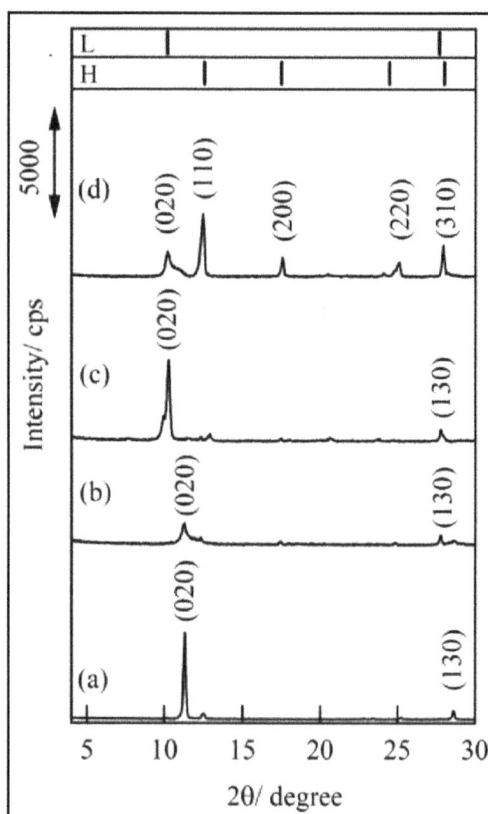

Figure 5.2: Powder X-ray Diffraction Patterns of the Catalyst;
(a) K/MnTO(0.6), (b) Li/MnTO(0.6), (c) Na/MnTO(0.6), (d) H/MnTO(0.6);
L = lepidocrocite phase, H = Hollandite phase

Table 5.2: X-ray Diffraction Parameters for K/MnTO(0.6) and
A/MnTO(0.6) (A = Li, Na, H) Catalysts

Entry	Catalyst	2θ/degree	d_{020}/nm	$d_{010}{}^a$/nm	CS^b
1	K/MnTO(0.6)	11.30	0.78	1.56	0.81
2	Li/MnTO(0.6)	11.28	0.78	1.56	0.81
3	Na/MnTO(0.6)	10.28	0.86	1.72	0.97
4	H/MnTO(0.6)	10.22	0.86	1.72	0.97

[a] Calculated from basal spacing (d_{020}), [b] CS = basal spacing (d_{010}) – layer thickness (0.75 nm)

amount of Mn after the exchange reaction, it is suggested that this decrease of Mn content causes a partial structure change of the catalyst, from the layered to the tunnel structure. On the other hand, layered structures such as demonstrated in the parent K/MnTO(0.6) were dominantly seen for the Li/MnTO(0.6) and Na/MnTO(0.6) catalysts. The widest CS value (CS = basal spacing (d010) – layer thickness (0.75 nm)) (Gao, 2009) was observed for Na/MnTO(0.6) catalyst since it showed the widest basal spacing (d010) of 1.72 nm (CS = 0.97 nm), whereas Li/MnTO(0.6) displayed the same basal spacing (d_{010}) as K/MnTO(0.6) of 1.56 nm (CS = 0.81 nm). The H/MnTO(0.6) catalyst also showed a wide CS value of 0.97 nm, however, this catalyst was a mixture of layered (lepidocrocite) and tunnel (hollandite) structures.

TG-DTA and BET Analyses

TG-DTA analysis was performed to estimate the water content of the catalysts (Table 5.3). Desorption of water molecules in the interlayer of layered titanates occurs below 120°C (Izawa, 1982). Among the catalyst, the highest water content was observed for Na/MnTO(0.6) catalyst with 0.15 mmol g^{-1}, which supports the wide CS value of this catalyst due to water molecules in the interlayer. It was previously reported that a dried sample of the Na+-exchanged layered titanate was observed to rehydrate rapidly in air and explains the origin of water in the molten salt exchange product (England, 1983). In the case of H/MnTO(0.6) catalyst, a lower water content of 0.09 mmol g^{-1} was obtained. Meanwhile, K/MnTO(0.6) and Li/MnTO(0.6) catalysts show trace amount of water as 0.03 and 0.02 mmol g^{-1}, respectively. The surface areas

Table 5.3: Surface Properties of K/MnTO(0.6) and
A/MnTO(0.6) (A = Li, Na, H) Catalysts

Entry	Catalyst	Surface Area^a/ m^2 g^{-1}	Crystalline Size^b/ nm	Water Content^c/ mmol g^{-1}
1	K/MnTO(0.6)	4.2	44	0.03
2	Li/MnTO(0.6)	9.2	29	0.02
3	Na/MnTO(0.6)	4.3	37	0.15
4	H/MnTO(0.6)	4.7	22	0.09

[a] Determined by BET analysis, [b] Determined by XRD analysis using the Scherrer Equation, [c] Determined by TG-DTA analysis

of all catalysts estimated by BET method are also presented in Table 5.3. Although their water content was almost the same, the Li/MnTO(0.6) catalyst showed a higher surface area compared to the parent K/MnTO(0.6) catalyst, presumably due to its smaller crystalline size.

Benzylic Oxidation of Alkyl Aromatics

The benzylic oxidation was first tested for diphenylmethane using K/MnTO catalysts with various Mn/Ti ratios (Table 5.4). From all of the K/MnTO catalysts, K/MnTO(0.6) gave the highest catalytic activity with 35 per cent conversion and 57 per cent selectivity toward the ketone product, benzophenone (entry 3). The K/MnTO(0.1) and K/MnTO(0.3) catalysts on the other hand, showed lower conversions and selectivity of 27 per cent and 21 per cent, respectively (entries 1 and 2). The byproduct besides benzohydrol most probably exists as a peroxide intermediate, diphenylmethane hydroperoxide (Leod, 2010). The higher activity of K/MnTO(0.6) catalyst seems to be assisted by its layered structure that allows easy mobility of substrates in the interlayer, enhancing the access of substrates towards the Mn active sites. Oxidants such as hydrogen peroxide and molecular oxygen were examined for the catalytic reaction; however, conversions were very low in both cases (entries 4 and 5). Moreover, a control reaction without the presence of the catalyst did not proceed well (entry 6).

Table 5.4: Oxidation of Diphenylmethane Catalysed by Various K/MnTO Catalysts

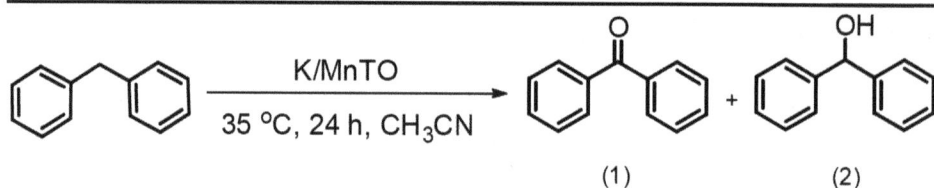

Entry	Catalyst	Mn Loading Amount/mmol g^{-1} cat.	Conv./ per cent [a]	Sel./per cent [a,b] (1)	(2) and (3)[c]
1	K/MnTO (0.1)	1.1	26	27	73
2	K/MnTO (0.3)	2.5	29	21	79
3	K/MnTO (0.6)	2.8	35	57	43
4[d]	K/MnTO (0.6)	2.8	5	60	40
5[e]	K/MnTO (0.6)	2.8	3	100	0
6	Blank	–	3	–	–

Reaction conditions: diphenylmethane, 0.3 mmol; K/MTO catalyst, 0.05-0.10 g; 70 per cent (v/v) TBHP, 2.5 eq; CH_3CN, 3 ml; reaction temperature, 35 °C; reaction time, 24 h; [a] Determined by an internal standard method, [b] Based on product (1), [c] Presumably diphenylmethane hydroperoxide as byproduct, [d] 5 eq H_2O_2 as oxidant, [e] 0.1 MPa O_2 as oxidant.

Effect of Cation Exchange

Results of the benzylic oxidation of diphenylmethane using cation exchanged A/MnTO(0.6) (A = Li, Na, H) catalysts are presented in Table 3.5. The Na/MnTO(0.6) catalyst showed a lower catalytic activity than the parent K/MnTO(0.6), with only 29 per cent conversion and 45 per cent selectivity for benzophenone (entry 1). This low activity is predicted due to the formation of a swollen phase in the catalyst structure, caused by the presence of water molecules in the interlayer (Sasaki, 1995). Meanwhile, the proton exchanged H/MnTO(0.6) catalyst showed a lower conversion of 32 per cent, although a higher selectivity of 69 per cent toward the ketone was obtained (entry 2). Among all of the Mn catalysts, the catalytic activity was best seen for Li/ MnTO(0.6) catalyst with 47 per cent conversion and 62 per cent benzophenone selectivity (entry 3). This yield of carbonyl product is higher than that observed for the parent K/MnTO(0.6) which show 57 per cent selectivity (entry 4). Besides the fact that a lower water content and higher surface area were present in the Li/MnTO(0.6) catalysts, enhanced catalytic activity might be aided by the higher charge density of Li cations, enabling stronger electrostatic interaction between the host and interlayer guest molecules. Increasing the amount of Li/MnTO(0.6) catalyst raised the selectivity to 80 per cent toward the ketone product (entry 5). Furthermore, the Li/MnTO(0.6) catalyst was able to assist the benzylic oxidation of ethylbenzene in good selectivity (entry 6).

Table 5.5: Oxidation of Diphenylmethane Catalysed by K/MnTO and Various Cation Exchanged A/MnTO(0.6) (A = Li, Na, H) Catalysts

Entry	Catalyst	Mn Loading Amount/mmol g^{-1} cat.	Conv./ per cent [a]	Sel./per cent [a,b] (1)	(2) and (3)[b]
1	Na/MnTO(0.6)	2.7	29	45	55
2	H/MnTO(0.6)	2.5	32	69	31
3	Li/MnTO(0.6)	2.8	47	62	38
4	K/MnTO (0.6)	2.8	35	57	43
5[d]	Li/MnTO(0.6)	2.8	45	80	20
6[e]	Li/MnTO(0.6)	2.8	50	70[f]	30[f]

Reaction conditions: diphenylmethane, 0.3 mmol; K/MnTO and A/MnTO(0.6) catalyst (A = Li, Na, H), 0.05 g; 70 per cent (v/v) TBHP, 2.5 eq relative to diphenylmethane; CH_3CN, 3 mL; reaction temperature, 35 °C; reaction time, 24 h. [a] Determined by GC analyses using an internal standard method. [b] Based on product (1), [c] Presumably diphenylmethane hydroperoxide as byproduct, [d] 0.1 g catalyst, [e] ethylbenzene as substrate at 65 °C. [f] (1) benzaldehyde, (2) 1-phenylethanol, and (3) the corresponding hydroperoxide.

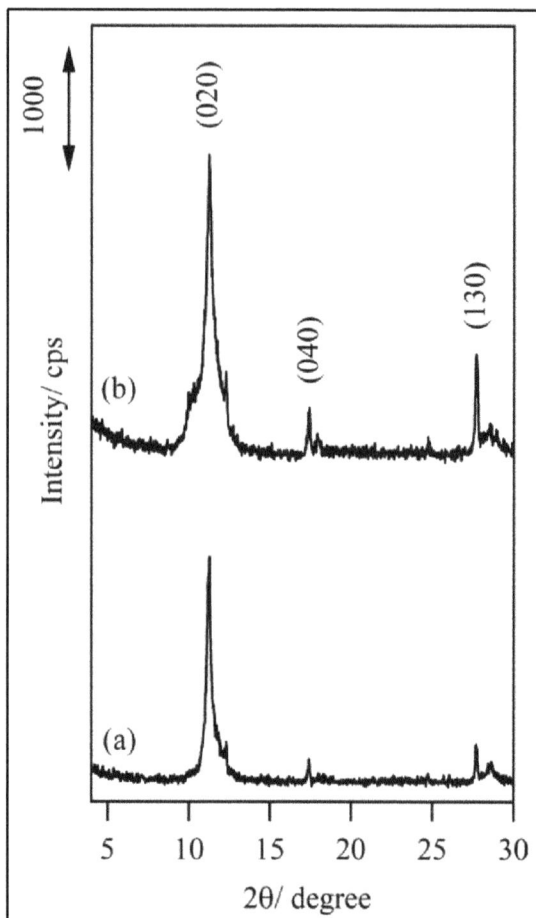

**Figure 5.3: Powder X-ray Diffraction Patterns of the Catalyst;
(a) Fresh Li/MnTO(0.6) and (b) Recovered Li/MnTO(0.6)**

Recycle of the Catalyst

Catalyst recycling tests were performed using Li/MnTO(0.6) as the catalyst. After the first oxidation reaction, the recovered Li/MnTO(0.6) catalyst was analysed by XRD as shown in Figure 5.3. The d_{002} peak of the recovered catalyst was observed at the same position ($2\theta = 11.2$) of that in the fresh, indicating that the CS value of Li/MnTO(0.6) catalyst was maintained even after the catalytic reaction. In addition, the recovered catalyst was analysed by ICP-AES spectroscopy, and elemental analysis data revealed that the Mn and K contents did not change after the reaction. These results confirm that there were no leaching of Mn spesies during the oxidation and the interlayer K^+ and Li^+ were preserved. The catalyst was tested for at least three runs and did not show any significant loss of catalytic activity, maintaining its selectivity toward the desired aromatic ketone (Figure 5.4).

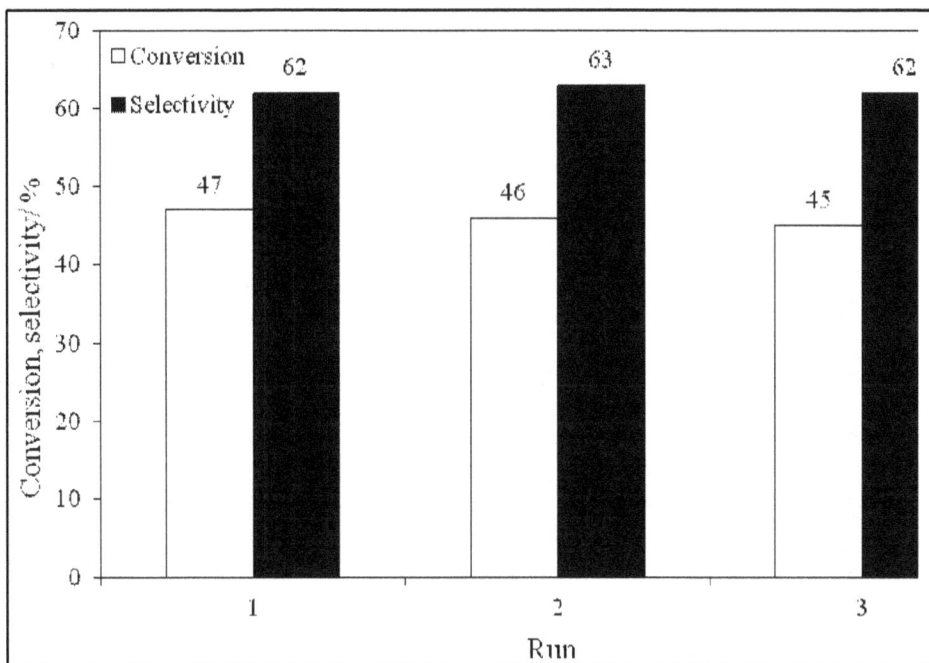

Figure 5.4: Recycle of Li/MnTO(0.6) Catalyst

Reaction conditions: diphenylmethane, 0.3 mmol; Li/MnTO(0.6) catalyst, 0.05 g; 70 per cent (v/v) TBHP, 2.5 eq relative to diphenylmethane; CH_3CN, 3 mL; temperature, 35 °C; reaction time, 24 h. [a] Determined by GC analysis using an internal standard method. [b] Selectivity based on benzophenone

CONCLUSIONS

A nano-structured Mn-incorporated titanate (K/MnTO) catalyst having cation-exchangeable properties was prepared by adjusting an amount of Mn/Ti ratio used in the synthesis. The formation of a layered structure was obtained using a Mn/Ti ratio of 0.6 whereas a tunnel structure was formed when Mn/Ti ratios of 0.1 and 0.3 were applied. The CS value of layered K/MnTO(0.6) catalyst was tuned via a cation exchange reaction of the interlayer K^+ using alkali metals in molten salts or proton exchange in acidic media (A/MnTO(0.6) catalyst, A = Li, Na, H). All of the Mn catalyst exhibited good catalytic activity for the mild benzylic oxidation of diphenylmethane using TBHP as the oxidant, with the Li/MnTO(0.6) catalyst displaying the highest selectivity toward the aromatic ketone due to its lower water content and higher surface area. Preservation of the Mn and K content after the oxidation reaction implies that the Mn spesies in the titanate framework was highly stable, giving reusability of the catalyst for additional runs.

REFERENCES

1.   Adilina, I. B., Hara, T., Ichikuni, N., Kumada, N., Shimazu, S., 2013. Recyclable Pd-incorporated perovskite-titanate catalysts synthesized in molten salts for the

liquid-phase oxidation of alcohols with molecular oxygen. *Bull. Chem. Soc. Jpn.* 86 (1): 146152.

2. Adilina, I. B., Hara, T., Ichikuni, N., Shimazu, S., 2012. Oxidative cleavage of isoeugenol to vanillin under molecular oxygen catalysed by cobalt porphyrin intercalated into lithium taeniolite clay, *J. Mol. Catal. A: Chem.*, 361-362: 72.

3. Armarego, W. L. F., Chai, C. L. L., 2005. *Purification of Laboratory Chemicals*, Elsevier Inc., Massachusetts.

4. Carter, M. L., Withers, R. L., 2005. A universally applicable composite modulated structure approach to ordered BaxMyTi8"yO16 hollandite-type solid solutions. *J. Solid State Chem.* 178: 1903.

5. Centi, G., Perathoner, S., 2008. Catalysis by layered materials: A review. *Micropor. Mesopor. Mat.* 107: 3.

6. Cullis, C. F., Ladbury, J. W., 1955. Kinetic studies of the oxidation of aromatic compounds by potassium permanganate. Part III. Ethylbenzene, *J. Chem. Soc.* 2850.

7. England, W. A., Birkett, J. E., Goodenough, J. B., Wiseman, P. J., 1983. Ion exchange in the Csx[Ti2"x/2Mgx/2]O4 structure. *J. Solid State Chem.* 49: 300.

8. Gao, T., Fjellvag, H., Norby, P., 2009. Protonic titanate derived from CsxTi2"x/2Mgx/2O4 (x = 0.7) with lepidocrocite-type layered structure. *J. Mater. Chem.* 19: 787.

9. Hara, T., Hatakeyama, M., Kim, A., Ichikuni, N., Shimazu, S., 2012. Preparation of clay-supported Sn catalysts and application to Baeyer–Villiger oxidation. *Green Chem.* 14: 771.

10. Izawa, H., Kikkawa, S., Koizumi, M., 1982. Ion exchange and dehydration of layered sodium and potassium titanates, Na2Ti3O7 and K2Ti4O9. *J. Phys. Chem.* 86: 5023.

11. Jana, S.K., Kubota, Y., Tatsumi, T., 2007. High activity of Mn-MgAl hydrotalcite in heterogeneously catalyzed liquid-phase selective oxidation of alkylaromatics to benzylic ketones with 1 atm of molecular oxygen. *J. Catal.* 247: 214.

12. Lee, C., Um, M., Kumazawa, H., 2000. Synthesis of Titanate Derivatives Using Ion-Exchange Reaction, *J. Am. Ceram. Soc.* 83: 1098.

13. Leod, T. C.O. M., Kirillova, M. V., Pombeiro, A. J. L., Schiavon, M. A., Assis, M. D., 2010. Mild oxidation of alkanes and toluene by tert-butylhydroperoxide catalyzed by an homogeneous and immobilized Mn(salen) complex. *Appl. Catal. A Gen.* 372: 191.

14. Pinnavaia, T. J., 1983. Intercalated clay catalysts. *Science*, 220: 365.

15. Sasaki, T., Watanabe, M., Hashizume, H., Yamada, H., Nakazawa, H., 1996. Macromolecule-like Aspects for a Colloidal Suspension of an Exfoliated Titanate. Pairwise Association of Nanosheets and Dynamic Reassembling Process Initiated from It. *J. Am. Chem. Soc.* 118: 8329.

16. Sasaki, T.,Watanabe, M., Michiue, Y., Komatsu, Y., Izumi, F., Takenouchi, S., 1995. Preparation and Acid-Base Properties of a Protonated Titanate with the Lepidocrocite-like Layer Structure. *Chem. Mater.* 7: 1001.

17. Selvaraj, M, Park, D. W., Kawi, S., Kim, I., 2012. Selective synthesis of benzophenone over two-dimensional mesostructured CrSBA-15. *Appl. Catal. A Gen.* 415– 416: 17.

18. Suresh, A. K., Sharma, M. M., Sridhar, T., 2000. Engineering aspects of liquid phase air oxidations of hydrocarbons. *Ind. Eng. Chem. Res.* 39: 3958.

19. Tusar, N. N., Laha, S. C., Cecowski, S., Arcon, I., Kaucic, V., Glaser, R., 2011. Mn-containing porous silicates as catalysts for the solvent-free selective oxidation of alkyl aromatics to aromatic ketones with molecular oxygen. *Micropor. Mesopor. Mat.* 146: 166.

20. Wiberg, K. B., Evans, R. J., 1960. The kinetics of the chromic acid oxidation of diphenylmethane. *Tetrahedron*, 8: 313.

21. Yamaguchi, N., Shimazu, S., Ichikuni, N., Uematsu, T., 2004. Synthesis of Novel Nano-structured Clays: Unique Conformation of Pillar Complexes. *Chem. Lett.* 33: 208.

22. Xu, Z., Inumaru, K., Yamanaka, S., 2001. Catalytic properties of metal loaded silica-pillared manganese titanate for CO oxidation. *Appl. Catal. A Gen.* 210: 217.

23. Xu, Z., Kunii, K., Fukuoka, H., Yamanaka, S., 1999. Protective Oxidation of a Layer Structured Manganese Titanate, RbxMnxTi2-xO4 (x = 0.75), in Acidic Solutions. *Chem. Lett.*, 927.

Chapter 6

Introduction to Iran Nanotechnology Initiative

Hojat Hajihoseini* and Farhad Abbasi

Iranian Research Organization for Science and Technology (IROST),
Tehran 13135 - 115, Iran
*E-mail: hajihoseini@irost.ir

ABSTRACT

This paper outlines the recent nano-technologies programs of the Islamic Republic of Iran. The report is organized in six sections. After a brief introduction and definition in the first and second section, in the third section the history of nanotechnology development in Iran is presented.

In Section two, briefly, the background history is mentioned. Then the Iran Nanotechnology Initiative Council is introduced in nest section. In section fourth, the nano-science and nano-technology situation in Iran are evaluated based on the selected indicators.Finally, the paper is ended by presenting the conclusion.

Keywords: *Nanotechnology, Iran, Initiative.*

INTRODUCTION

The earliest, widespread description of nanotechnology referred to the particular technological goal of precisely manipulating atoms and molecules for fabrication of macro scale products, also now referred to as molecular nanotechnology. A more generalized description of nanotechnology was subsequently established by the National Nanotechnology Initiative, which defines nanotechnology as the manipulation of matter with at least one dimension sized from 1 to 100 nanometers (Drexler, 1992).

Because of the variety of potential applications (including industrial and military), governments have invested billions of dollars in nanotechnology research.

New technologies that are currently developing or will be developed over the next five to ten years, and which will substantially alter the business and social environment include information technology, wireless data communication, man-machine communication, on-demand printing, bio-technologies, and advanced robotics and nanotechnologies.

These technologies now are growing and have significant role on the progress and rapid development of countries. The positive trends of publishing articles or patent registration in these areas show this progress in Iran. Recently in Iran, there have been paid attentions to the formation of emerging technologies in Iran. This has been occurred on policy making and planning and also on institutionalization. Some of these considerations are;

☆ Defining the priorities on emerging technologies

☆ Establishing initiative councils for each new technology by Iran President Deputy on S&T

The progress of advanced technologies in Iran is faced with some challenges. The most important of them are as follow:

☆ Weakness on demand side policy stimulation

☆ Lack of active market for their products

☆ Lack of general consensus

☆ Deficiency on vertical and horizontal policies

☆ Weaknesses on commercialization processes

☆ Lack of competition within the sectors.

RESEARCH METHOD

This study as a descriptive analysis is based on the recently statistical report published by Iran Nanotechnology Initiative Council (INIC). The research provides a holistic view on Iranian nano-technology status.

Background History

Over the three decades there has been a wave of interest in facilitating and fostering R&D-based businesses among the Iranian scholars, government, private and public industries and institutions (Farhad, 2012).

In August 2009, Iran announced a 'comprehensive plan for science' focused on higher education and stronger links between industry and academia. The establishment of a US$2.5 million centre for nanotechnology research is one of the products of this plan. Other commitments include boosting R&D investment to 4 per cent of GDP, and increasing education to 7 per cent of GDP by 2030 (The Royal Society, 2011).

The government's attention to nanotechnology in Iran started in 2001, when the Iranian President Mohammad Khatami made Technology Cooperation Office (TCO) responsible for coordination of developmental activities for nanotechnology in the country. Nanotechnology policy was studied in Technology Cooperation Office (TCO). In 2003, after extensive studies and analysis, TCO recommended creation of a council and was given the task of defining a direction for nanotechnology development in Iran. Additionally, the TCO concluded that nanotechnology development in Iran requires national initiative, proposed the National Iranian Nanotechnology Initiative Program (NINI) that was subsequently approved by Iranian cabinet in July 2005(Sepehr, 2009).

INIC was officially established in 2013, having as its main objective the development and promotion of Nanotechnology in Iran. The "Future Strategy" Plan, a ten years Nano initiative plan, was approved by the government cabinet in July 2005. The aim of the program was to position Iran among the top 15 countries in the field of nanotechnology and consists of 33 action plans in the following categories:

- ☆ Public Awareness
- ☆ Human Resource Development
- ☆ Infrastructure Development
- ☆ Industrial Production and Commercialization
- ☆ International Collaborations
- ☆ Policy and Evaluation

IRAN Nanotechnology Initiative Council (INIC)

INIC is affiliated with the President Deputy of Science and Technology. Beside the general instruction of President Deputy of Science and Technology, the INIC Board of Trustees is the Maine policy making body of INIC. Under the general governance of the President Deputy of Science and Technology, the Secretary General is another main body on INIC. Head of secretariat is working with General Secretary.

There are several technical and supporting departments under the secretariat. They are including:

- ☆ Commercialization development department
- ☆ Industrial development, department
- ☆ Tech-Market service corridor department
- ☆ Technology development department
- ☆ International cooperation department
- ☆ Human resources development department
- ☆ Science and technology infrastructures department
- ☆ Public awareness department.

Time Frames of the Future Strategy at INIC are following:

- ☆ The first program of Nano technology was developed for 3 years in 2006-2008

☆ The second programme was developed for 3 years in 2009-2011

☆ The third programme was developed for four years in 2012-2015

Public Knowledge Promotion on Nano-Tech was the main master plan in the recent years. This includes the following programme:

☆ Politicians and high ranking decision makers

☆ Nano club for children

☆ Student nanotech educational exhibitions

☆ Nanotech sections In high school books

☆ Programmes on TV and radio

☆ Monthly newsletter, No. 12, Vol. 185

☆ Industrialists knowledge promotion, (Workshops, newsletters, leaflets and Industrial show)

Iran's Nano-science and Technology indicators

Student Nanotech Educational Exhibitions

☆ High school students have been trained about nanotechnology by nano-club activities (2008-2011) the number of trained students are 148000 people.

Post Graduate Training Programmes

☆ 34 universities engaged in M.Sc. programmes

☆ 15 universities running Ph.D. programmes

☆ Subjects of specialties: chemical engineering medicine, chemistry, physics, polymer, biotechnology

Horizontal Approach

☆ Centers: 105 universities and research institutes

☆ Human Resources Development

☆ Scientists: 16391 scientists and 2587 faculty members

☆ Students: Total number of PhD and MSc is 14555 people

☆ PhD: total No. of finished projects: 1173and number of ongoing projects are 1398

☆ M.Sc. total No. of finished projects : 7399 and number of ongoing projects are 4585

Vertical Approach Priorities are

☆ Energy, oil, gas and petrochemicals, solar cells, health, DDS and diagnostic kits

☆ Water and environment construction publications

☆ Published books: International books are 29 and the number of national books is 123

Patents Numbers

The Iran Nanotechnology Initiative Council (INIC) established in 2003 launched a program me to encourage nanotechnology researchers to protect their inventions in the country as well as abroad (Ghazinoory, 2010).

Since 2003, 113 inventions have been registered abroad in the field of nano-technology by Iranian researchers. The Figure 6.2 shows that it is increasing from 12 patents registered in 2007 to 25 in 2012.

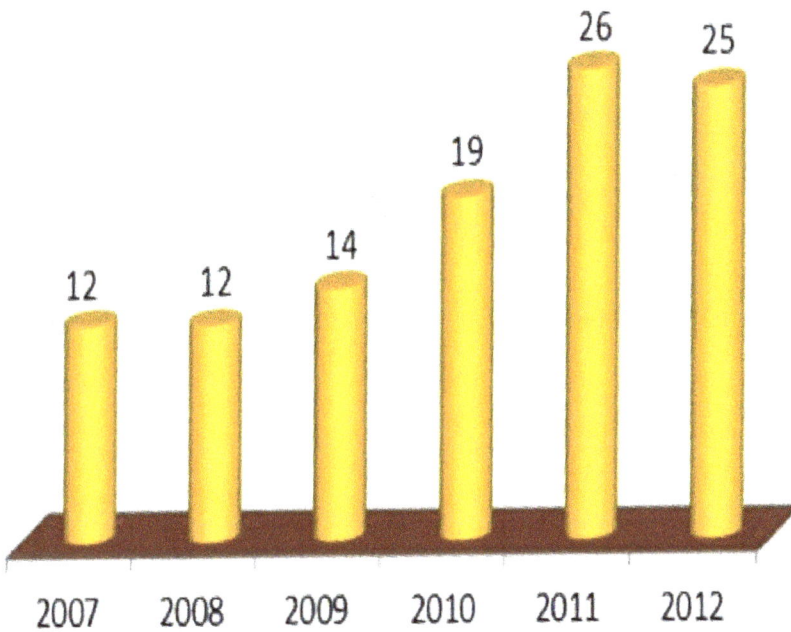

Figure 6.1: International Patents (INIC)

International Collaborations

Iran through INIC has international collaboration with some international bodies such as ECO, UNIDO. The headquarter of Eco-Nano Network (10 countries with 450 million population) is coordinated by INIC in Iran. INIC has collaboration with UNIDO International Center on Nanotechnology for Water Treatment. INIC also is the active member of ANF. INIC has Joint programs with India and Russia in the area of nanotechnology development. Iran has a MOU with Brazil and various joint International conferences with different scientific entities

Start-up Companies

Over the last three decades there has been a wave of interest in facilitating and fostering R&D based businesses among the Iranian scholars, government, private and public industries and institutions (Farhad *et al.*, 2012).

In the field of nano technology, more than 100 start-up have been established by Iranian entrepreneurs. The total areas of working of start-up companies is showed in Figure 6.2.

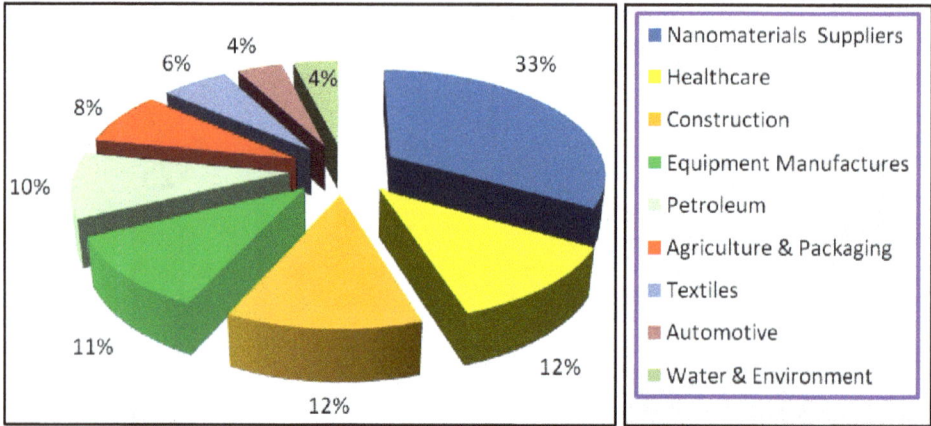

Figure 6.2: The Number of Start-up Companies and their Related Area (INIC)

The number of manufacturing companies are 266.The area of manufacturing firms are; healthcare, construction industry, agriculture and packaging, petroleum and related industries, textile industry, automotive industry and water and environment.

As showed in Figure 6.3, the biggest portion of the figure is allocated to nonmaterial's suppliers with 33 percentage share. It shows that nonmaterial's is one of the most important activities within the nano-manufacturing companies. The second rank related to healthcare activities with 18 per cent of total manufacturing

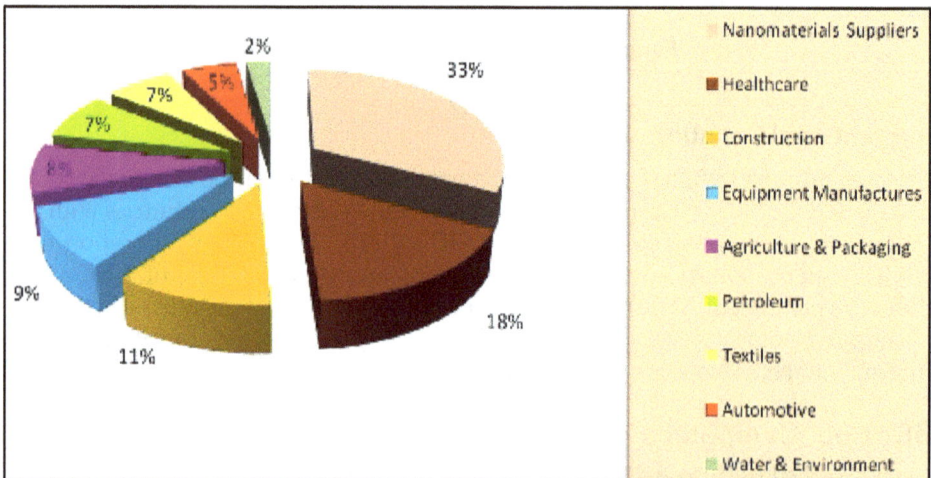

Figure 6.3: The Number of Manufacturing Companies (INIC)

firms. The least portion is allocated to water and environment with 2 per cent of total activities.

INFRASTRUCTURES DEVELOPMENT

IRAN Nanotechnology Laboratory NETWORK (INLN)

INLN network shares more than 852 equipment from 57 research centers throughout I.R.IRAN. These research centres are located in Tehran, Isfahan, Hamadan, Karaj, Yazd, Tabriz, Birjand, Zahedan and Kashan.

Iran Nanotechnology Standardization Committee (ISIRI/TC229)

Iran Nanotechnology Standardization Committee is established in 2006. The ISIRI is the P-member of the ISO/TC229 and the elected member of the Chairman Advisory Group (CAG) in ISO/TC229. This committee published 7 national nano-standards and another 5 currently under review. Also the Committee was Published 1 international standard (ISO/TR11360). Iran Nanotechnology Standardization Committee established Nano Standardization Committees at the Ministry of Health and Agriculture. The Committee was established Nano-Safety Network.

Tech-Market Services Corridor

In order to support nanotech commercialization in Iran, the Corridor was established at 2010 with the aim to provide wide range of services to start-ups, SMEs and large scale industries. These services are including:

- ☆ Nano-Scale Audit
- ☆ Intellectual Property (IP)
- ☆ Technology Readiness Level (TRL)
- ☆ Assessment, Business plan (BP)
- ☆ Licensing and, Standard, Tech-Monitoring
- ☆ Venture capital
- ☆ Market evaluation
- ☆ Legal advisory and
- ☆ International marketing

Technical aspects of Tech-Market Services Corridor are: nano-scale, technology level, documentation, patenting, technology monitoring, technology transfer, technology guaranty fund, market requirement and monitoring and market aspects of Tech-Market Services Corridor are: business planning, production advisory, venture capital, standards and certificates, financing Local marketing, global marketing.

Nano-science Papers

The trend of ISI nano publications of Iran between 2000-2012. It shows the increasing number of papers from 59 in 2000 to 3650 papers in 2012.

Based on NANO STATISTICS site, the number of ISI Articles in the field of nano-science and nanotechnology, during the period of the end of July, 2013 and 20 of Sept.

2013 has been 2173.and 2,663 respectively. As Table 6.1 shows that Iran has saved its international rank in the 8th rank after the South Korea, Japan and France among 101 countries.

Table 6.1: Number of ISI Articles

Rank	Country	Nano-article	Share (per cent)	Rank	Country	Nano-article	Share (per cent)
		End of July, 2013				20 of Sept. 2013	
1	China	16366	30	1	China	20,463	30.2
2	USA	9856	18.1	2	USA	12,231	18.1
3	India	3822	7.0	3	India	4,687	6.9
4	Germany	3430	6.3	4	Germany	4,277	6.3
5	South Korea	3374	6.2	5	South Korea	4,260	6.3
6	Japan	3199	5.9	6	Japan	4,030	6.0
7	France	2314	4.3	7	France	2,938	4.3
8	Iran	2173	3.9	8	Iran	2,663	3.9
9	UK	1823	3.4	9	UK	2,279	3.4
10	Spain	1708	3.1	10	Spain	2,133	3.2

CONCLUSIONS

Based on the annual report issued by INIC, the rank of Iran nanotechnology is growing rapidly at the stage of knowledge creation. But the process of commercialization and bringing the knowledge to the market is not well developed. The report shows that the engine of nanotechnology progress at the stage of knowledge creation in Iran is some incentive from the government of Iran. Therefore, the government should make some other policies and planning to stimulate the market to use the nano-products.

ACKNOWLEDGMENTS

The authors would like to acknowledge NAM S&T Centre, RISTEK and Indonesian Society for Nanotechnology for organizing the International workshop on Nanotechnology (IWON) 2013. We need to offer our special thanks to the Iran Nanotechnology Initiative Council (INIC) authorities.

They would also like to thank Dr. Akbari, the IROST's president for facilitation of this visit.

REFERENCES

1.   Abbasi, Farhad; Attar, Hooman; Hajihoseini, Hojat, 2012. Commercialization of new technologies: The case of Iran, *International Journal of Technology Management and Sustainable Development*, Volume 11, Number 2, 1 June 2012, pp. 191-202(12)

2.   Drexler-K.Eric, 1992. Nanosystem: Molecular machinery and computing, New York, John Wiley and Sons.

3. http://www.ingentaconnect.com/content/intellect/tmsd/2012/00000011/00000002/art00005

4. Ghazinoory, Sepehr; Saber Mirzaei, and Soroush Ghazinoori., 2009. A model for national planning under new roles for government: Case study of the National Iranian Nanotechnology Initiative Science and Public Policy (2009) 36 (3): 241-249 doi:10.3152/030234209X427095 ory *et al.,* 2009a).

5. Ghazinoory, S., Abdi M. and k. Bagheri., 2010. Promoting Nanotechnology patenting: A new experience in national innovation system of Iran, Journal of Intellectual Property Rights. Vol. 15, November 2010, pp 461-473.

6. http://www.nano.ir/index.php?lang=2

7. The Royal Society, 2011. Knowledge, Networks and Nations: Global scientific collaboration in the 21st century, RS Policy document 03/11, Issued: March 2011 DES2096, ISBN: 978-0-85403-890-9.

8. Sawahel W., 2009. Iran: 20-year plan for knowledge-based economy. University World News.

9. http://statnano.com/

10. www.inic

Chapter 7

Madagascar Nanotechnology Initiative Programme

Raoelina Andriambololona, H. Andrianiaina*,
H. Rakotoson and T. Ranaivoson

Institut National des Sciences et Techniques Nucléaires (INSTN),
Madagascar
*E-mail: hery_andrianiaina5@yahoo.fr

ABSTRACT

Nanosciences and Nanotechnology are now developing considerably around the world, and covering many domains which are used to find issue on many topics. Madagascar has the opportunity to have all natural resources used in most of nanotechnology research and industrial application domains, but not were utilized. Since some decades the business related to mining activities is considerably increasing, and many companies from developed countries (Canada, Australia, China, etc.) began to exploit and export all their productions (zircon and titanium, for instance) only abroad. Mineral such as is titanium could be used in the domain of energy conversion and storage using solar cells, or in other applications. This would fits with the governmental program to reduce reliance on the expensive thermal power plants. The government, through the Ministry of Higher Education and Scientific Research has initiate a program and has just created the CORANANO (Commission RAOELINA ANDRIAMBOLOLONA pour la Nanotechnologie) to lead any related activities, to sensitize and educate peoples for the benefits but also the risks of the nanotechnology. The program has just started in Madagascar, and it was identified that some Research and Development activities could be started.

Keywords: *Madagascar business, Madagascar economy, Nanotechnology, Photovoltaic, Solar cells, Titanium.*

INTRODUCTION

The science of Nanotechnology is developing very fast around the world, and converging to find issue on many topics. Madagascar has the opportunity to have all natural resources used in most of nanotechnology research and industrial application domains. Since some decades the economy and business of Madagascar are more centered on mineral resources: coal, bauxite, industrial beryl, garnets, chromate, graphite, zircon and titanium. And the program of Madagascar in matters of energy is to reduce reliance on the expensive thermal power plants (more expensive imported fuel), and expansion of electricity supply by using renewable energy. Solar energy would gives power to remote regions which don't have power grids. Small rooftop photovoltaic systems are used and still imported from abroad. Titanium dioxide is used in dye-sensitized solar cells, which are a type of chemical solar cell (also known as a Gratzel cell).

MATERIALS AND METHODS: MADAGASCAR INITIATIVE

Madagascar Nanotechnology Initiative

This year (2013) Madagascar, through the Ministry of Higher Education and Scientific Research and the TInstitut National des Sciences et Techniques NucléairesI (INSTN) has decided to launch a national program to evaluate all issue and benefit for the country with Nanotechnology. Through the Tarrêté Ministériela n° 6221/2013-MESupReS on 21st March 2013, the committee, namely CORANANO (for

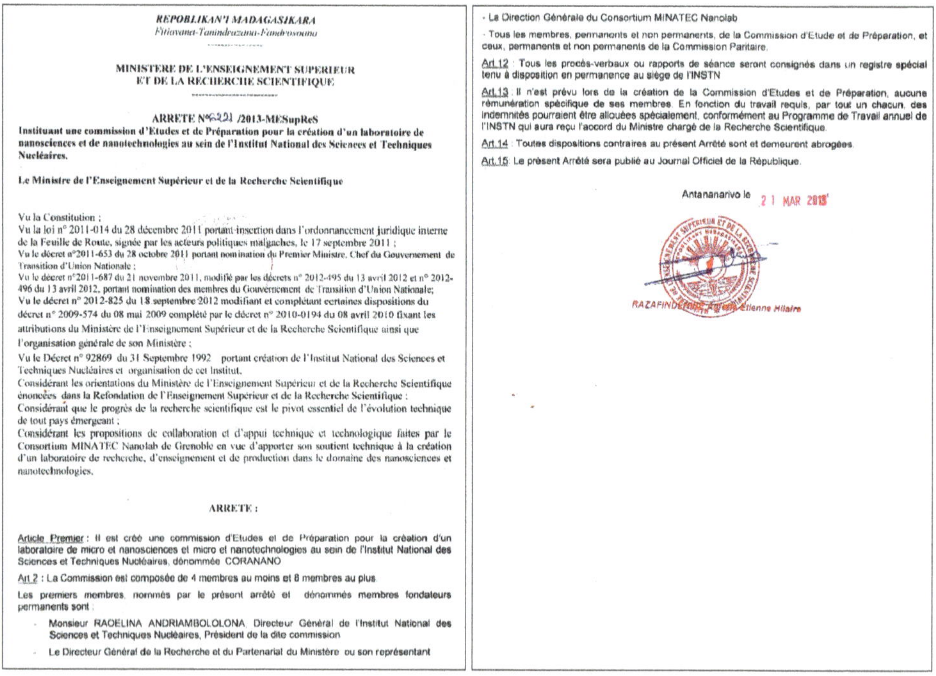

Figure 7.1: Ministerial Decree for the Creation of CORANANO

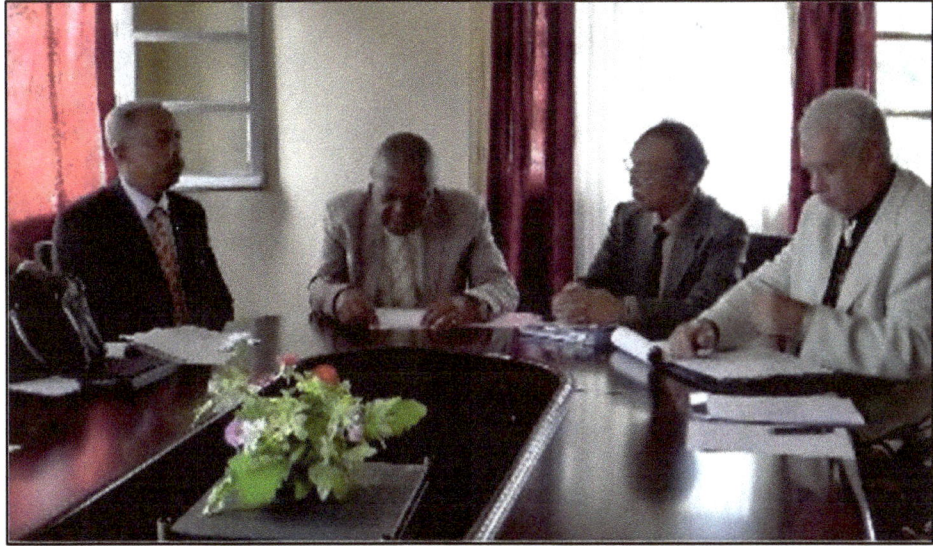

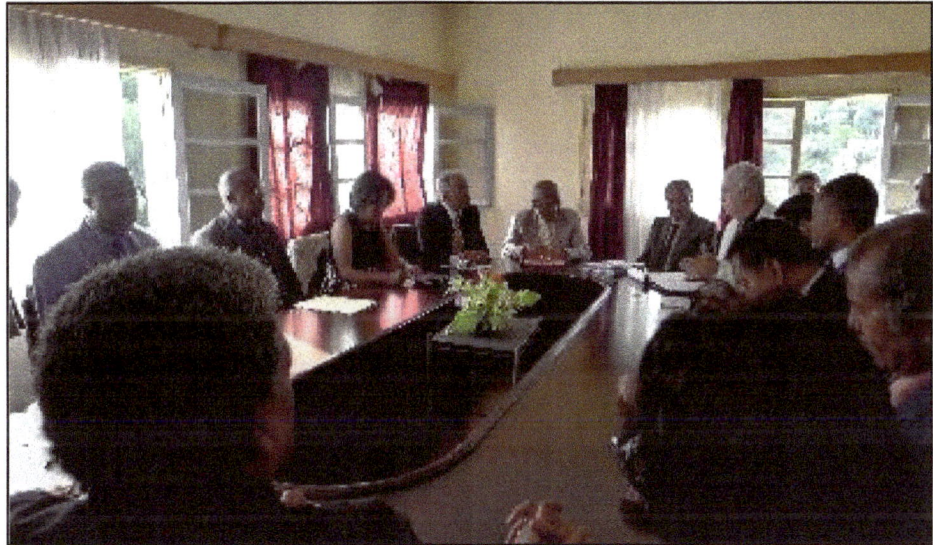

**Figure 7.2L The Minister (Higher Education and Scientific Research)
Launching the Meeting of the CORANANO**

Commission RAOELINA ANDRIAMBOLOLONA pour la Nanotechnologie) was created as the leader related to this new domain for the country.

The CORANANO has launched its first meeting on 15th April 2013. Many representatives of the Government and from Research Centres honored the event by their presence.

Sensitization

Series of conferences on Nanotechnology are scheduled through SIRA (Séminaire Interdisciplinaire RAOELINA ANDRIAMBOLOLONA), which is a platform created

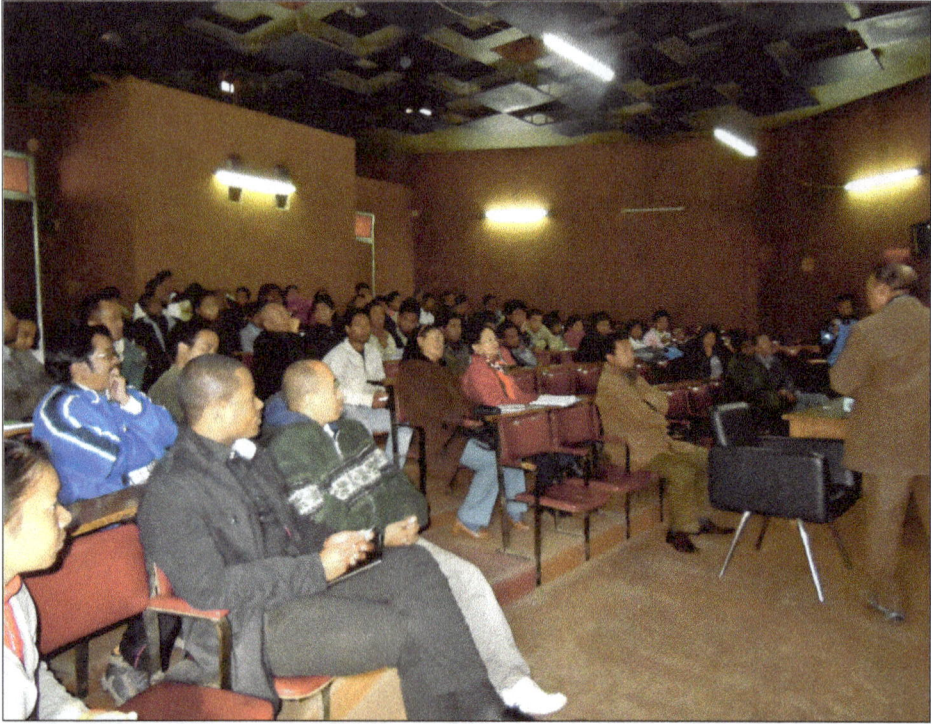

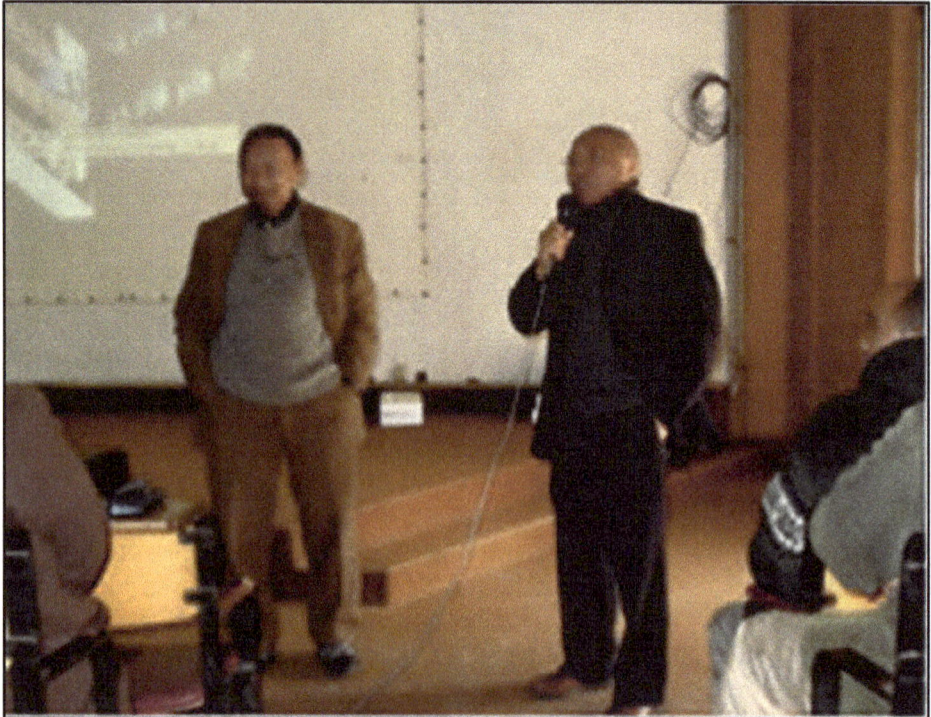

Figure 7.3: Conference Presentation Made by Pr. RAOELINA ANDRIAMBOLOLONA (Executive President of CORANANO)

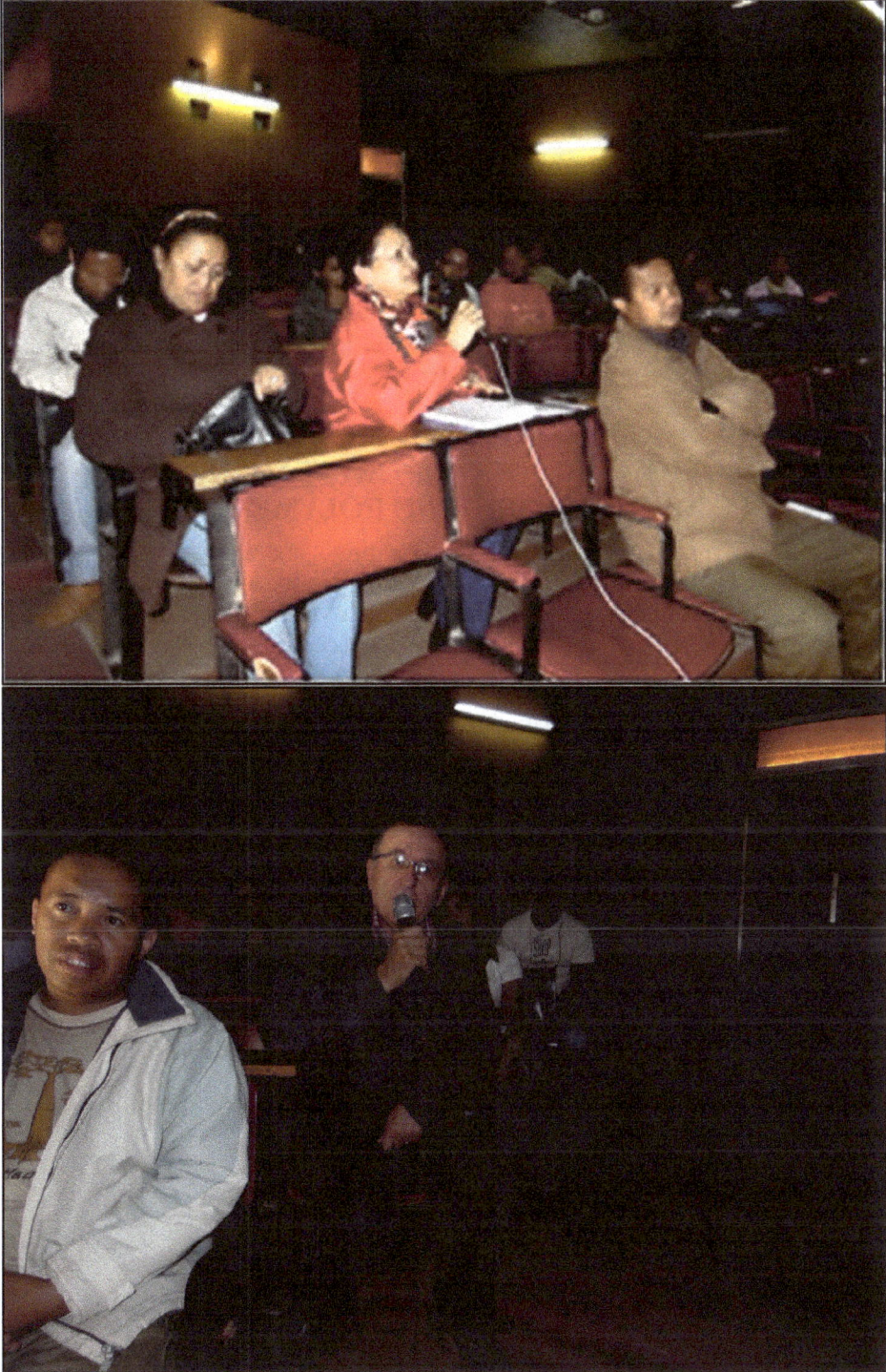

Figure 7.4: Peoples are Very Interested with this New Technology

by INSTN since many years intended to disseminate information related to any research activities.

The first, inaugural one was on July 13th which gave some basic overview of nanoparticles and nanomaterials.

Assessment and Recommendations

- ☆ Young scientists were the majority of attendees of all workshop
- ☆ Young scientists were sensitized, and many very enthusiast to get involved in Nanotechnology activity
- ☆ The start-up of initiative for collaborative research activities was discussed and planned in order to get benefit on using available resources and putting on more added-value.

RESEARCH AND DEVELOPMENT PROJECT ON SENSITIZATION OF NANO-CRISTALLINE TiO$_2$ BY AVAILABLE NATURAL ORGANIC POLYMERS

One result from the series of workshop is the collaborative program from the INSTN-Madagascar (Institut National des Sciences et Techniques Nucléaires) and some researchers from the university of Antananarivo. The main area of interest is the use of nanotechnology for "green" energy, specially based on natural organic polymers.

Research Project on the Use of Locally Available Natural Organic Polymer for DSSC

The main object is to find a good and reliable candidate for the Dye material to be used as sensitizer for solar cell. For the technology known as "Nano-Crystalline Dye Sensitized Solar Cell" (DSCC), most of the material used as semiconductor do not absorb spectrum of visible light. The method to attach these colored dyes and sensitize the semiconductor has to be defined for better collection and transport of electron, thus the current.

Some locally abundant natural organic colored materials are identified to be a potential candidate for the task, and will be subject to be studied and evaluated: Sepia ink (from *Sepia Officinalis*).

a) Project Activity to Theoretically Study of the Sepia Ink Structure

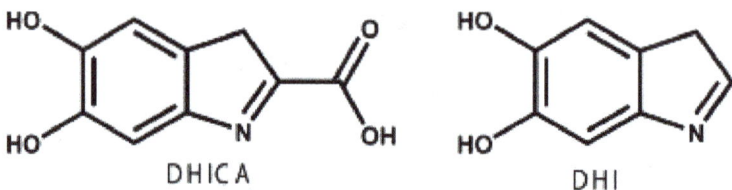

DHICA   DHI

Sepia ink is a copolymer of DHICA and DHI

The main targets are to define the right model and for simulation determination of:

- ☆ Electronic coupling between the **dye molecule** (copolymer of DHI and DHICA: IMIM or HMHM) and the TiO_2 semiconductor
- ☆ Molecular adsorption of Copolymer on TiO_2 semiconductor
- ☆ Location of the **highest occupied molecular orbital (HOMO)** and the **lowest occupied molecular orbital (LUMO)** Energy compared to **TiO_2 band gap** (enhancing Visible light absorption? electron-hole recombination probability?)
- ☆ Project activity to Chemically determination of the sensitization process of TiO_2 by Eumelanin (*Sepia ink*).

CONCLUSIONS

Many possibilities could be done and some project activities which can be started are identified. The one very promising and fits with the governmental programme related to energy planning, is in the domain of energy conversion and storage using solar cells. Another field deals with water treatment.

As Nanotechnology is a multi-disciplinary and multi-domain field of activities, working in pool is avoidable. Madagascar has just lunch a nanotechnology initiative, and still not has adequate facilities for nanotechnology. However for the beginning theoretical prediction by simulation and limited physic-chemical studies can be started.

AKNOWLEDGEMENTS

We wish to extend our great appreciation to

- ☆ Pr. RAOELINA ANDRIAMBOLOLONA, Executive President of CORANANO, Director General of INSTN-Madagascar for all his support and allowing participation to this symposium,
- ☆ His Excellency ARTANTO SALMOEN WARGADINATA, Minister, Republic of Indonesia Embassy in Madagascar, for his support and taking in charge our air fare ticket, which allow us to join this symposium
- ☆ The NAM S&T for organizing this symposium and allow us to get acquainted with this network, and information sharing.
- ☆ The RISTEK for hosting the symposium in Indonesia

REFERENCES

1. http://www.ehow.com/list_7388737_madagascar_s-energy-sources.html#ixzz2c3FqtvxP (accessed 15 Sep.2013).

2. http://www.theodora.com/wfbcurrent/madagascar/madagascar_economy.html (accessed 24 Sep.2013). Madagascar Economy 2013

3. http://www.worldtitaniumresources.com/ (accessed 25 Sep. 2013)

4.   Shun Yu, Sareh Ahmadi, Marcelo Zuleta, Haining Tian, Karina Schulte, Annette Pietzsch, Franz Hennies, Jonas Weissenrieder, Xichuan Yang, and Mats Göthelid, 2010. Adsorption geometry, molecular interaction, and charge transfer of triphenylamine-based dye on rutile TiO_2(110). In: *Journal of Chemical Physics*, Vol. 133, Issue 22.

Chapter 8

Nanotechnology Contribution as Economic Driver in Malaysian Economic Transformation Programme

Abdul Kadir Masrom

National Nanotechnology Directorate,
Ministry of Science, Technology and Innovation, Putrajaya, Malaysia
E-mail: akadir@mosti.gov.my

ABSTRACT

The Economic Transformation Programme (ETP) was launched on 25 September, 2010 by Malaysian 6th Prime Minister Datuk Seri Najib Abdul Razak, formulated as part of Malaysia's National Transformation Programme. It is a comprehensive economic transformation plan with an ultimate goal is to propel Malaysia's economy and turn it into a high income economy by the year 2020, targeting GNI per capita of US$15,000. This will be achieved by attracting US$444 billion in investments which will, in turn, create 3.3 million new jobs. The program will lift Malaysia's Gross National Income (GNI) to US$523 billion by 2020 that can be achieved through the implementation of 12 National Key Economic Areas (NKEAs), representing economic sectors which account for significant contributions to GNI. The 12 National Key Economic Areas (NKEAs) are Oil, Gas and Energy; Palm Oil and Rubber; Financial Services; Tourism; Business Services; Electronics and Electrical; Wholesale and Retail; Education; Healthcare; Communications Content and Infrastructure; Agriculture; and Greater Kuala Lumpur/Klang Valley. Malaysian Government recognized that Nanotechnology is a key enabling technology that will generate new sources of economic growth. It is perceived as a singular scientific discovery that has the potential to create a wealth of innovative products and solutions across a vast array of fields. Malaysia's involvement in nanotechnology started back as early as year 2001 when nanotechnology was included as one of priority research area under Intensified Research in Priority Area (IRPA) and Malaysian involvement in nanotechnology forum at international level started in year 2003, when the country became a member of the Asia Pacific Nanotechnology Forum which was initiated by Japan. The current Prime Minister, Datuk Seri Mohd. Najib bin Tun Abdul Razak are the main forces and drivers for nanotechnology development in Malaysia as through his strong support, National Nanotechnology Initiatives was proposed and approved by the Cabinet in 2006. In year 2009, Prime Minister Datuk Seri Mohd. Najib identified nanotechnology as an important growth engine for the new economic policy he introduced that will stimulate and accelerate development of home grown nano science, engineering and technology into beneficial technologies. Going by global trends, nanotechnology will impact all 12 NKEAs in varying degrees. Nanotechnology will soon be manifested in the materials, tools, components, services and end-products of all 12 sectors. In this paper, the author would like to share challenges in developing nanotechnology as one of the growth engine and how nanotechnology was positioned to fit with Malaysian ETP. The author also present the high impact nanotechnology R&D for National Key Economic Area (NKEA) and review on how NanoMalaysia Program impacting our 18 identified Entry Point Project (EPP) as well as presenting our strategic approach to jumpstart the NT industry by aligning NT to national socio-economic planning initiatives comprises of New Economic Model (NEM) and Economic Transformation Programme (ETP).

Keywords: Economic transformation program, National key economic area.

INTRODUCTION

Malaysian Economic Transformation programme launched on September 21, 2010 is an initiative by the Malaysian government to turn Malaysia into a high income economy by the year of 2020. It is managed by the Performance Management and Delivery Unit (PEMANDU), an agency under the Prime Minister Department of Malaysia. It is a comprehensive economic transformation plan to propel Malaysia's economy into high income economy. The program will lift Malaysia's Gross National Income (GNI) to US$523 billion by 2020, and raise per capita income from US$6,700 to at least US$15,000, meeting the World Bank's threshold for high income nation (PEMANDU, 2010). It is projected that Malaysia will be able to achieve the targets set if GNI grows by 6 per cent per annum. Set to revitalize Malaysia's private sector, the 60 per cent of the blueprint's investment would derived from private sector, 32 per cent from government linked companies and the remaining 8 per cent from the government. Various sectors for development have been identified and are called *National Key Economic Areas (NKEA)*. The Economic Transformation Programme (ETP) is a focused, inclusive and sustainable initiative that will transform Malaysia into a high-income nation, driven by private sector investments. The ETP has two key thrusts - focus, through the 12 NKEAs, and competitiveness, to be delivered by the Strategic Reform Initiatives (SRIs). It is driven by 12 National Key Economic Areas (NKEAs): Oil, Gas and Energy; Palm Oil and Rubber; Financial Services; Wholesale and Retail; Tourism; Business Services; Electrical and Electronics; Communications Content and Infrastructure; Healthcare; Education; Agriculture; and Greater Kuala Lumpur/Klang Valley. The Six Strategic Reform Initiatives (SRIs) namely Public Finance; Government's Role in Business; Human Capital Development; Public Service Delivery;

Competition, Standards and Liberalisation and Narrowing Disparities (Bumiputera SMEs) were launched in 2011 to help boost Malaysia's global competitiveness. Entry Point Projects outlined within the 12 NKEAs are catalytic in nature and will lead Malaysia towards achieving a high-income nation status with a per capita income of RM48,000 (USD15,000) and create more than 3.3 million new jobs by 2020, throughout the country (PEMANDU, 2010).

Malaysia will have to balance between opportunities and risks that will be encountered in making nanotechnology a strategic growth area for the country. The proposed approach is to leverage upon sectors where we already have relatively strong market positions and to be in line with the ETP and the NKEA. This is where early markets for nanotechnology will be created. Nanotechnology, by virtue of its technological convergence qualities, is the common underlying denominator between our socio-economic goals and technological needs. In 2007, the Malaysian Industry Government Group for High Technology (MIGHT) produced a report detailing six priority areas to focus Malaysian's nanotechnology players (MIGHT, 2007). Malaysia has undergone a decade of continuous R&D activities and developmental initiatives that validate the benefits of nanotechnology. This was evidenced by the launch of the Malaysian Nanotechnology Initiatives in 2006; establishment of the National Nanotechnology Directorate (NND) and the National Nanotechnology Statement in 2010; and the incorporation of NanoMalaysia Berhad (NMB) as the commercial entity for the development of the nanotechnology industry in Malaysia. These are significant Malaysian nanotechnology milestones to date. As we recognized nanotechnology as the next new growth area that will ensure prosperity for Malaysia, we need to seize this opportunity to ride on the coming wave of technological evolution. NND was given authority and responsibility in formulating national nanotechnology policy and blueprint aims at providing favorable conditions for industrial innovation in nanotechnology to ensure that research and technological development is translated into affordable and safe wealth-generating products and processes and ensuring Malaysian will not be left behind in the fast moving nanotechnology. Future nanotechnology development need to be comprehensively integrated into the economy as it require high readiness, effective strategic planning and widespread investments by business, education, labour and government. There are need to educate policy makers and government official to ensure widespread understanding of the numerous benefits from applications of nanotechnology, its strategic economic value for the nation, and its role in maintaining our global competitiveness. Comprehensive social and industry-wide adoption will lead to a positive impact on national productivity and an enhanced quality of life.

Nanotechnology in Malaysia

Nanotechnology is fast emerging and marks the beginning of a new wave of technologies that will redefine, reshape and eventually transform economies and societies on a global scale. Nanotechnology was considered as a key enabling technology that will generate new sources of economic growth may well shape the sustainability and wealth of nations, organizations and entire industries for Malaysia in the future. It is a continuation of the next chapter in the acceleration of advanced technology and, perhaps more importantly, it may point towards the transformation of the future global economy.

A mind-boggling array of nano-enhanced products is now trickling into the global market, however Malaysia has yet to figure prominently in this new technology and product paradigm, despite a looming global market worth up to USD3 trillion by 2020, the nation just cannot afford to ignore nanotechnology. The Malaysian GDP stood at USD237.8 billion in 2010, an impressive amount generated by industries, products and services that will yet be made redundant without nano-technological inputs by 2020. By then, all cutting edge products, materials and instruments will incorporate nanotechnology in one form or the other. In a nutshell, Malaysia needs to incorporate nanotechnology as a primary, new growth engine.

Nanotechnology R&D in Malaysia started way back in year 2001 when the Intensification of Priority Areas (IRPA) program of the Eight Malaysia Plan (8MP) funded under IRPA by then Ministry of Science, Technology and Environment (MOSTE) (later known as Ministry of Science, Technology and Innovation, MOSTI) that spans from 2001 to 2005 identified and include nanotechnology as one of the 14 research priority areas and was categorized as Strategic Research (SR). SR projects are medium term project for a maximum period of 60 months with potential to enhancing future competitive socio-economic development or new breakthroughs with commercial potential. During 8MP, MOSTE has awarded about RM160 million to nanotechnology related projects.

However, the development of nanotechnology during that period suffers from some shortfalls mainly due to lack of linkages between projects, no definitive plan to realized and develop nanotechnology industry, lack of direction and roadmap on nanotechnology R&D and lack of efforts to promote awareness in nanotechnology. All the short falls can be link to one major factor – lack of lead agency in the government to steer nanotechnology development that can provide initiatives and plans. During implementation of Ninth Malaysia Plan (9MP) spans from 2006 to 2010, Malaysian government has taken a serious concern over the development of nanotechnology. During preparation of the Third Industrial Master Plan (IMP3) that spans for 15-years period from 2005-2020, nanotechnology was recognized as the new emerging field. In 2006, in the budget speech, The Prime Minister Datuk Sri Abdullah Ahmad Badawi among other words stated that; "To further strengthen and diversify the sources of economic growth, the Government will intensify its efforts to encourage the private sector to venture into new areas with high growth potential and competitive edge. These include modern methods for agriculture, biotechnology, *nanotechnology*, high technology manufacturing as well as services, especially ICT, education and tourism" (BERNAMA, 2006). Following that, nanotechnology has been included as a one of the priority area under Intensified Research and Prioritised Area (IRPA) for Eight and Ninth Malaysia plan and poised to position the country in the long term to nurture a nanoscience research and develop world class nanotechnology research.

The national nanotechnology progress makes a major landmark in 2006 with the launch of the National Nanotechnology Initiatives which is intended to advance nanotechnology and related sciences by clustering local resources and knowledge between Malaysian researchers, industry and the government. The Mission of NNIM is Nanotechnology for Sustainable National Development of Science, Technology, Industry and Economy. Among the main functions of NNIM are:

1. Integrating all existing local nanotechnology activities
2. To coordinate and plan the R&D and C activities
3. To prepare a platform for commercialisation and transfer of new technology to generate economic return for the general public
4. To develop educational resources, skilled labour, expertise and nanotechnology infrastructure
5. To provide facilities and nanotechnology research support services.

In one of his speech in 2009, PM Dato' Sri Najib Tun Razak has again made a strong statement to support nanotechnology development. Among others he stated that "Nanotechnology development would be given priority and be made one of the resources of the country's economic model. .... Thus, it is important for Malaysia to not be left behind in the field of nanotechnology and we have decided to give it importance…" (BERNAMA, 2009). With the launch of NNIM in 2006, MOSTI was entrusted to spearhead the planning and development of national nanotechnology agenda with immediate tasks to be implement by MOSTI include plan for establishment of National Nanotechnology Centre and drafting National Nanotechnology Policy. To further strengthen the commitment from the government, National Nanotechnology Directorate was established in July 2010. The National Nanotechnology Statement was released with five major themes, Vision 2020, and the specific goal attaining a developed nation status by 2020, is directly contingent upon establishing a vibrant local nanotechnology sector.

National Nanotechnology Directorate (NND)

The New Economic Model (NEM) unveiled by Malaysian Prime Minister in 2010 embarks on knowledge-based economy through knowledge creation, wealth generation and societal well-being. The government through various measures wants Malaysia not just a consume technology, but also become a contributor, and this makes MOSTI become lead ministry to fulfilling these agendas execute through various action plans on R&D and C of strategic area including biotechnology, ICT and nanotechnology. To show government commitment to developing further nanotechnology in the country, government has established National Nanotechnology Directorate (NND) under the auspices MOSTI in 2010 to facilitate, guiding and spearheading nanotechnology development in Malaysia by acting as a central coordination agency. The establishment of NND was timely as it coincided with the start of planning for 10th Malaysia Plan (10MP) span from 2011 to 2015 and due to pressing needs to steer and coordinate research funding and to build research capacity for Malaysia for the coming 10th Malaysia Plan. The NND's mandates are:

☆ To develop national capability and capacity through the development of policies, infrastructure, facilities, and early education in nanosciences
☆ To boost human capital in the field

☆ To plan and coordinate Research, Development and Commercialisation activities in Malaysia

☆ To plan and coordinate activities that contribute to the development of nanotechnology-based industries

☆ To facilitate the positioning of Malaysia's nanotechnology industries and products in the global supply and value chain

The NND helped accelerate various key activities related to nanotechnology through initiatives such as:

☆ The launch of the National Nanotechnology Statement (NNS) in 2010

☆ Establishment of National Nanotechnology Centers of Excellence in 2011

☆ The incorporation of NanoMalaysia Berhad in 2011

☆ Development of the NanoMalaysia Centre in Iskandar Malaysia in 2013

National Center of Excellence in Nanotechnology

Under the 9th Malaysia Plan and up till 2010, the MOSTI had invested about RM140 million on research and development grants dedicated to nanotechnology research consisted of more than 100 projects implemented by 16 research centers focused on nanotechnology research involving 450 researchers. For the short term strategy, NND has identified and create a database for researchers in various area of nanotechnology with specific expertise and preparing a plan for upgrading and equipping nanotechnology laboratories as well as to prepare a comprehensive human resource development program for producing competence nanotechnologist. NanoMalaysia program introduced by NND is a master plan program spanning from 2010 to 2020 and consisting of 29 key programmes that will ensure a sustainable momentum for the nanotechnology industry by building and reinforcing all elements within the national nanotechnology ecosystem. With a robust and integrated ecosystem in place, nanotechnology will be transformed from a nascent, emerging industry into a major growth area that may worth up to 1 per cent of the GNI by 2020. To realize this target, NND has identified five centers out of 16 centers to be upgraded into NanoMalaysia Center of Excellence (CoE) for nanotechnology research. These CoEs support nanotechnology R&D and provide shared facilities and human capital training and is expected to contributes in increase talents with high knowledge in nano science and technology and to commercialise local products. The five NanoMalaysia COEs are:

1. Institute of Micro Engineering and Nanoelectronics (IMEN), UKM: It focuses on Nanoelectromechanical Systems (NEMS) and Lab-on-Chips for the biomedical industry

2. Institute of Nanoelectronics and Engineering (INEE), UNIMAP: Focuses on Nano DNA Chips for medical diagnostics. It has established five research groups namely nanobiochips, photonics, non-volatile memory devices, novel devices and smart sensor (Hashim, 2009)

3. Centre for Innovative Nanostructures and Nanodevices (COINN), UTP: Focuses on Solar energy

4. NEMS/MEMS Research Laboratory, MIMOS: Focuses on Self-Powered Breath Sensors for Intelligent Wearable and Healthcare Monitoring Systems

5. Enabling Science and Nanotechnology Research, Ibnu Sina Institute for Fundamental Science Studies (IIFS), UTM: Focuses on Novel Functional Nanomaterials: Synthesis and Computational Design

All five Nanotechnology Centre of Excellence are well positioned to become the key catalyst for Malaysia's Nanotechnology Development and Commercialization. In line with the national aspiration of making Nanotechnology the enabling engine for the new economic growth, all Nanotechnology CoE are focusing on incorporating nanotechnology to its technology development platforms which are expected to directly contribute towards the National Key Focus Areas (NKEAs).

MIMOS is one of the agency under MOSTI with current Nano-related R&D activities include the development of its top-down and bottom-up Nanofabrication, Nanomaterial processing and Nano devices testing facilities. MIMOS' sensor systems and solutions technology platform roadmap from 2011 to 2015, developed in line with global market growth expectations, is focused on enhancing its sensors and micro energy devices are incorporating Nanotechnology based elements to ensure higher sensitivity, better responses, lower power consumption, smaller size, increased robustness, flexibility and energy storage capacity applicable for industries such as aquaculture, environmental, health, safety and defence. MIMOS' Nanotechnology CoE includes state-of-the-art cleanrooms that houses an array of Nanofabrication equipment, capable of processing up to eight inch wafers and a comprehensive laboratory for Nano characterisation and analysis.

NanoMalaysia BHD

On the 14th of February 2011, the National Innovation Council convened and agreed that a nanotechnology commercialization agency was needed. NanoMalaysia Berhad was then incorporated as Company Limited by Guarantee (CLG) in August 2011 under Section 24, Company Act 1965 to take the lead in commercialization of nanotechnology products. As a commercial vehicle set up by the National Nanotechnology Directorate (NND), NMB act as a business entity entrusted with nanotechnology commercialization activities and support the operations of the NanoMalaysia Centre. Its goal is to have the nanotechnology industry contribute 1 per cent of Malaysia's GNI by 2020. Some of its roles include:

1. Managing commercial facilities at NanoMalaysia Centre and other approved Strategic Infrastructure and Facilities for the NND

2. Pre-commercialization and commercialization of nanotechnology products

3. Bringing in venture funds and international investments in nanotechnology

4. International linkages and networking

National Nanotechnology Centre

The Senai Hi-Tech Park, located in Johor's Iskandar Malaysia economic zone, has been chosen to house National nanotechnology center to be known as

NanoMalaysia Center (NMC), the first complex of its kind in Malaysia. The development of the centre is part of the NanoMalaysia Master Plan Program. The new complex will be developed under a private-public partnership (PPP) concept and should be completed and started it operation in 2016. NMC would become "a one-stop center" for nano science and technology activities and provide a missing link between technology and market. NMC is designed not only to provide a workplace for nanotechnology researchers, but is part of a plan to form other new companies through technology entrepreneurship incubators and assist downstream industries by providing commercialisation platforms including technology incubator facilities. It will be managed by NND with the incorporation of NanoMalaysia Bhd as commercial vehicle. NMC will work closely with NanoMalaysia Berhad (NMB), to provide a common platform for universities, research centres and industries aimed at building collaborations towards a concerted effort in developing the nation's Nanotechnology capabilities. The centre aimed to create the critical mass of entrepreneurs and to facilitate the creation of new nanotechnology based firms. This also involves establishing NMC as the gateway for international collaboration in state-of-art Nanotechnology research. It will also provide the infrastructure and facilities with conducive environment for translational and downstream nano research activities as well as a work place for nanotechnologists and scientists. As part of its intentions, NMC strives to become the preferred shared facility in Nano testing and characterization, and full scale manufacturing of Nano-based products. The target is that, when it will be operated fully, the center will be able to generate from RM100-150 million ($33-39 million) in business.

Nanotechnology as the Next Economic Growth Driver for Malaysia

In 1991, the YAB Prime Minister of Malaysia declared that Malaysia would be a developed nation by the year 2020. This would have been achieved by sustaining a growth momentum of 7 per cent per annum (1997 projection). However, the regional financial crisis that hit Asia in 1997 had substantially impacted the trajectory of targets set by Vision 2020. To re-generate growth and fulfil the 2020 goal, current PM Dato' Seri Najib Tun Razak announced new initiatives for the Malaysian economy in 2010 for the coming decade. Malaysia has not wavered from its original target of becoming a high income nation by the year 2020. This will be achieved via implementation of the New Economic Model (NEM) and the introduction of Economic Transformation Programme (ETP), which, will lift the national per capita income to between USD15,000 and USD20,000. To realise this goal, Malaysia has to fundamentally change its worldview and innovation capabilities. There is an urgent need to identify a sustainable driver of real growth up till 2020 and beyond. Achieving reasonable growth is a challenge by itself. With the global economy still reeling from meltdowns in the Developed World, Malaysia must identify niche areas that will serve as new engines of growth – one that provides premium income and harnesses its natural assets. Growth will be powered by the 12 National Key Economic Areas (NKEA).

The NKEAs were selected based on their expected contributions to Malaysia's GNI by 2020. High technology such as nanotechnology together with biotechnology and ICT will be the key driver to attain high income status. Nanotechnology was identified as a "high growth generator," is pivotal to Malaysia becoming a developed nation by 2020. Therefore, a sound policy is needed to enable the nation to retool key innovation fundamentals by 2020. Malaysia needs nanotechnology to move up the global high-technology value chain. Malaysia government recognised that nanotechnology will touch all aspects of economics: wages, employment, purchasing, pricing, capital, exchange rates, currencies, markets, supply and demand. Nanotechnology may well drive economic prosperity or at the least be an enabling factor in shaping productivity and global competitiveness. Lagging behind in this sector is not an option. The NEM is primarily supported by the Economic Transformation Programme (ETP) which details revenue generation through 12 National Key Economic Areas (NKEAs). They are Oil, Gas and Energy; Palm Oil and Rubber; Financial Services; Tourism; Business Services; Electronics and Electrical; Wholesale and Retail; Education; Healthcare; Communications Content and Infrastructure; Agriculture; and Greater Kuala Lumpur/Klang Valley (Figure 8.1). Going by global trends, nanotechnology will impact all 12 NKEAs in varying degrees. Nanotechnology will soon be manifested in the materials, tools, components, services and end-products of all 12 sectors.

Nanotechnology provides unparalleled opportunities for existing Malaysian companies in key industrial sectors. It will help them move up the value chain by

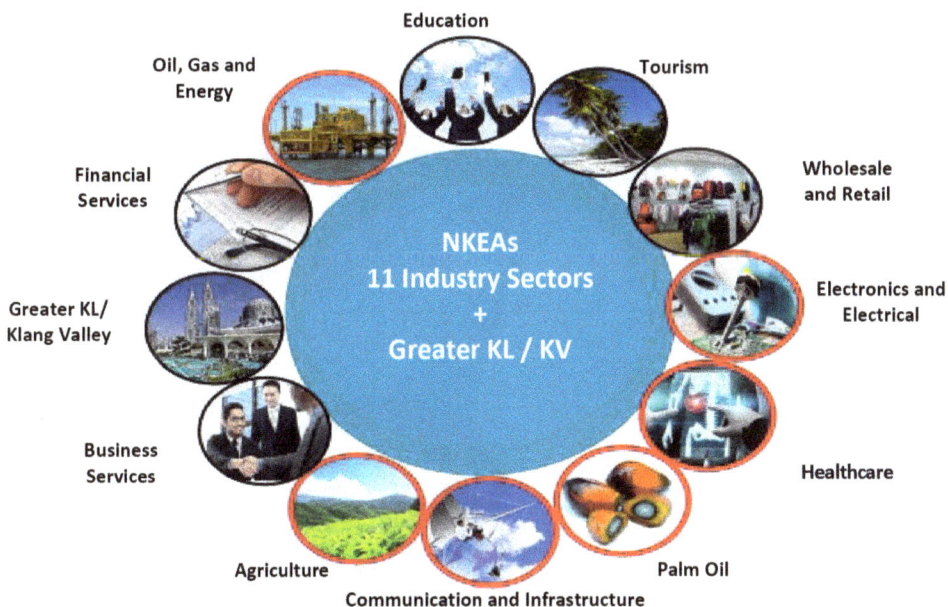

Figure 8.1: The 12 National Key Economic Areas (NKEAs) under Economic Transformation Program

(*Source*: Un-published Report: National Nanotechnology Policy and Strategic Direction Study, MOSTI, Malaysia, 2012)

generating premium products and services. Identifying future products and markets will be crucial to local nanotechnology undertakings. As shown in Figure 8.2, nanotechnology is the crux upon which the following areas will be impacted:

☆ **High value additions:** Sectors such as food and agriculture; medical and healthcare; energy and environment; and electronic devices and systems will need nano-level augmentation to either introduce new products or improve current ones. These core NKEA sectors will be impacted by nanotechnology

☆ **Leveraging upon existing key markets:** Nano-augmented products – in the sectors described above – will create an initial momentum for the development of the local nanotechnology sector. It is important that initial momentum is created within mature sectors that enjoy a large global market

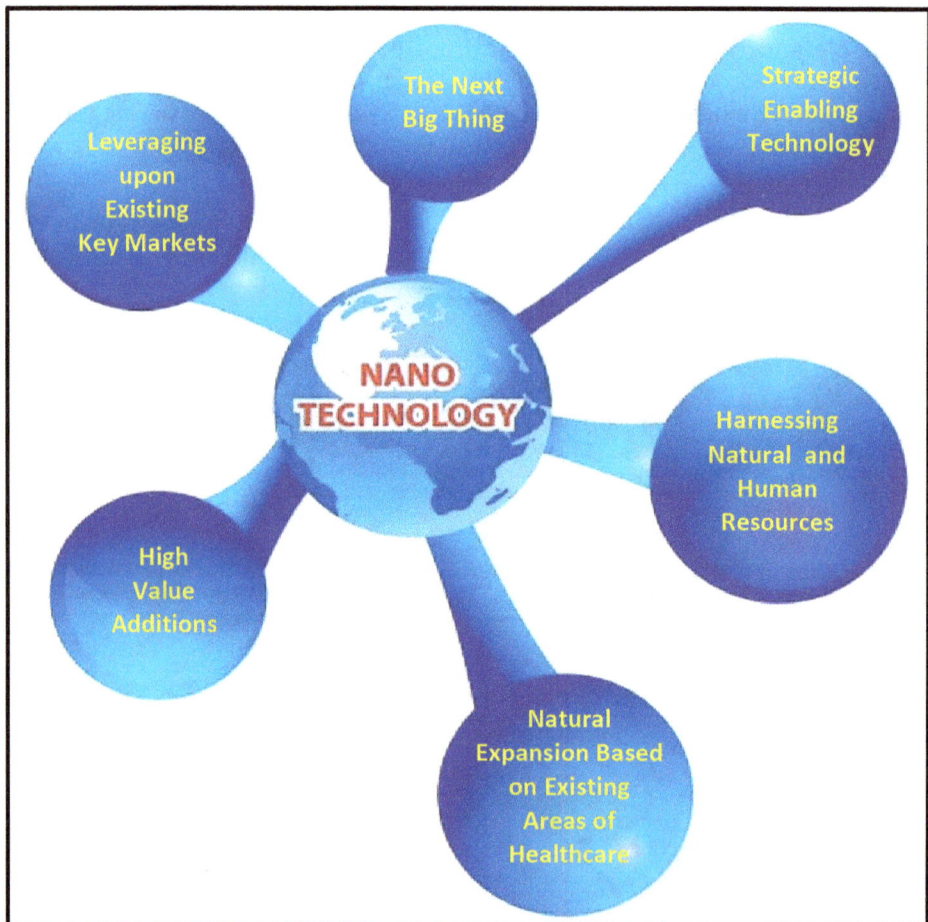

Figure 8.2: Impact of Nanotechnology on the New Economic Model (NEM)
(*Source*: Un-published Report: National Nanotechnology Policy and Strategic Direction Study, MOSTI, Malaysia, 2012)

☆ **Natural expansion based on existing areas of strength:** After initial momentum is attained, the introduction of additional Nano products for wider industrial applications is a natural outcome

☆ **Next big thing:** No other sector has the capacity to either to create new products or augment existing ones in exponential terms. Without nanotechnology, current product lines will only witness incremental improvements and will be redundant in a few years' time

☆ **Strategic enabling technology:** Nanotechnology is poised to impact every product line in the future – from mundane plastics to new drug delivery systems

☆ **Harnessing our current natural and human resources:** Natural Resources such as oil and gas, and our biodiversity potentials need new technological solutions to either extract dwindling reserves or to harness new possibilities from the abundant local flora and fauna. Malaysia also has an expanding skilled human resource base that will benefit greatly from the introduction of nanotechnology.

Jumpstarting Nanotechnology

Nanotechnology as a key economic enabler will help the nation attain a high income status. By re-engineering products and services at the most fundamental level, it is poised to add untold value into future revenue streams. The ultimate goal here is to ensure a better quality of life for the *people*. Malaysian is ready to jump into the "nano-fray." Various national-level initiatives have contributed to Malaysia's current state of nanotechnology readiness.

Coupled with activities at organisational levels, primarily in the academia and industry, Malaysia is in a prime position to harness new potentials in nanotechnology. With all the foundations in place, the country needs a primary route to jumpstart nanotechnology. This route will accelerate the impact of nanotechnology for the nation's socio-economic well-being.

Nanotechnology's contribution to 1 per cent of the GNI by 2020 will be partly achieved through native technological capabilities and by leveraging on existing economic sectors where we already possess a market presence. Four key economic clusters have been identified as the Jumpstart Sectors of nanotechnology (Figure 8.3). They are:

☆ **Food and Agriculture** - Malaysia has traditionally been an agriculture-based nation. Even today, its plantation sector is a major contributor to the gross national income. Nano-biotechnology can help increase agricultural productivity, boost pest-resistance and improve food quality. Considering the global outlook in the food and agriculture sector, the application of nanotechnology may avert a major food crisis worldwide.

☆ **Energy and Environment** - Malaysia has abundant natural energy sources in the form of solar, biomass, natural gas, petroleum, tidal wave and wind. The biggest challenge is to bring energy from source to consumers in the most cost-effective, safest and convenient manner. There is a need for higher

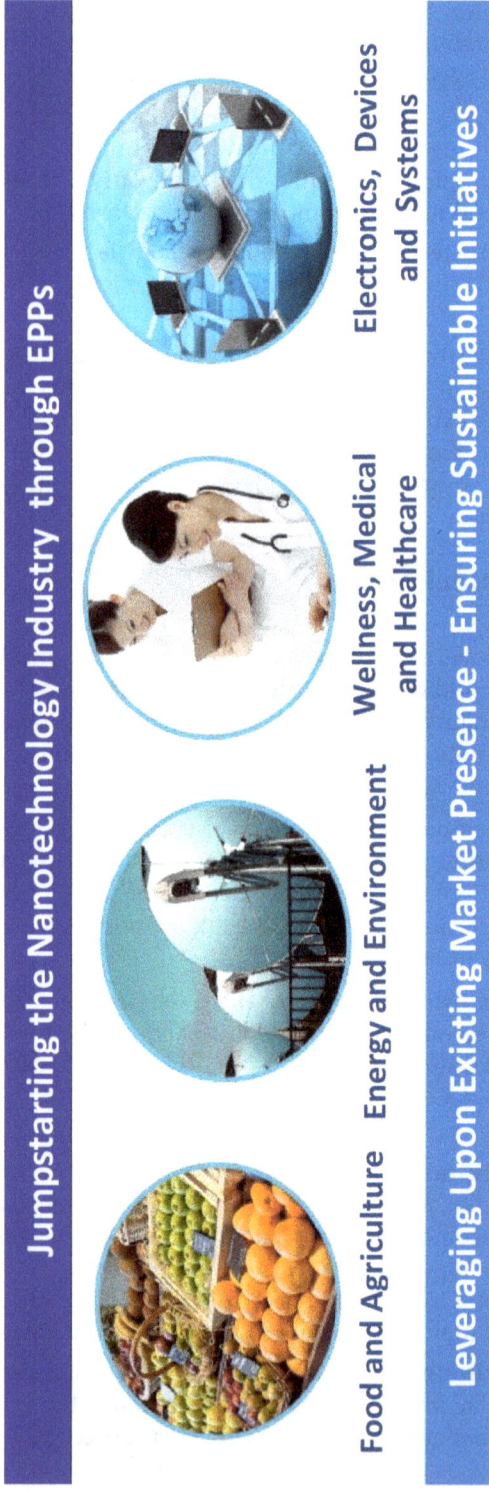

Jumpstarting the Nanotechnology Industry through EPPs

Food and Agriculture   Energy and Environment   Wellness, Medical and Healthcare   Electronics, Devices and Systems

Leveraging Upon Existing Market Presence - Ensuring Sustainable Initiatives

Figure 8.3: The Four Key Jumpstart Sectors for Nanotechnology Based on EPPs

(*Source:* Un-published Report: National Nanotechnology Policy and Strategic Direction Study, MOSTI, Malaysia, 2012)

degree of portability, longer usage periods, higher energy outputs and a sustainable supply of energy sources. Further developments in the energy sector will be contingent on nanotechnology, as conventional technology has breached the limits of energy processing and storage capacity. Nanotechnology may be the panacea for the rapid depletion of traditional energy sources. It also fulfills the general sustainability criteria through increased energy efficiency and savings

☆ **Wellness, Medical and Healthcare** - In the area of healthcare, the NKEA's anticipated GNI impact has been increased to RM42.2 billion, with over 260,000 new jobs to be created by the year 2020. (Source: PEMANDU) There are now 13 EPPs under the Healthcare NKEA as compared to only six identified earlier.This increase reflects the growing importance of the medical and healthcare industry to Malaysia's economic growth. It is therefore appropriate to leverage upon the medical and healthcare industry's strengths to introduce nanotechnology product and solutions. Future drug delivery systems and anti-cancer treatment, among others, will be dependent on breakthroughs in nanotechnology.

☆ **Electronics, Devices and Systems** - The Malaysian Electronics and Electrical sector (E and E) is an important contributor to the economy. In 2009 alone, it accounted for 6 per cent of Malaysia's gross national income (GNI), 522,000 jobs, representing more than 40 per cent of total manufacturing labour and 41 per cent of Malaysia's total exports. The electrical and electronics (E and E) industry is the largest single contributor to the manufacturing sector, accounting for 26.1 per cent of total manufacturing output (Source: EPU, Pemandu). Malaysia's world-class electronics industry is the top sectorial employer and exporter within the manufacturing sector. The E and E industry is also Malaysia's most liberalised sector. The future of E and E will be shaped by developments in nanotechnology. With established players and a strong global presence, the E and E sectors can jumpstart expansions in Nano electronics and Nano photonics etc.

The above four core clusters will jumpstart Malaysia's strategic entry into the emerging nanotechnology sector. Malaysia has done reasonably well in these sectors with conventional technology; now it has the opportunity to explore value-added alternatives through nanotechnology. In developing nanotechnology into a new, high potential sector for the country, we have to take cognisance of the overriding national agenda – achieving Vision 2020 through the Economic Transformation Programme (ETP). The ETP is activated through a number of Entry Point Projects (EPPs) within the 12 NKEAs. The nanotechnology development strategy evaluates and identifies nanotechnology-ready EPPs to support the NKEAs. The EPPs are appropriate avenues to jumpstart nanotechnology in high potential areas.

Nanotechnology Commercialisation

The research, development and commercialisation aspects of nanotechnology are probably its most crucial components. This is where the integration of resources will ultimately produce world-class products and services that will generate income for the nation. Malaysia needs a sound human capital development program, world-class infrastructure and funding to deliver strategic outcomes. Malaysia will have to balance between opportunities and risks that will be encountered in making nanotechnology a strategic growth area for the country. The proposed approach is to leverage upon sectors where we already have relatively strong market positions. This is where early markets for nanotechnology will be created. Sectors where Malaysia has a strong lead or presence are palm oil, oil and gas, and electrical and electronics.

These sectors are appropriate sector to jumpstart local nanotechnology commercialisation initiatives. These areas will create the initial wave of products to position Malaysia as an emerging niche player in the global marketplace, and generate enough technological momentum for more innovative nanotechnology products down the line. Research and development projects therefore need to be identified and created to support the technological needs of products and solutions envisaged for the above-mentioned areas. A roadmap spanning the period till 2020 will recommend ways to

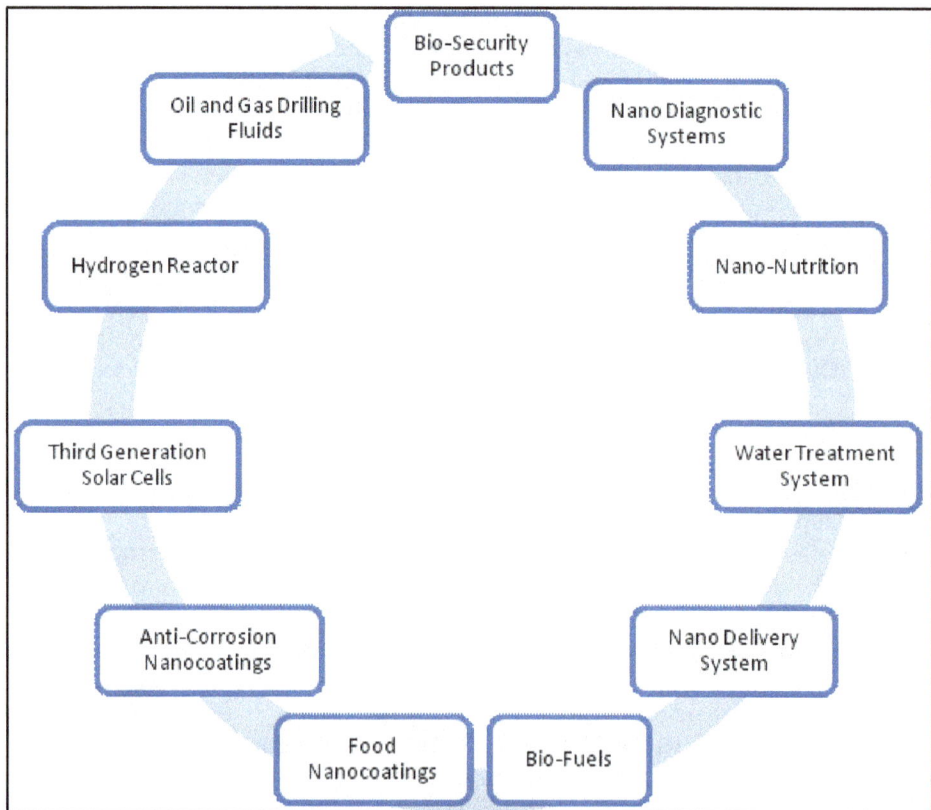

Figure 8.4: The 11 High Impact Projects Proposed to Jumpstart the Nanotechnology Commercialisation Process that will Impact 18 EPPs

(*Source*: Un-published Report: National Nanotechnology Policy and Strategic Direction Study, MOSTI, Malaysia, 2012)

jumpstart sectors that are the mainstays of our economy i.e. oil and gas, palm oil, electrical and electronics, ICT, and transportation equipment.

The Economic Transformation Programme (ETP) has identified 12 key economic areas that will generate an increase in GNI by more than RM1.0 trillion by 2020. The main ETP initiatives will be initially driven by 133 Entry Point Projects (EPPs), drawn from the 12 economic areas. From these 12 economic areas, four have been identified to benefit directly from the nanotechnology development plan. From these four areas, 18 EPPs may benefit from nanotechnology. Based on the needs of these 18 EPPs, 11 high impact projects have been proposed to jumpstart the nanotechnology commercialisation process. The 11 nanotechnology projects outlined have the potential to create significant impacts for a number of NKEA Entry Point Projects. All 11 projects were found to be suited for local adaptation and global export. These projects as shown in Figure 8.4, upon closer scrutiny, were also found to be the perfect platforms for 18 EPPs as shown in Figure 8.5.

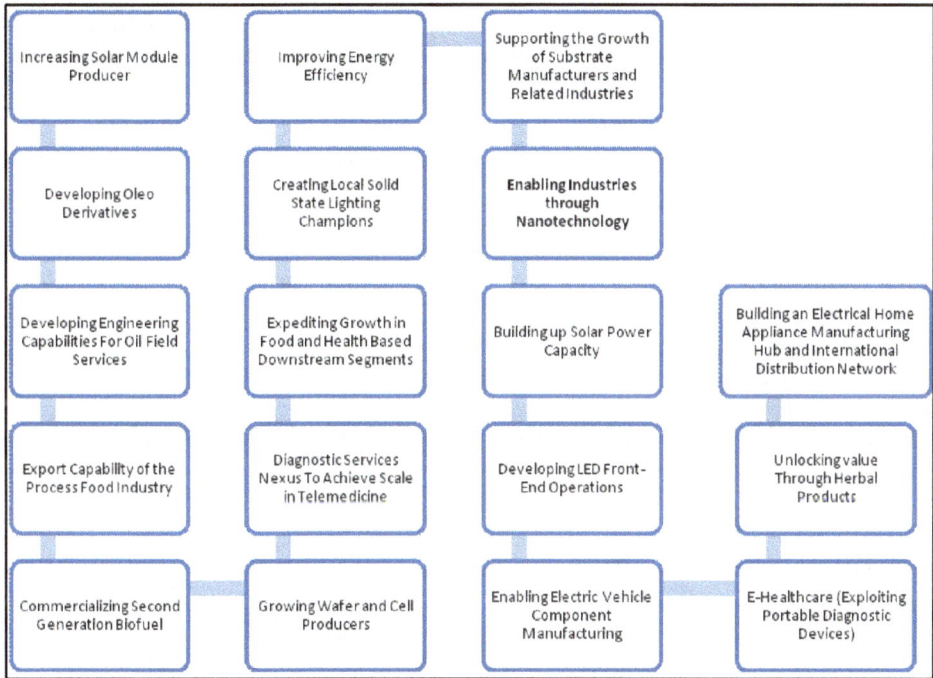

Figure 8.5: Relevant 18 EPPs to Initiate High Impact Projects in Nanotechnology
(*Source*: Un-published Report: National Nanotechnology Policy and Strategic Direction Study, MOSTI, Malaysia, 2012)

CONCLUSIONS

Nanotechnology provides a stimulating and somewhat awesome challenge to meet. Fast moving radical technologies are reshaping the marketplace and society. Technology will continue to drive global and domestic GDP. Competition will be fuelled increasingly by fast breaking innovations in technology. If the proliferation of today's technologies to form new business models is any indication of the speed and power of change in the economy, future nanotechnologies will make for an even more dramatic paradigm shift. Much of the growth in the Malaysian economy towards realising vision 2020 of turning Malaysia into high income economy will been in high-technology, high-value industries, with information technology, biotechnology and nanotechnology be a main driver. Recognizing the promise of research at the nanoscale as one of the important economic driver for Malaysian Economic Transformation Program (ETP), the government mandate to research under the National Nanotechnology Initiative Malaysia (NNIM) spearhead by National Nanotechnology Directorate (NND) involves an expectation for significant outcomes—that a federal investment in nanotechnology-related R&D programs will lead to results that increase the Malaysian capacity to effectively address national priorities, meet economic needs, and advance societal interests. In addition to improving our fundamental quality of life as a result of positive developments in nanotechnology-related medicine, energy production, national security, environmental protection, and education, the commercialization and adoption of new technologies resulting from nanoscale R&D are expected to yield a positive economic return in the form of benefits such as the creation of businesses, jobs, and trade with projected contribution of 1 per cent to Malaysian Gross National Income (GNI) by 2020.

ACKNOWLEDGEMENTS

The author would like to acknowledge Ministry of Science, Technology and Innovation (MOSTI) and Malaysia government for their support.

REFERENCES

1. The Sun Daily, M'sia may set up nanotechnology initiative, 5 July 2005

2. BERNAMA, Malaysia To Invest In Nanotechnology, Central Region News, April 27, 2006

3. BERNAMA, Malaysia To Upgrade Six Nanotechnology Centres, Tuesday, September 19, 2006

4. MIGHT, 2007. Identification of Business and R&D Opportunities in the Application of Nanotechnology in Malaysia, Malaysia: Malaysian Industry-Government Group for High Technology (Report of limited circulation).

5. BERNAMA, Government to establish national innovation centre, Kuala Lumpur, Oct 29, 2009 (Bernama)

6. Hashim, U. *et al.*, 2009. Nanotechnology Development Status in Malaysia: Industrialization Strategy and Practices. *Int. J. Nanoelectronics and Materials*, 2(1), 119-34.

7. Malaysia's Transformation Story: From Message to Passage, YB Senator Dato' Sri Idris Jala Minister in the Prime Minister's Department and Chief Executive Officer, PEMANDU Invest Malaysia 2011- 12 April, 2011

9. National Nanotechnology Directorate (NND), National Nanotechnology Policy and Strategic Direction Study, National Nanotechnology Directorate, Ministry of Science, Technology and Innovation. 2012(Internal Unpublished Report).

10. PEMANDU, 2013 PEMANDU Homepage available at http://etp.pemandu.gov.my/

Chapter 9

A Review of Nano-Biomaterials and Nano-Carrier Drug Delivery Research at the Centre for Biomedical and Biomaterials Research

Archana Bhaw-Luximon, Roubeena Jeetah,
Nowsheen Goonoo, Anisha Veeren, Yeshma Jugdawa
and Dhanjay Jhurry*

ANDI Centre of Excellence for Biomedical and Biomaterials Research,
MSIRI Building, University of Mauritius, Réduit, Mauritius
*E-mail: djhurry@uom.ac.mu

INTRODUCTION

This paper will present a review of research undertaken at Centre for Biomedical and Biomaterials Research (CBBR) in biomaterials and drug delivery areas.The engineering of biocompatible and biodegradable polymers plays a central role in the development of new nanomaterials suitable for scaffold or drug delivery applications. This has been the main focus of the research thrusts at CBBR for the past years. CBBR has developed a new family of poly(ester-ether)s by copolymerization of dioxanone and its methyl analogue, methyl dioxanone,By varying the content of methyl dioxanone in the copolymer or by using blends of the homopolymers, the physico-chemical, mechanical and biological properties of the copolymers can be adjusted to meet specific tissue engineering applications. The elaboration of nanofibrous mats based on these copolymers or blendshave proved to be quite promising for cell growth and proliferation.In the area of controlled drug delivery, various block and graft copolymers based on PEG, polylysine or a polysaccharide in association with a hydrophobic poly(ester-ether) or poly(ester) have been tailored by our group. These copolymers self-assemble in aqueous solution into nanomicelles whose properties can be tuned to encapsulate and release various drugs such as anti-inflammatory, anti-TB and anti-cancer in a controlled manner. The biosafety of these systems make them quite promising for use as nanocarriers.As will be discussed, the success of scaffolds or drug delivery devices depends largely on the ability to match the requirements for healthy cell growth or diseased-cell destruction with the engineered-materials properties.

Keywords: Nano-biomaterials, Nano-carrier drug delivery, Biomedical and biomaterial research.

Biomaterials and Scaffolds for Tissue Engineering

The main objective of this thrust is to engineer polymer-based scaffolds for tissue engineering applications. Scaffolds for tissue engineering applications should be biocompatible, biodegradable, porous, possess appropriate mechanical properties (Goonoo *et al.*, 2013).

Although poly(dioxanone) (PDX) was introduced in 1981, the development of that family of poly(ester-ethers) has remained almost a virgin area. Mimicking the PLGA family, we have reported on the synthesis of a dioxanone analogue namely D,L-3-methyl-1,4-dioxan-2-one(MeDX) (Lochee, 2009 and 2010) and its copolymerization with dioxanone or blending with polydioxanone to produce either films or electrospun nanofibres, thus opening up new perspectives for these materials.

Random P(DX-*co*-MeDX) copolymers and diblock copolymers consisting of PCL and P(DX-*co*-MeDX) have been synthesized by ring-opening polymerization of DX and MeDX and used to produce nanofibrous mats (Wolfe, 2011). The incorporation of MeDX units in the diblock copolymers influenced both thermal properties and degradation kinetics through phase mixing of segments (Goonoo, 2012). Hydrolytic degradation studies indicated that degradation occurred via bulk erosion and that the copolymers with higher mole per cent of MeDX degraded faster.

Blend films of semi-crystalline PDX and amorphous PMeDX have been prepared and their mechanical performance, thermal and degradation behavior investigated (Goonoo, 2014a). Mechanical tests showed overall reduced tensile properties of the blends withincreasing weight percent of PMeDX due to a decrease in crystallinity. Blends were immiscible over the whole range of compositions. Low amounts of PMeDX, within 15 weight per cent could act as plasticizer to high molar-mass-PDX. Hydrolytic degradation studies showed that blend films with higher PMeDX content degraded faster.

Electrospunnanofibrous mats of PDX/PMeDX blends were fabricated in varying weight ratios of the two components (Goonoo, 2014b). AFM images of fibresshowed higher degree of heterogeneity with increasing PMeDX content in the fibres (Figure 9.1). PMeDX had reduced plasticizing effect in the fibres compared to films. Fibres were significantly more thermally stable as compared to blend films. Electrospun

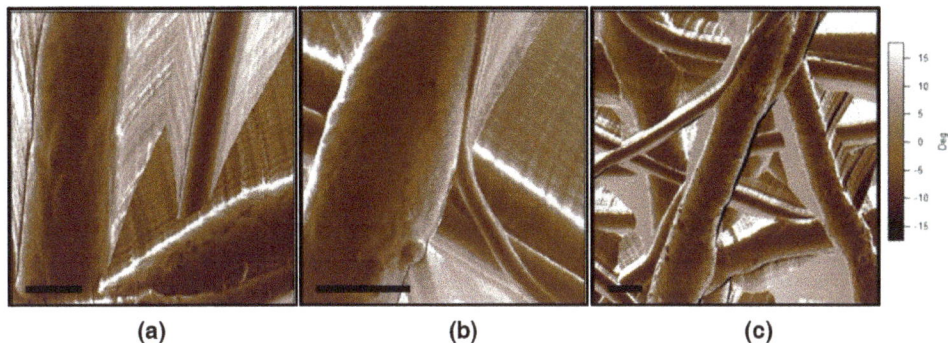

Figure 9.1: AFM Phase Images of Electrospun (a) 100/0, (b) 93/7 and
(c) 85/15 PDX/PMeDX scaffolds (Scale bar = 500 nm)

(*Source*: Reproduced from Goonoo *et al.* Biomater. Sci., 2014, 2, 339
with permission from The Royal Society of Chemistry)

PDX/PMeDXnanofibrous scaffolds had good biocompatibility as confirmed by cell viability studies with human dermal fibroblasts (HDF) (Figure 9.2). These poly(ester-ether) materials – copolymers, blend films and blend nanofibres – are interesting candidates for applications in tissue engineering or for drug delivery applications.

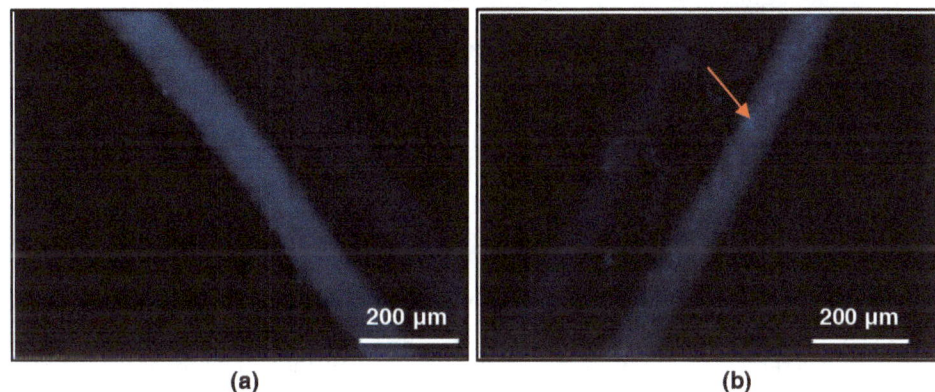

Figure 9.2: Fluorescence Microscopy Images of HDFs on PDX/PMeDX Scaffolds
After (a) 1 and (b) 7 days

(*Source*: Adapted from Goonoo *et al.* Biomater. Sci., 2014, 2, 339 with permission
from The Royal Society of Chemistry)

Drug Delivery Systems

Nanoparticle sustained drug delivery systems offer several advantages over conventional delivery such as maintenance of optimum therapeutic concentration of drug in the blood or cell, elimination of frequent dosing and better patient compliance. Consequently, they are good candidates for more efficient drug release devices. As block copolymer micelles attract increased interest as drug nanocarriers, there is a growing need for tailor-made biodegradable polymers whose size and surface properties can be intelligently designed not only to achieve long circulation times in the blood and site-specific drug delivery but also to exploit physiological or biochemical features of infectious diseases. Most polymeric self-assembled nano carrier systems are based on amphiphilic block copolymers (ABCs) with a hydrophilic PEG shell and a biodegradable hydrophobic core such as polycaprolactone or polylactide. A vast majority of systems in clinical trials or on the market are thus PEG-based targeting mainly cancer (Table 9.1).

Table 9.1: Examples of Nanomicelle-Based Polymer Therapeutics in the Market and Clinical Development

Sub Class	Examples	Composition	Status
Block copolymer	SP1049C	Doxorubicin block copolymer micelle	Phase I/II
micelles	NK 105	Paclitaxel block copolymer micelle	Phase II
	NK-6004	Cisplatin block copolymer micelle	Phase II
Self assembled polymer conjugate nanoparticles	IT-101	Polymerconjugated-cyclodextrinnano-particle-camptothecin	Phase II
	CALAA 01	Polymer-conjugatedcyclodextrin-nanoparticle-si RNA	Phase II

Our group has focused on engineering novel amphiphilic block copolymers based on biodegradable synthetic polymers or biopolymers (Scheme 1).

Novel Amphiphilic Self-Assembled Block and Graft Copolymers

PEG-*b*-poly(Dioxanone-co-Methyl Dioxanone) Copolymers

Our novelty in this area has been the development of a novel class of poly (ester-ether)s namely PEG-*b*-poly(Dioxanone-co-Methyl Dioxanone) copolymers (MPEG-*b*-P(DX-*co*-MeDX) and P(DX-*co*-MeDX)-*b*-PEG-*b*-P(DX-*co*-MeDX)). Adjustment of the dioxanone to methyldioxanone ratio gives a range of copolymers whose properties (physicochemical and biological) can be tuned to meet specific biomedical requirements. The efficacy of these copolymers to encapsulate and release anti-inflammatory (Jeetah, 2012) or anti-TB drugs (Jeetah, 2014) has been tested. Tuberculosis remains a major plague of the African continent. However, only a few studies report on the use of block copolymer micelles to encapsulate anti-TB drugs.

The block copolymers self-assembled in aqueous solutions with diameters in the range of 120-300 nm and with critical micelle concentration (CMC) values of the order of 10^{-4}M. The drug-free copolymer micelles were found to be non-hemolytic and showed no erythrocyte agglutination between concentration ranges of 0.125mg/ml to 1 mg/ml. Biocompatibility of the micelles was determined using brine shrimp lethality assay. The copolymer micelleswere highly safe, fully biocompatible and had no toxicity profile at 200 µg/ml (<50 per cent mortality) (Jeetah, 2014).

Anti-tubercular drugs rifampicin (RIF), isoniazid (INH) and pyrazinamide (PZA) were encapsulated into the amphiphilic diblock/triblock copolymers. Rifampicin was found to have the highest binding constant with our nanomicellar systems and it achieved a higher encapsulation in single or dual loading with the other drugs. The drug loading achieved was 45-74 per cent for single-loaded RIF micelles, 42-79 per cent for dual-loaded RIF-INH micelles, 26-28 per cent for PZA and 17-25 per cent

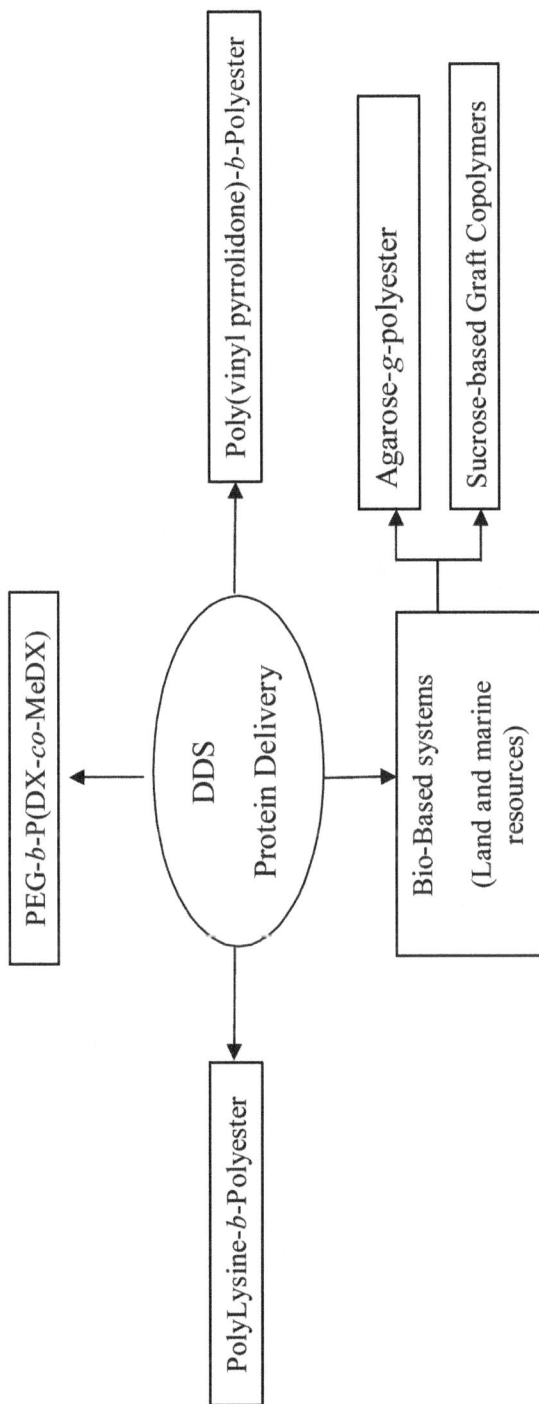

Scheme 1: Amphiphilic Block and Graft Copolymer Systems Engineered by CBBR

for INH. TEM images (Figure 9.3) confirmed the encapsulation of drugs within the hydrophobic core of the micelle.The drug-containing nanoparticles gave rise to sustained release profiles which could be tuned by modifying the MeDX content in the copolymers. Sustained release was observed for 9 days for rifampicin, 5 days for PZA and 4 days for INH. The drug-loaded micelles were stable up to two months when the lyophilized micelles were reconstituted in dextrose solution. Single-loaded micelles were found to be more stable than dual-loaded micelles (Jeetah, 2014).

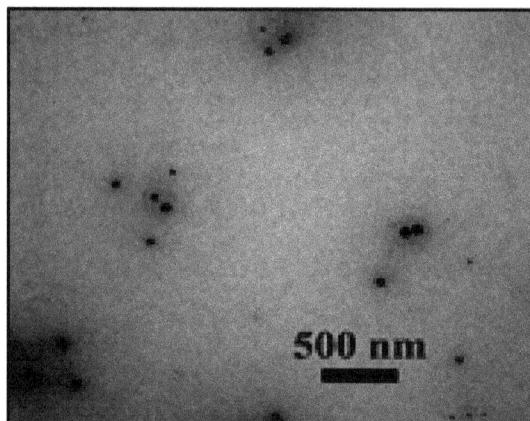

Figure 9.3: TEM Micrographs of MPEG-*b*-P(DX-*co*-MeDX),
per cent DX: per cent MeDX = 70:30 rifampicin/isoniazid-loaded micelles in water

PEG Replacement in Copolymers

Polymer-drug-cell interaction and polymer-drug compatibility play crucial roles in increasing efficacy of drugs. The chemical structure of PEG offers limited possibilities of modification to increase efficacy or drug compatibility. Hydrophilic bio-based polymers could offer interesting alternatives to PEG due to their biocompatibility and availability of functional groups for drug interaction and chemical modification.

PolyLysine-*b*-Polycaprolactone Copolymers

As a replacement of PEG, we have prepared polyLysine-*b*-polycaprolactone (PolyLys-*b*-PCL) copolymers, another type of ABCs (Scheme 2) (Veeren, 2012). The amino groups of lysine can be interesting for targeting or drug-conjugation. Various novel di-or tri-block copolymers with hydrophilic PEG and/orpolylysine in association with hydrophobic polycaprolactone segments namely PEG-*b*-PolyLys and PEG-*b*-PolyLys-*b*-PCL, have been synthesized and characterized.Poly(Lys-*g*-Glu)-*b*-PCL has been successfully synthesized where D-gluconolactonewas grafted on the NH$_2$ group of PolyLys. These copolymers self-assemble in waterto form micelles in the size range 165 to 365 nm and CMC from 0.1 mg/ml to 2 mg/ml. Both micelle size and CMC showed a strong dependency on the hydrophobic chainlength. The encapsulation of ketoprofen and rifampicin in the different copolymerfamilies was assessed and encapsulation efficiency determined using UV Spectroscopy.The per

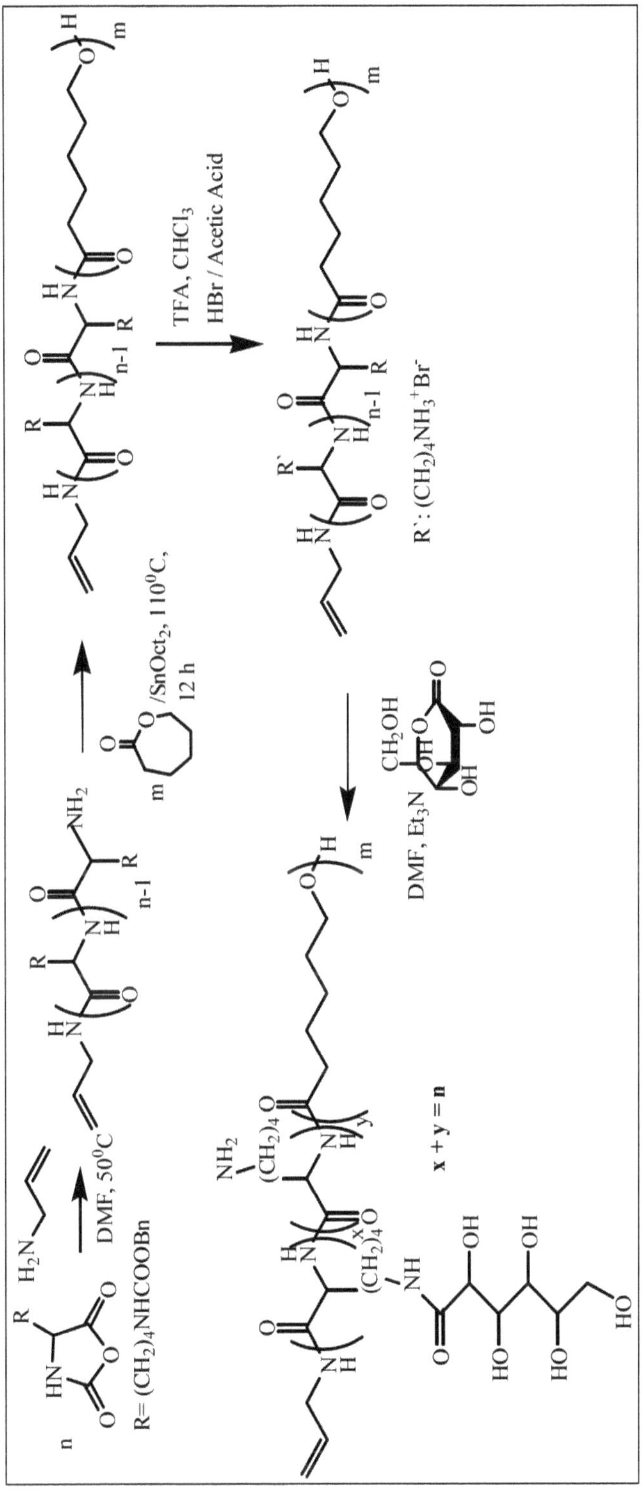

Scheme 2: Synthesis of di-block Poly(Lys-*g*-Glu)-*b*-PCL

(*Source:* Adapted from Veeren *et al.* Macromol.Symp. 2012, 313-314, 59 with permission from John Wiley and Sons)

cent drug loaded was found to depend on the interaction between drug and copolymer system. Both drugs showed chemical conjugation with PolyLyssegment and physical entrapment in the PCL hydrophobic core. Higher encapsulation efficiency was obtained with rifampicin (17–70 per cent).

PVP-based Copolymers

Engineering of amphiphilicpoly(vinyl pyrrolidone)-*b*-polycaprolactone (PVP-*b*-PCL)diblock copolymers with varying chain lengths by Atom Transfer Radical Polymerisation (ATRP) using bromo-polycaprolactone as macroinitiator and copper(I) bromide/bipyridine catalytic system has been achieved (Veeren, 2013). The copolymers were found to self-assemble in solution into core-shell micelles with sizes varying from 150 to 205 nm and critical micelle concentration of the order of 10^{-5} to 10^{-6} M.

Anti-TB drugs were successfully loaded singly (RIF or PZA) and in dual combination (RIF and INH) into the PVP-*b*-PCL nanoparticles. It was observed that the percentage drug loading varied in the order RIFPZA>INH and that it increases with increase in hydrophobic chain length and decreases with increase in hydrophilic chain length (Figure 9.4).

The release profiles of both single and dual drug-loaded micelles have been studied *in vitro* under physiological conditions (Phosphate buffer solution, pH = 7.4

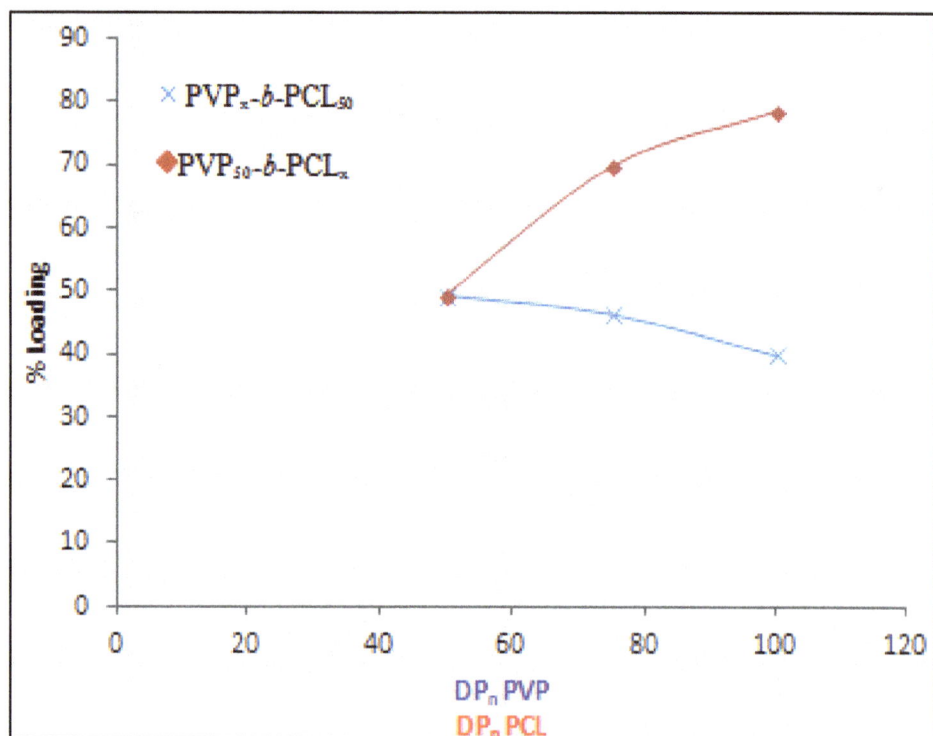

Figure 9.4: Plot of DP$_n$ PCL and PVP against per cent Loading
(***Source***: Reproduced from Veeren*et al. Eur. Polym. J.* 2013, *49*, 3034 with permission from Elsevier)

and 37°C). Release kinetics of the loaded micelles was studied using the zero-order model and Higuchi model respectively. Sustainable release of the anti-TB drugs and close to zero-order kinetics was achieved over a period of 11 days for both single and dual loaded micelles. A higher drug release is noted as the hydrophilic chain length increases with a maximum of 55 per cent release after 10 days for a PVP_{100}-b-PCL_{50}. On the other hand, the percentage drug release decreases with increase in hydrophobic chain length as depicted in Figure 9.5a. For singly loaded micelles, PZA is found to be released at a slightly faster rate than RIF while in dual combination, INH was found to release faster than RIF (Figure 9.5b).

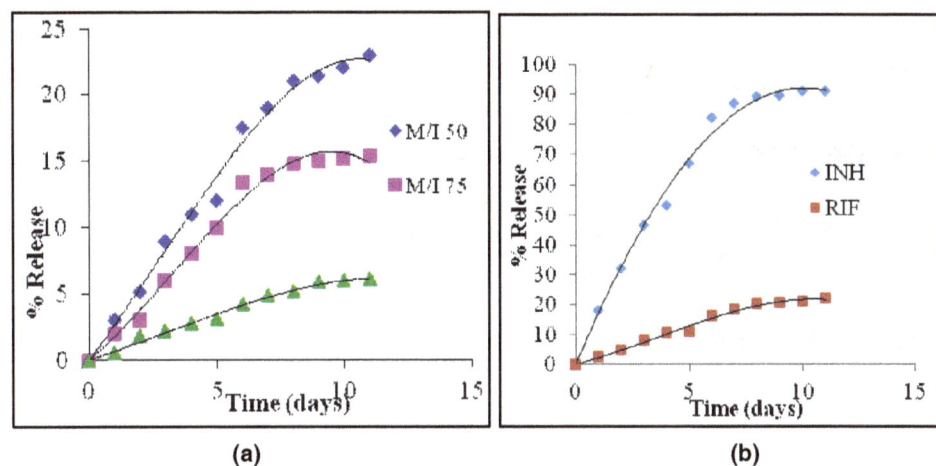

(a)   (b)

Figure 9.5: Plot of per cent Release of (a) RIF (Single loading) Against Time (Days) of PVP_{50}-b-$PCL_{50,75,100}$(b) RIF and INH (Dual loading) Against Time (Days) of PVP_{50}-b-PCL_{50}
(Source: Reproduced from Veeren *et al. Eur. Polym. J.* 2013, *49*, 3034 with permission from Elsevier)

Oligoagarose-g-polycaprolactone copolymers

We have also engineered graft copolymers based on marine polysaccharides. Our oligoagarose-*g*-polycaprolactone copolymers (HO-OligoAga-*g*-PCL)organize into spherical micelles and we have successfully loaded different drugs into the hydrophobic core (Bhaw-Luximon, 2011). Agarose-based systems present the unique advantage of having galactose end groups, which can play a key role in cell targeting. Well-defined oligoagarose-*g*-polycaprolactone copolymers ofvarying polycaprolactone (PCL) chain lengths have been synthesised using protection/deprotection chemistry. The graft copolymers showed amphiphilicbehaviour with spherical micelles in the size range 10 to 20 nm (Figure 9.6). Ketoprofen was loaded into the core of the micelles. The drugloading efficiency was shown to increase with the length of thehydrophobic PCL chain: 2 per cent for PCL10 and 5.5 per cent for PCL15.Sustained drug release was observed over a period of 72 h and wasfaster with shorter PCL chains.

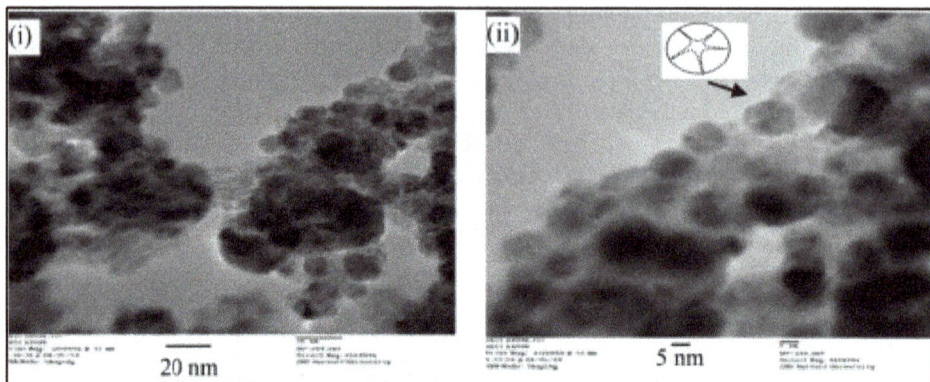

Figure 9.6: TEM Images of (i, ii) HO-OligoAga-*g*-PCL$_{10}$

(*Source*: Adapted from Bhaw-Luximon *et al.* Polym. Chem., 2011, 2, 77
with permission from The Royal Society of Chemistry)

Poly(sucrose)-*g*-Polycaprolactone Copolymers

CBBR recently filed a patent on a method of preparation of bio-amphiphilic polymers from sucrose that self-assemble into core shell micelles (Jhurry, 2013). The invention describes the preparation of novel amphiphilic graft copolymers consisting of sucrose-ether polycondensates onto which biodegradable polymer chains such as polyesters, poly(ester-ether)s or polypeptides have been covalently grafted (Scheme 3). This invention also includes the application of the prepared amphiphilic sucrose-

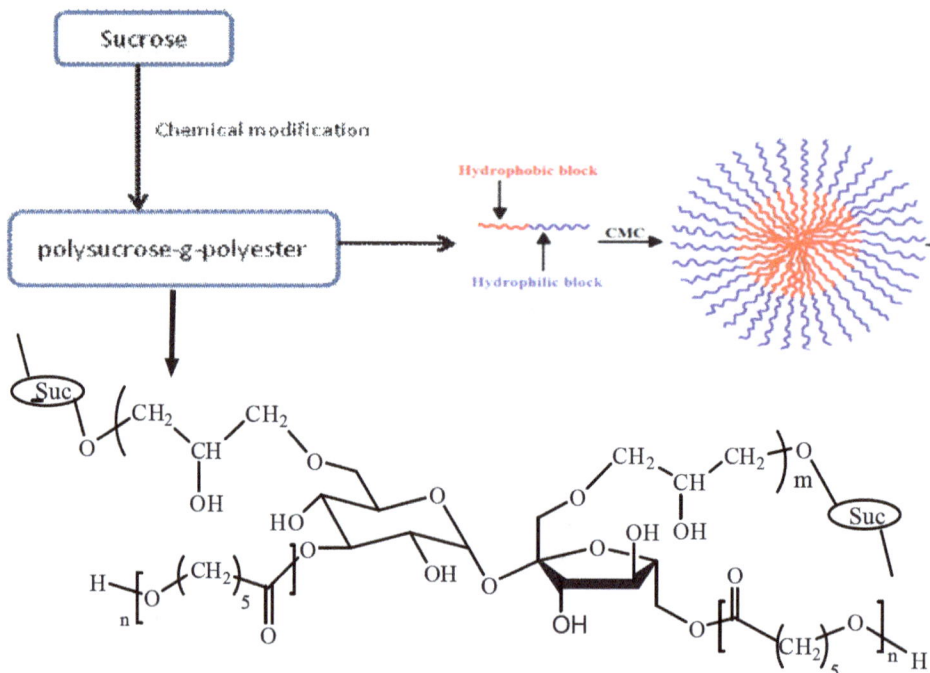

Scheme 3: Bio-amphiphilic Copolymers from Sucrose

ether polycondensates for drug or protein encapsulation and release. Anti-inflammatory, anti-TB and anti-cancer drugs have been tested but this invention encompasses all BCS (Biopharmaceutics Classification System) Class II and IV drugs that are hydrophobic and require surfactants for their transport. The sucrose-based polymeric micelles here disclosed allow a better solubility, enhanced bioavailability of the drug when administered, a prolonged circulation and a prolonged delivery.

CONCLUSIONS

CBBR is the focal point in Mauritius for active research in nanotechnology/nanomedicine. We have given in this article an overview of the main research thrusts and findings in the areas of biomaterials and drug delivery. Our expertise in engineering tailor-made polymers can certainly be extended to applications other than health such as development of nanofiltration membranes for water purification. The issue of research commercialization remains a daunting challenge. It is an area where we are putting a lot of emphasis and we welcome with enthusiasm the meeting organised by NAM S&T with focus on *'Transferring nanotechnology concept towards business perspectives'*. CBBR also offers high level postgraduate training not only restricted to locals but we welcome students from the big Indian Ocean region. The Centre has been recently recognized as a COMESA Regional Centre of Excellence for Polymers.

ACKNOWLEDGEMENTS

We thank the Tertiary Education Commission,Mauritius, for PhD fellowships to RJ, NG, AV and YJ. We are most grateful to our international collaborators Prof. Gary L. Bowlin (University of Memphis, USA), Prof. Viness Pillay (WITS University, South Africa), Dr. Daniel Wesner and Prof. Holger Schönherr (University of Siegen, Germany) for their assistance with analytical techniques not available at CBBR. DJ is most grateful to NAM S&T Centre for inviting him and sponsoring his participation at the International Workshop on Nanotechnology (IWON) 2013, Serpong, Indonesia.

REFERENCES

1. Goonoo, N.; Bhaw-Luximon, A.; Bowlin, G.L.; Jhurry, D. 2013. An assessment of biopolymer- and synthetic polymer-based scaffolds for bone and vascular tissue engineering. *Polym. Int.*, *62*, 523.

2. Lochee, Y.; Bhaw-Luximon, A.; Jhurry, D.; Kalangos A. 2009. *Macromolecules.*, *42*, 7285.

3. Lochee, Y.; Jhurry, D.; Bhaw-Luximon, A.; Kalangos A. 2010. *Polym. Int.*, *59*, 1310.

4. Wolfe, P.S.; Lochee, Y.; Jhurry, D.; Bhaw-Luximon, A.; Bowlin, G.L. 2011. *JEFF*, *6*, 60.

5. Goonoo, N.; Bhaw-Luximon, A.; Bowlin, G.L.; Jhurry, D. 2012. *Ind. Eng. Chem. Res.*, *51*, 12031.

6. Goonoo, N.; Bhaw-Luximon, A.; Bowlin, G.L.; Jhurry, 2014. *Int. J. Polym. Mater. Polym. Biomater.*, *63*(10), 527.

7. Nowsheen Goonoo, ArchanaBhaw-Luximon, Isaac A Rodriguez, Daniel Wesner, HolgerSchönherr, Gary L Bowlin and DhanjayJhurry. 2014. *Biomater. Sci.*, *2*, 339.

8. Jeetah, R.; Bhaw-Luximon, A.; Jhurry, D. 2012. *J.Nanopart. Res.*, *14*, 1168.

9. Jeetah, R.; Bhaw-Luximon, A.; Jhurry, D. 2014. *J. Nanopharmaceutics Drug Delivery*, *1*, 240.

10. Veeren, A.; Bhaw-Luximon, 2012. A.*Macromol.Symp.*, *313-314*, 59.

11. Veeren, A.; Bhaw-Luximon, A.; Jhurry, D. 2013. *Eur. Polym. J.*, *49*, 3034.

12. Bhaw-Luximon, A.; Meeram, M. L.;Jugdawa, Y.;Helbert, W.; Jhurry, D. 2011. *Polym. Chem.*, *2*, 77.

13. Jhurry, D. and Bhaw-Luximon A. (granted Oct **2013**). *'A method of preparing an amphiphilic graft copolymer'*, SA Patent 2013/00961.

Chapter 10

Synthesis and Characterization of Leaf-Like CuO Nanostructures by Alkaline Precipitation Method

Lwin Thuzar Shwe[1]* and Phyu Phyu Win[2]

[1]Metallurgical Research Department,
[2]Nanotechnology Research Department,
Myanma Scientific and Technological Research Department,
Yangon, Myanmar
*E-mail: lwinthuzarshwe@gmail.com

ABSTRACT

Copper oxide nanostructures with leaf–like shape were successfully synthesized by simple and cost effective precipitation method using copper metal chips and sodium hydroxide as a stabilizing agent at different calcination temperatures. The synthesized products were characterized by X-ray Diffraction (XRD), Scanning Electron Microscopy (SEM) and Energy Dispersive Spectrometer of X-ray (EDX). X-ray diffraction indicated that the nanostructure product before calcination was orthorhombic $Cu(OH)_2$ and after calcinations was monoclinic CuO. SEM images showed that leaf-like nanostructures of monoclinic CuO were formed through orthorhombic $Cu(OH)_2$ nanowire bundles by heat treatment. It was found that bundles of copper hydroxide nanowires with an average width of 80-100 nm and length 3-5 μm and leaf-like shape nanostructures of copper oxide with 80 nm after calcinations at 150°C for 3 hr. The changes in morphology of CuO nanostructures were observed from leaf-like nanostructures to fiber-like structures and then to a more plate-like aggregate structures with increasing calcination temperatures. The particle size of CuO nanostructures was found to increase with increasing calcination temperatures.

Keywords: CuO, Copper oxide, Leaf-like nanostructures, Precipitation, Calcination.

INTRODUCTION

Copper oxide is a p-type semiconductor material and has a natural abundance of starting material. It is one of the important metal oxide which has attracted recent research because of its low cost, abundant availably as well as its peculiar properties (Nithyal, 2014). Recently, copper-based nanomaterials have received attention because of their applications in optoelectronic devices, catalysis and superconductor (Sambandam, 2010). Copper oxide nanoparticles are used in a wide range of applications such as gas sensors, magnetic storage media, lithium ion batteries, solar energy transformation, semiconductors and organic catalysis (Kim, 2008; Suleiman, 2013; Ritu, 2013; Jopnani, 2009; Giinter, 2004; Wang, 2003).

For synthesizing copper oxide nanoparticles, many efficient approaches have been carried out such as sonochemical preparation, alkoxidebased preparation, microwave irradiation, precipitation-pyrolysis and thermal decomposition (Giinter S, 2004; Wang W, 2003; Sabbaghi1 S, 2012). Various copper compound nanostructures, including nanotubes, nanowires, whiskers and nanosheets, have been grown directly by the chemical oxidation of copper foil in alkaline aqueous solutions with an oxidant additive or by the electrochemical anodization in alkaline solutions (Singh, 2009). Due-Duong L reported wire-like orthorhombic $Cu(OH)_2$ nanobundles were grown by electrochemical anodization of copper foil in aqueous NaOH (Duc-Duong, 2010). Instead of electrochemical anodization, the quick-precipitation is used because it is safe and environmentally friendly (Shahmiri, 2013). The use of the quick precipitation method is particularly more attractive because of its cost-effectiveness and simple operation (Ritu, 2013; Shahmiri, 2013).

In this paper, CuO nanostructures with leaf–like shape were synthesized by simple aqueous precipitation method using copper chips and sodium hydroxide as a stabilizer. The copper precursor solution was prepared by nitric acid dissolution of copper chips. The aim of the present work is to investigate the crystal growth of leaf-like nanostructures of CuO through $Cu(OH)_2$ nanowire bundles by heat treatment. Moreover, we study the effect of calcination temperatures on particle size, crystallinity and morphology of the nanostructures by characterizing X-ray diffraction (XRD), scanning electron microscope (SEM) and Energy Dispersive Spectrometer of X-ray (EDX).

EXPERIMENTAL PROCEDURE

Synthesis of CuO Nanomaterials

All chemical materials used in the experiment were analytical grade without any further purification and copper chips were provided by Copper Mine (Monywa) in Myanmar. Firstly, copper precursor solution (0.1 M) was prepared by dissolving 3.0 gm of copper metal chips in 6.0 ml of nitric acid. The reddish-brown copper metal chips were first oxidized, the solution was very concentrated and first a green color and then a greenish-brownish color. The Cu^{2+} product was initially coordinated to nitrate ions from the nitric acid, giving the solution first a green, and then a greenish-brownish color which was explained by Phathaitep and co-authors. Then 0.1 M precursor solution was obtained by diluting this copper solution with distilled water and changed to blue color solution. When the solution was diluted with water, water molecules displace the nitrate ions in the coordinate sites around the copper ions, causing the solution to change from greenish-brownish to a blue color (Sabbaghi, 2012; Phathaitep, 2005).

Sodium hydroxide solution (1 M) was added to this copper solution drop by drop under stirring at room temperature. The copper solution turned into light blue precipitate and gradually the blue color materials turned into gray and black color. Copper hydroxide nanostructures were precipitated at pH≈10. The resulting precipitate was filtered and washed several times with distilled water until free of nitrate ions and finally dried at ambient condition. The as-obtained materials were calcined for 3 hr at different temperatures of 150°C, 200°C, 300°C and 600°C, respectively. The black powder products were further characterized by XRD, SEM and EDX.

Characterization

X-ray Diffraction Analysis

The crystal structures of the samples were examined by X-ray diffraction, XRD (D8 Advance Bruker Co.,) with CuKα (λ = 1.54056 Å) in the 2θ range from 5° to 80° in steps of 0.03° with a count time of 0.4s. The crystallite sizes of the particles were calculated by using Scherrer's equation.

$$D = K\lambda/\beta\cos\theta \qquad [1]$$

where,

D is the crystallite size of the particles, K is a shape factor (K=0.9 in this work), λ is the wavelength of the incident X-ray (1.54056 Å, CuKα), θ is the diffraction angle and β is the full-width half maximum (Suleiman M, 2013; Sabbaghi S, 2012; Aparna Y, 2012; Manimaran R, 2013).

Scanning Electron Microscopy

The composition and morphology of the prepared nanoparticles were studied using scanning electron microscope (Carlzeiss AURIGA Crossbeam Work Station, FIB SEM) attached with energy dispersive analysis of X-ray (EDX).

RESULTS AND DISCUSSION

X-ray Diffraction Analysis

The crystalline structures of $Cu(OH)_2$ and CuO nanomaterials prepared at different calcination temperatures of 150°C, 200°C, 300°C and 600°C, were characterized by X-ray diffraction. Figure 10.1(a) shows the XRD pattern of as-obtained sample after the alkaline prepicitation of $Cu(NO_3)_2$ solution and formation of highly crystalline $Cu(OH)_2$ nanostructures. All peaks can be indexed to the orthorhombic $Cu(OH)_2$ in good agreement with JCPDS No (35-0505). It demonstrates that single crystalline nanowires, growing along the [100] direction parallel to the longest dimension, are predominantly laid on the (010) plane. The plausible mechanism for

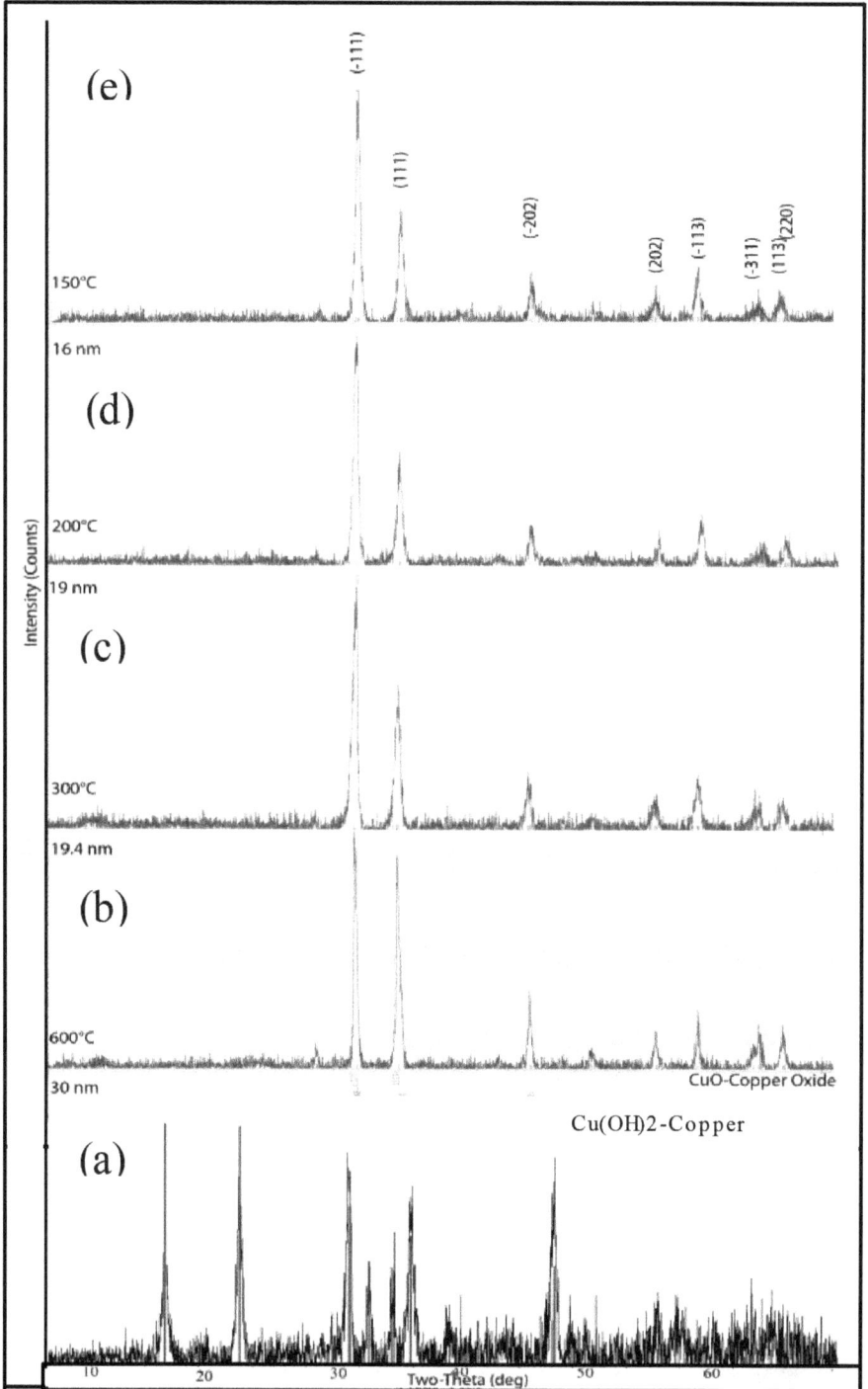

Figure 10.1: XRD Pattern of (a) Cu(OH)$_2$ Nanostructures and CuO Nanoparticles at different Calination Temperatures of (b) 150°C, (c) 200°C, (d) 300°C and (e) 600°C

the formation of nanowire bundle structures can be given on the ground of previous results obtained in the alkaline solution (Duc-Duong, 2010).

Figure 10.1(b-e) shows the XRD patterns of CuO nanoparticles after heat treatment at different temperatures. All of the diffraction peaks can be perfectly indexed to monoclinic CuO with lattice constants $a = 0.4689$nm, $b = 0.3428$nm, $c = 0.5142$nm and $\beta = 99°28$ and good to the Joint Committee on Powder Diffraction Standards (JCPDS No: 80-1268). The XRD patterns of calcined samples indicated that the nanomaterials obtained via our method consist of highly crystalline monoclinic structure of CuO. The intensity of the product at 150°C, 200°C, 300°C were not substantially different. The highest intensity of the product calcined at 600°C was found with the sharp diffraction peaks and the largest crystallite size.

Scanning Electron Microscopy Analysis

The SEM images of $Cu(OH)_2$ and CuO nanostructures synthesized at different calcination temperatures are shown in Figure 10.2. Figure 10.2(a-b) shows a large number of nanowire bundles of $Cu(OH)_2$ after alkaline precipitation at about pH 10. It is found that the nanobundles consist of several uniform nanowires with an average width of 80-100 nm and average length of about 3-5μm. After calcination at 150°C, consequently, it was observed that orthorhombic $Cu(OH)_2$ nanowire bundles were transformed into corresponding CuO leaf-like nanostructures with noticeable change in morphology during the thermal treatment.

SEM analysis was used to investigate the effect of different calcination temperatures on the morphology of CuO nanostructures. Figure 10.2(c-f) shows the morphology changes with heat treatment. It was observed that the leaf-like nanostructures changed to fiber like- structures and then to a more plate-like aggregate structures with increasing calcination temperatures.

Figure 10.2(c) shows the leaf-like CuO nanostructures with the particle size of about 80 nm at 150°C for 3 hr. When we increased the temperature to 200°C for 3 hr, fiber-like CuO nanostructure with the particle size of about 100 nm was obtained as shown in figure 2(d). When the calcinations temperature was increased to 300°C, the plate-like aggregate nanostructures of CuO with the particle size of about 150 nm at 300°C was found. At 600°C, a more aggregate nanostructure of CuO with average particle size of 190 nm was obtained. Heating of the materials helped in better crystallization of materials and in the formation of different nanostructures of CuO.

The atomic composition of the CuO nanostructures was determined using EDX analysis as shown in Figure 10.3. From the EDX result, the CuO nanostructures were comprised of Cu and O atoms with a Cu:O atomic ratio of 1:1.1, close to the stoichiometry of cupric oxide. The XRD pattern shown in Figures 10.1(b-e) clearly supports the existence of a monoclinic CuO phase. The CuO formation may becomes from the sequential dehydration process of $Cu(OH)_2$. The overall reactions involved in the preparation of CuO are shown below.

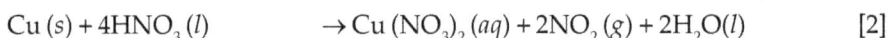

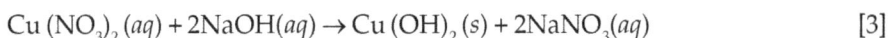

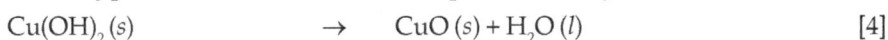

$$Cu\ (s) + 4HNO_3\ (l) \qquad \rightarrow Cu\ (NO_3)_2\ (aq) + 2NO_2\ (g) + 2H_2O(l) \qquad [2]$$

$$Cu\ (NO_3)_2\ (aq) + 2NaOH(aq) \rightarrow Cu\ (OH)_2\ (s) + 2NaNO_3(aq) \qquad [3]$$

$$Cu(OH)_2\ (s) \qquad\qquad \rightarrow \qquad CuO\ (s) + H_2O\ (l) \qquad [4]$$

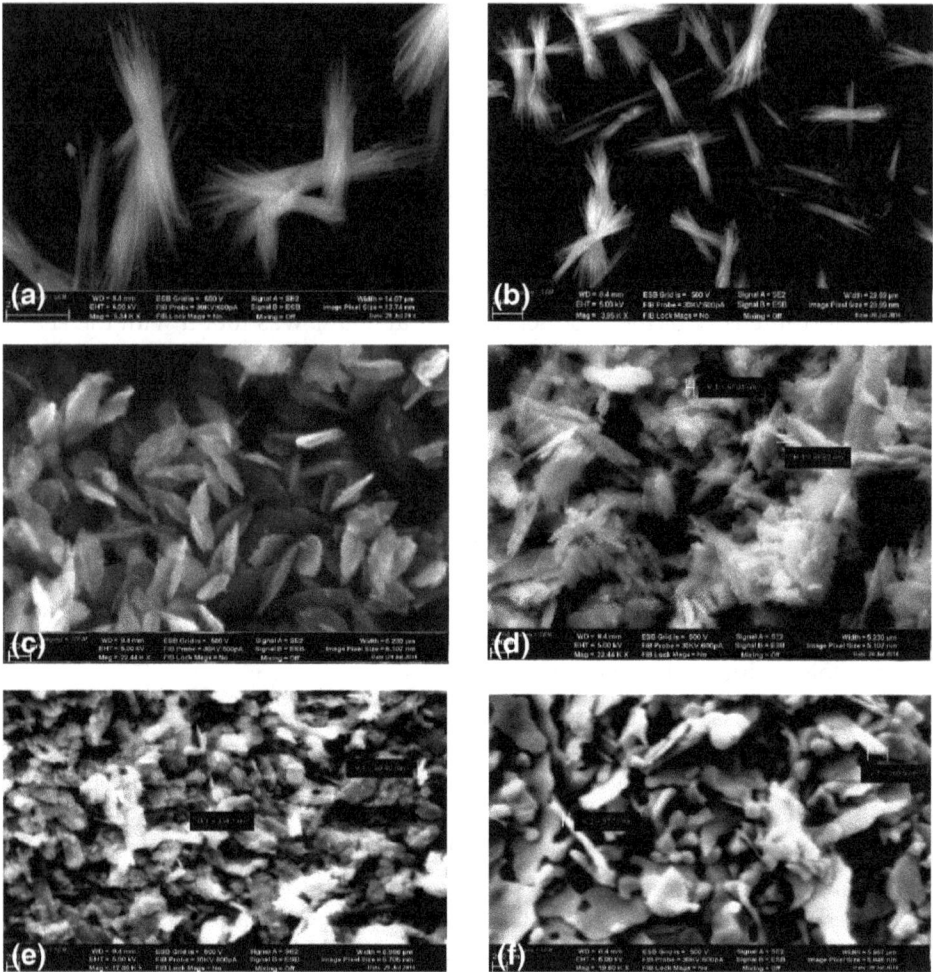

Figure 10.2: SEM Images: (a-b) bundles of Cu (OH)$_2$ nanowires, (c) leaf-like CuO nanostructures calcined at 150 °C, (d) flake-like CuO nanostructures calcined at 200°C, (e) plate-like aggregate structures of CuO calcined at 300 °C and (f) more aggregate plate-like nanostructures of CuO calcined at 600 °C

Effect of Calcination Temperature

To investigate the effect of temperature on size and morphology of nanostructures the as-obtained materials were further heated at different temperatures of 150°C, 200°C, 300°C and 600°C. Average crystallite sizes of the CuO nanomaterials were calculated using Scherer equation and average particle sizes were calculated from SEM images. By applying the Scherer equation, the average size of the crystal was calculated to be in the range of 16-30 nm. It can be seen that the intensity of the diffraction peaks, become sharpness and the crystallinity of the powders were enhanced with increasing temperature. Higher heating temperature led to larger particles size and more oxidize because of its high temperature which gives more

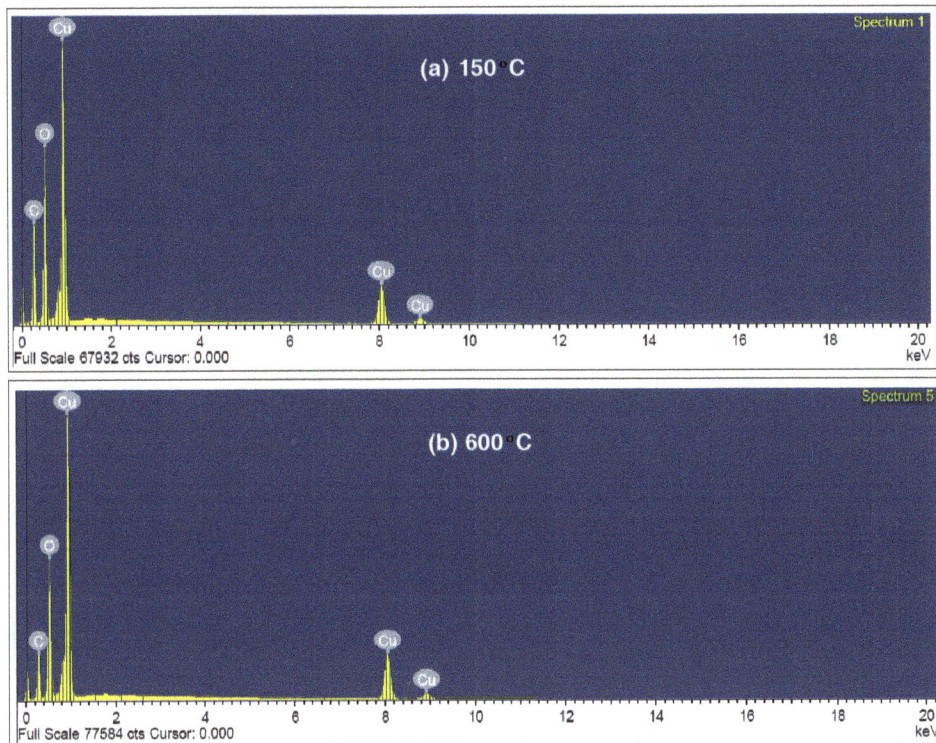

Figure 10.3: EDX Spectra of CuO Nanomaterials Calcined at 150 °C and 600°C

energy (Phathaitep R, 2005). It was clearly found that the average particle sizes and average crystallite sizes of synthesized nanomaterials were increased with increasing temperature as shown in Figure 10.4. This may be attributed to the agglomeration of the particles at high temperatures especially at 600°C. Average particle sizes of CuO nanostructures were also increased with temperature of heat treatment.

CONCLUSIONS

Leaf-like CuO nanostructures were successfully prepared by alkaline precipitation method using copper chips, nitric acid and caustic soda at different calcination temperatures of 150°C, 200°C, 300°C and 600°C. XRD pattern revealed copper oxide nanostructures have monoclinic structure. From EDX analysis the copper oxide nanomaterials are pure and free from impurities. It was found that changes in morphology of CuO nanostructures was from leaf-like nanostructures to fiber- like structures and then to a more plate-like aggregate structures with increasing calcination temperatures. Among them the size of CuO nanoparticles at the temperature of 150°C was obtained 80 nm in this research. Generally, the crystallite size and particle size of the powders increased with increasing calcination temperatures. This alkaline precipitation method is very promising and potential for large scale production.

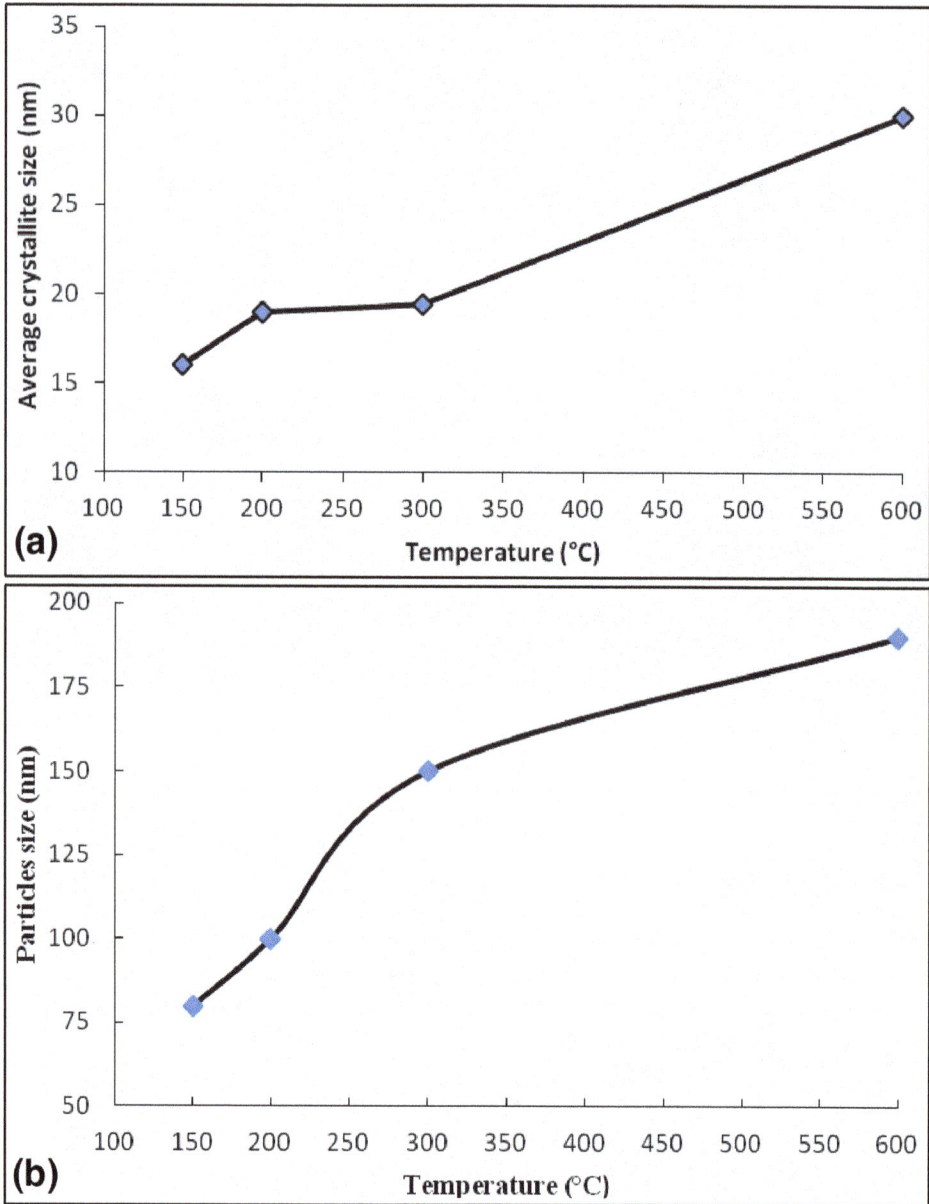

**Figure 10.4: Effect of Calcination Temperatures on
(a) Crystallite Size and (b) Particles Size**

ACKNOWLEDGEMENTS

This research is supported by Ministry of Science and Technology, Myanmar. We are grateful to Metallurgical Research and Development Centre for providing laboratory facilities and Dr. Aye Aye Toe, Dr. Myat Soe Aung from National Analytical laboratory and Mr. Myo Min Tun and Mr. Kyaw Naing Oo from Analytical Lab, Pyin Oo Lwin for taking keen interest in measuring of SEM.

REFERENCES

1. Aparna Y., Enkateswara Rao K.V., Srinivasa Subbarao P., 2012. Synthesis and characterization of CuO nanoparticles by novel sol-gel method, *IPCBEE*, Vol,48: 30.

2. Dinesh Pratap Singh., Animesh Kumar Ojha., Onkar Nath Srivastava., 2009. Synthesis of Different $Cu(OH)_2$ and CuO (Nanowires, Rectangles, Seed-, Belt-, and Sheetlike) Nanostructures by Simple Wet Chemical Route, *J.Phys.Chem*. C, 113(9), 3409-3418.

3. Duc-Duong L., 2010. Wire-like Bundle Arrays of Copper Hydroxide Prepared by the Electro-chemical Anodization of Cu Foil. *Bull Korean Chem. Soc*. Vol.31: No. 8 2283.

4. Giinter S., 2004. Nanoparticles: From Theory To application. WILEY-VCH Verlag GmbH and Co. KGaA, Weinheim, 8-10.

5. Jopnani N., Kushwaha S., Athar T., 2009. Wet synthesis of Copper oxide nanopowder international journal of green nanotechnology, *Mat. Sci. Eng*., 1: M67-M73.

6. Kim Y-S., Hwang I-S., Kim S-J., 2008. CuO nanowire gas sensors for air quality control in automotive cabin, *Sensors and Actuators*, B (135): 298-303.

7. Nithyal K., 2014. Preparation and Characterization of Copper Oxide Nanoparticles, International Journal of Chem Tech Research, *CODEN (USA): IJCRGG* ISSN: 0974-4290 Vol.6: No.3, 2220-2222.

8. Mahdi Shahmiri., 2013, Effect of pH on the Synthesis of CuO Nanosheets by Quick Precipitation Method, WSEAS TRANSACTIONS on ENVIRONMENT and DEVELOPMENT, Vol. 9:2.

9. Manimaran R., Palaniradja K., Alagumurthi N., Sendhilnathan S., Hussain J., 2013. Preparation and characterization of copper oxide nanofluid for heat transfer applications, *Appl. Nanosci*., 1-5.

10. Miss Ritu., 2013. A Simple and effective method of the synthesis of nanosized CuO particles, *Int. Chem. Res*., 3 (i-3): 10-17.

11. Phathaitep R., Sombat K., Supab C., 2005. CuO nanowires by oxidation reaction, *Special Issue on Nanotechnology* 4: 1-5.

12. Sabbaghi S., Heydari O., Parvizi M. R., Saboori R., Sahooli1 M., 2012. Effect of temperature and time on morphology of CuO nanoparticle during synthesis, *Int. Nano-dimens*. 3 (1): 69-73.

13. Sambandam A, Shihe Y., 2010. Emergent methods to synthesize and characterize semiconductor CuO nanoparticles with various morphologies – an overview, *J. Experi. Nanosci*., 2 (1-2): 23-56.

14. Suleiman M., Mousa M., Amjad H., Belkheir H., Taibi. H., Ismail W., 2013. Copper (II)-oxide nanostructures: synthesis, characterizations and their applications–review, *Mater. Environ. Sci.* 4 (5): 792-797.

15. Wang W., Oomman K., Chuanmin R.,2003. Synthesis of CuO and Cu_2O crystalline nanowires using $Cu(OH)_2$ nanowire templates, *Mater. Res.*,18.

Chapter 11
Copper Nanoparticle Preparation and its Characterization

Htain Lin Aye[1], Supab Choopun[2]
and Torranin Chairuangsri[3]

[1]*Metallurgy Research Department, Ministry of Science and Technology*
No. 6, Kabaraye Pagoda Rd., Yankin Tsp., Yangon, Myanmar
[2]*Physics Department, Faculty of Science,*
[3]*Industrial Chemistry Department, Faculty of Science,*
Chiang Mai University, 50200, Thailand
E-mail: [1]*htainlinaye@gmail.com;* [2]*supab99@gmail.com;*
[3]*chato@chiangmai.ac.th*

ABSTRACT

Nd:YAG laser ablation on copper target was carried out to produce nanoparticles in distilled water, ethanol and acetone. The particles were characterized by UV-Vis spectroscopy, dynamic light scattering (DLS-Zeta-sizer Nano-S) and transmission electron microscopy (TEM). Maximum absorption peaks of colloids were about 620, 590 and 585 nm in distilled water, ethanol and acetone, and their colours were light-green, light-brown and dark-yellow, respectively. DLS resulted all produced particles in colloids were in the range of 1-100 nm and they had narrow size distribution. TEM revealed that spherical nanoparticles were observed in distilled water and acetone, but those in ethanol were not cleared. Regarding of the selected area electron diffraction pattern (SADP), the nanoparticles in distilled water and ethanol were mainly copper oxide, whereas those in acetone were both copper and copper oxide. Almost of copper nanoparticles in ethanol were precipitated after a day, whereas a week in distilled water. In acetone, a stable colloid was obtained for a long time.

Keywords: Laser ablation, Nanoparticles, Copper Nanoparticles, Distilled water, Ethanol, Acetone.

INTRODUCTION

Nanoparticles were useful in a number of applications in physics, chemistry, engineering and biology as they had a large surface to volume ratio and unique properties (Patil, 1987; Nawathey, 1989; Becker, 1998; Yang, 2007; Semaltianos, 2010). Nanoparticles could be synthesized by laser ablating on a solid target that lay in a gaseous or a liquid environment as the form of nanopowders or colloids. Size, size distribution, shape, composition and structure of produced nanoparticles from each target material were dependent not only on the choice of laser parameters but also their environments *i.e.* vacuum or controlled gas or liquid (Becker, 1998; Amikura, 2008). It was also shown that copper and copper oxide nanoparticles were obtained with the average size of 30 nm in water and 3 nm in acetone by Nd:YAG laser (1064 nm wavelength) ablation on copper target with the pulsed energy of 130 mJ/pulse, pulse duration of 10 ns, repetition rate of 10 Hz (Tilaki, 2007a). And, formation of zinc oxide nanoparticles was achieved by pulsed Nd:YAG laser (355 nm wavelength) ablation with the laser energy of 50 mJ/pulse, pulse duration of 5 ns and repetition rate of 10 Hz from a zinc metal target in different liquid environments in which the average particle size of 14-20 nm in water with isopropanol solvent and around 100 nm in acetone were obtained (Thareja, 2007). It had been known that round and multi-twined crystalline particles of copper and copper oxide were produced in decane and distilled water from copper and copper oxide metal target by Nd:YAG laser (532 nm wavelength) ablation with the pulse energy of 184-210 mJ/pulse, pulse duration of 6 ns and repetition rate of 1 Hz (Amikura, 2008; Ho, 2008). Above studies indicated atomic compositions of produced nanoparticles were identical or different to those of their source metals chose. They also suggested these composition changes were dependent on the effect of solvents. In addition, it had been shown that producing noble and alloy metal nanoparticles could be synthesized by laser ablation operating with various laser parameters in liquids (Kabashin, 2003; Andrei, 2003; Pyatenko, 2004; Tarasenko, 2006; Tiliki, 2006; Lin, 2006; Tilaki, 2007b). It was suggested that above studies were succeeded on producing nanoparticles by operating with various laser wavelengths, high laser energy, low repetition rate and short pulse duration. Former studies had been used high laser parameters on producing metal nanoparaticles in liquids. In addition, copper nanoparticles had been produced separately for different conditions (Simakin, 2004; Tarasenko, 2005). Therefore, further investigations of producing nanoparticles operating with low laser parameters on metal target in different liquid carrier media were necessary to be proved. In this study, Nd:YAG laser ablation (1064 nm wavelength) on copper target was carried out to produce nano-sized particles in distilled water, ethanol and acetone. The laser was operated with the laser energy of 3 mJ/pulse, pulse duration of 3 ns and repetition rate of 30 kHz on the copper target which was immersed at 3 mm (9.55 ml) distance from the surface of liquid.

EXPERIMENT

The target with dimension of 12 mm × 12 mm were cut from a 2-mm thick copper sheet (ADVENT Research Materials Ltd, Oxford, England) which was proved to contain 99.9 wt. per cent Cu. The target was washed with ethanol and distilled water in sonicator for several hours in order to exclude its superficial oxide layer and to prevent the simultaneous oxidation. Distilled water, absolute ethanol with 99.9 per cent purity (BEC-Thai Co., Ltd) and AR grade Acetone 99.9 per cent purity (BEC-Thai Co., Ltd) were used as laser ablation media. Firstly, Nd:YAG laser (Kevron Marker Laser machine) beam was focused to start ablation as the scanning area of 10 mm × 10 mm on the metal target. Then, nanoparticles were fabricated as shown in Figure 11.1 by laser operating (fundamental wavelength of 1064 nm) at the laser energy of 3 mJ/pulse and 30 kHz on the surface of a cleaned copper target which was placed at the bottom of glass vessel in which the liquid was filled to a desired height of 3 mm (9.55 ml) for 7 min. During laser ablation, small plasma plume containing ions, atoms and very tiny particles was occurred above the target surface by confining effect of liquid carrier media. The particles were observed as colloidal nanoparticles indicating by visible apparent colours in liquids. It was obvious the colours of colloidal solutions were changed differently by changing different liquid carrier media within the laser ablation process. Light-green, light-brown and dark-yellow colours were appeared in distilled water, ethanol and acetone, respectively, while the laser ablation was occurred. One fact was noted while the laser ablation; a few volume of the colloids was becoming less than initial for acetone as it could be evaporated and flown in air. After the laser ablation process, the absorption spectra of colloids were measured immediately by UV-Vis spectroscopy (CARY-50). Along with the absorption spectroscopy, DLS (Zeta-sizer Nano-S) was used to analyse the size and size distribution of the nanoparticles in colloids. Their morphology was analysed by using transmission electron microscopy (TEM, JEOL-2010, Electron Microscopy

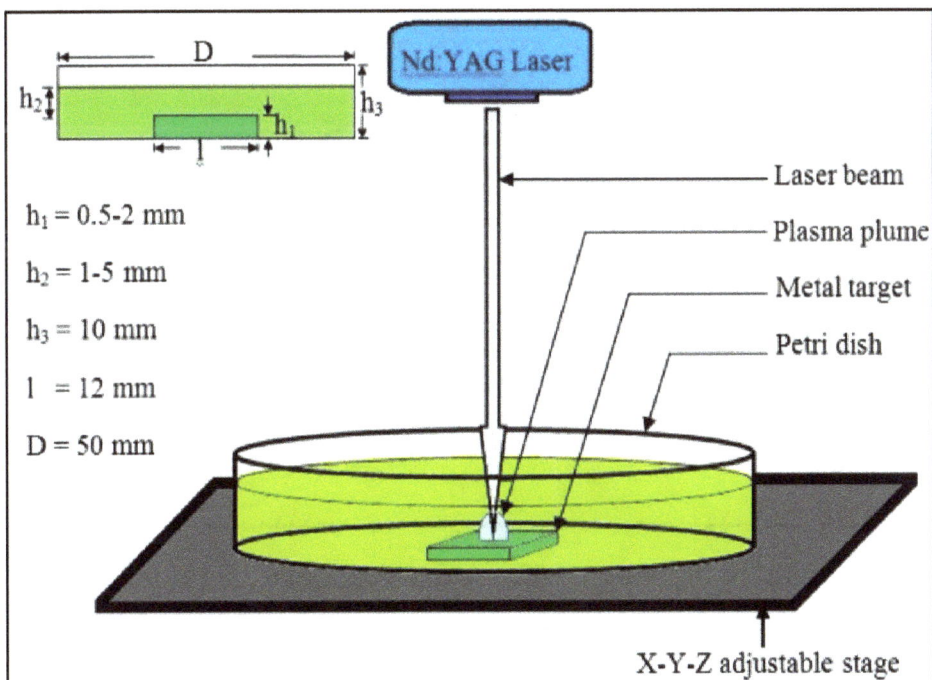

$h_1 = 0.5\text{-}2$ mm

$h_2 = 1\text{-}5$ mm

$h_3 = 10$ mm

$l = 12$ mm

$D = 50$ mm

Figure 11.1: Laser Ablates on Metal Target in Liquid

Research and Service Centre (EMRSc), Chiang Mai University) which was operated at 200 kV.

RESULTS AND DISCUSSION

Optical Absorption Spectra

Because of the sensitivity of the optical properties of metal nanoparticles resulting from the surface plamon resonance, UV-Vis spectral characterization was a useful measurement for monitoring the size and shape changes of nanoparticles in the liquid (Becker, 1998; Tiliki, 2006; Amikura, 2008). The maximum absorption peak of the spectrum was appeared by the presence of average size of the nanoparticles in colloid and its position is tending to relevant with the particle size. It also could be realized the higher the liquid dipole movement, the more the maximum absorption peak to ultraviolet region (Pyatenko, 2004; Tilaki, 2007b). In Figure 11.2, the absorption spectra of copper nanoparticles in distilled water, ethanol and acetone were presented and their maximum absorption peaks, were about 620, 590 and 585 nm, respectively.

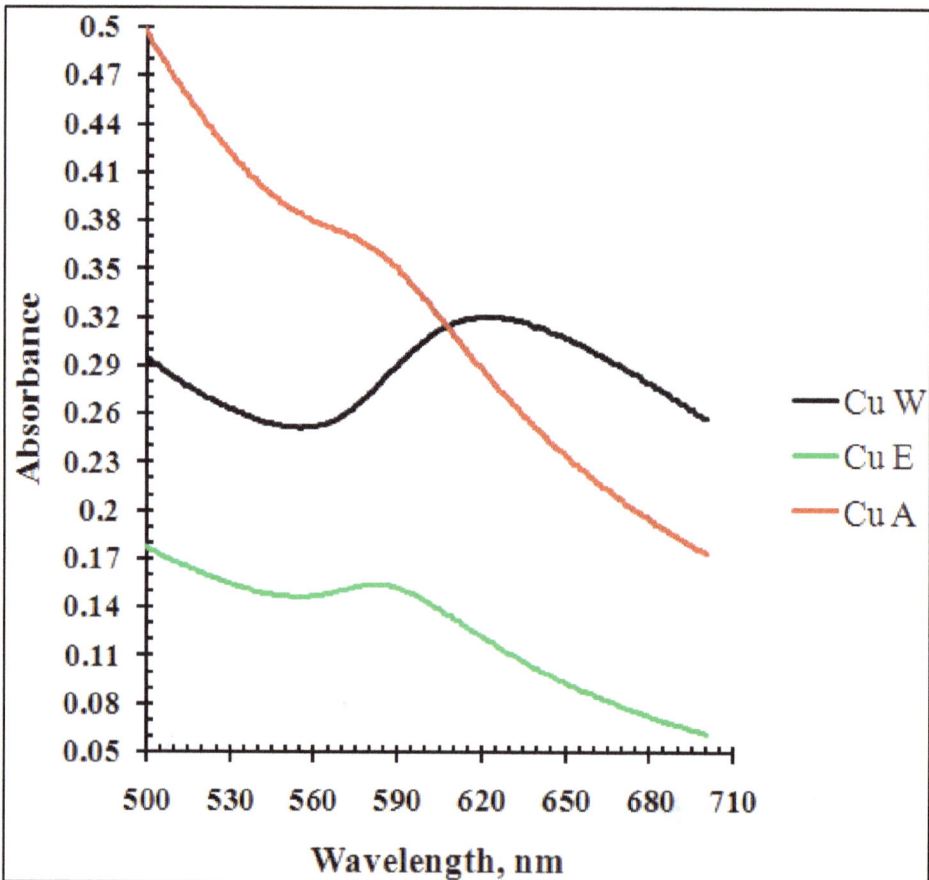

Figure 11.2: Absorption Spectra of Colloidal Copper Nanoparticls in Distilled Water (Cu W), Ethanol (Cu E) and Acetone (Cu A)

The maximum absorption peak of copper nanoparticles in ethanol could be seen not affected by the dipole moment effects of liquid medium, it was clearly realized that the value of maximum peak for ethanol was showed between distilled water and acetone, even ethanol had lower dipole movement than others. It was also noticed that the lowest absorbance of spectrum was observed in ethanol due to the ions, atoms and other tiny particles in colloids in which their growth first and precipitate rapidly in ethanol and the optical laser was touched very fine particles only in UV-Vis spectroscopy. The presence of the single surface plasmon peak implied that the observed nanoparticles were nearly spherical (Bohren and Huffman, 1983; Pyatenko, 2004; Lin, 2006; Tilaki, 2007b). Copper nanoparticles in distilled water showed light-green and suspended nanoparticles were precipitated in a week. In ethanol, nanoparticles precipitated after a day and appeared as a light-brown colour. A stable colloidal suspension of nanoparticles was obtained only in acetone, at least for 9 months.

Dynamic Light Scattering

The size distribution in the case of distilled water, ethanol and acetone were presented at Figures 11.3 (a), (b) and (c). The average size of nanoparticles in distilled water, ethanol and acetone were 37, 85 and 10 nm. Hence, it could be noticed that the concentration of nanoparticles in acetone was more appeared and finer than in others. These results were related to the dipole moment effects of liquid carrier media. Due to the interaction of liquid environment molecules and charge nanoparticles in plume, electrical double layers were formed surrounding of the surface of the nanoparticles (Tiliki, 2006; Tilaki, 2007; Tarasenko, 2007). Higher dipole moment of surrounding molecules culminated in stronger bonds between these molecules and surface of primarily synthesized nanoparticles in plume, prohibiting the growth mechanism. Therefore, finer copper nanoparticles were synthesized in acetone than in distilled water and ethanol. Plume – nanoparticles interaction depended on the attractive and repulsive forces between the nanoparticles and plume species that caused growth or aggregation by the attractive van der Waals force or electrostatic repulsive force due to the overlapping field of the electrical double layers (Tilaki, 2006). The sizes of ablated nanoparticles were also depended on the confinement effect of the liquid during laser ablation. High polar molecules of liquid formed stronger bond to the surface of the nanoparticles, therefore the electrostatic repulsive forces due to overlapping fields of the electrical double layers of the nuclei and species in the plume prevented further growth (Tilaki, 2006 and 2007). It was suggested that nanoparticles produced in an increase in the dipole moment of the surrounding liquid molecules (*e.g.* acetone) tended to decrease the size. The average size in the case of distilled water was comparable, but in the case of acetone was somewhat larger than those reported by Tilaki (2007) using the same laser source, but different operation with higher laser energy (130 mJ/pulse) and repetition rate (10 Hz). It was anticipated to get as much as minimum average nanoparticle size and narrow size distribution of the ablated particles due to both a relatively low ablation threshold and the absence of target heating effects by operating laser energy 3 mJ/pulse with pulse duration 3 ns at the liquid height of 3 mm (9.55 ml) for all solvents. The mechanism of laser ablation in liquid was explained by Yang (2007). In brief, a dense

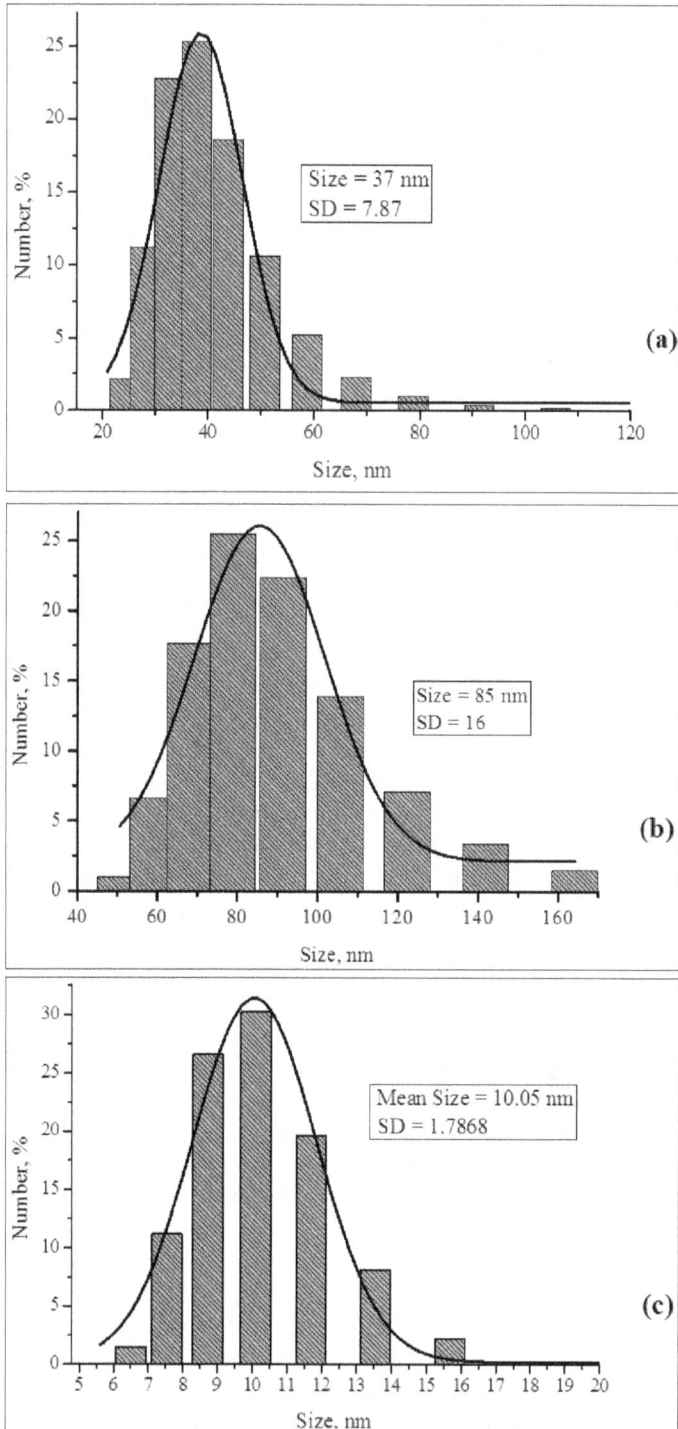

Figure 11.3: Mean Size and Size Distribution of Copper Nanoparticles in Distilled Water (a), Ethanol (b) and Acetone (c)

cloud of plume including copper atoms was accumulated in the laser spot of the copper target during the ablation. The plume was composed of a number of small copper atoms that were aggregated dramatically due to the density of fluctuation to form embryonic nanoparticles. That aggregation continued significantly with slower rate even after the ablation process had been finished. These consecutive nanoparticles growth was slow, random, and uncontrollable because both ablated atoms and embryonic nanoparticles diffuse through the solution toward each other to form larger clusters.

TEM Examination

The nanoparticles were mostly spherical in agreement with the results from optical absorption spectroscopy. Narrow size distribution, some agglomeration and welded ligament were observed in the case of distilled water in Figure 11.4 (a). Two types of particles were observed, one was larger spherical particles and the other was

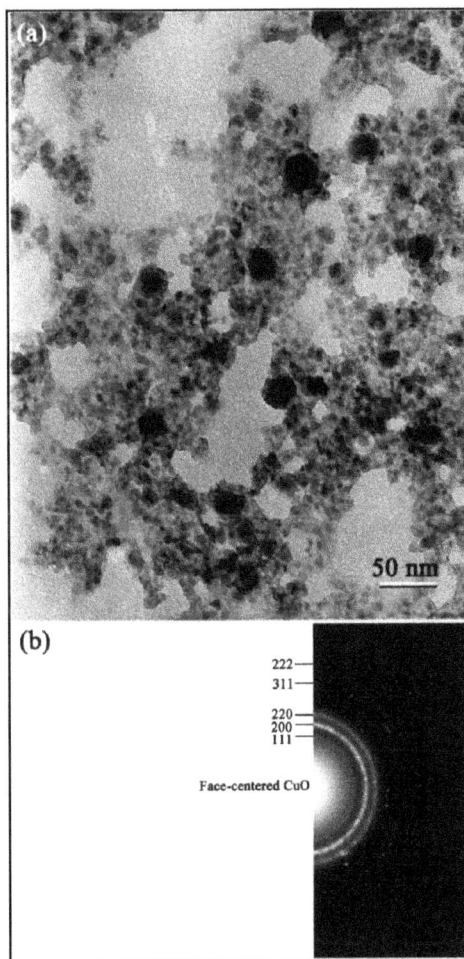

Figure 11.4: Bright-Field TEM Images (a) and SADP (b) in Distilled Water

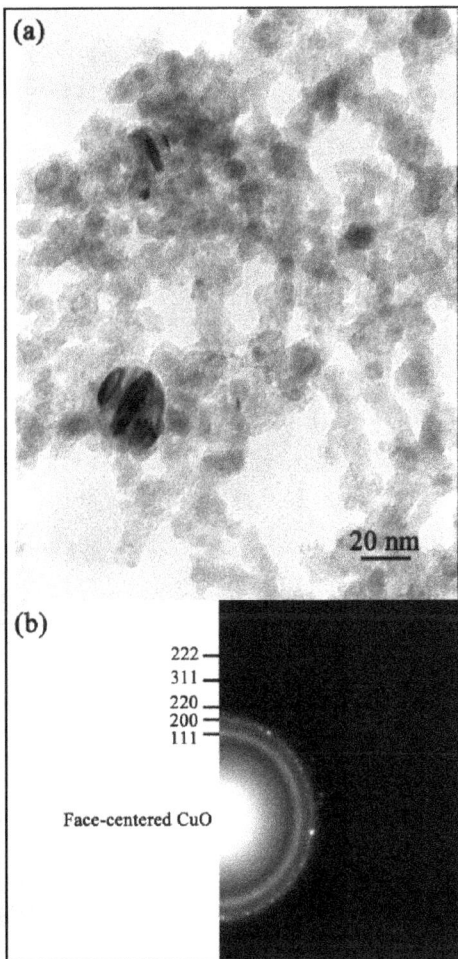

Figure 11.5: Bright-Field TEM Images (a) and SADP (b) in an Ethanol

smaller particles with unclear outlines. Corresponding selected area diffraction pattern (SADP) as shown in Figure 11.4 (b) revealed that nanoparticles in distilled water were mainly of copper oxide as the oxidation affects of copper in water.

It was not as similar as spherical those of particles obtained in distilled water and acetone. Two types of particles were also observed, one was larger spherical

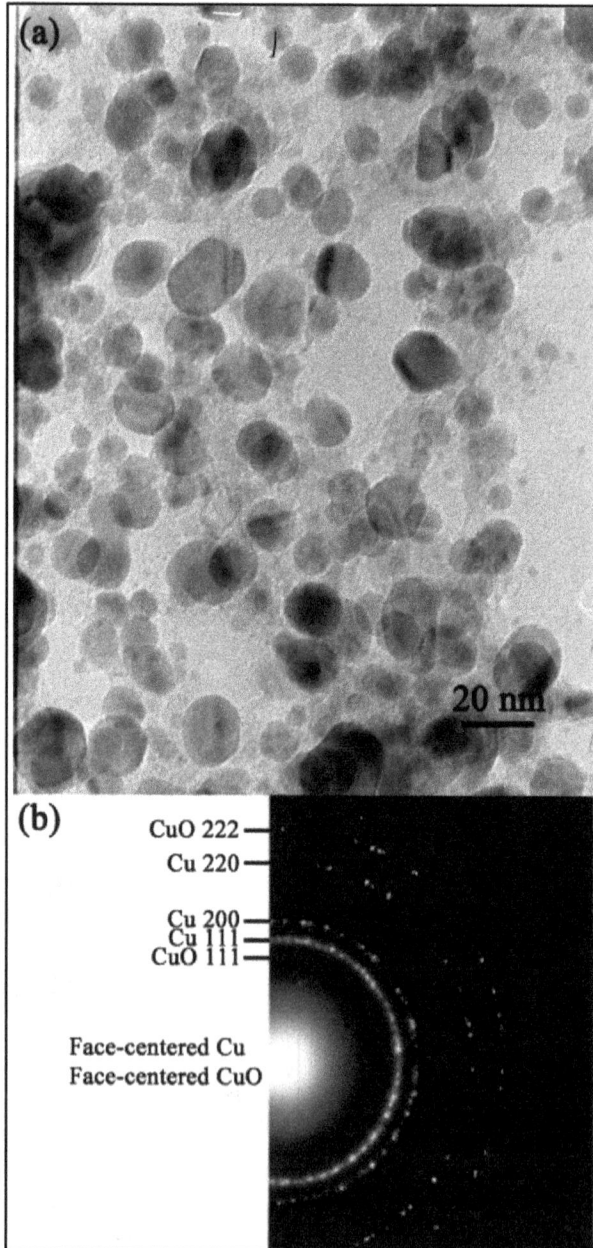

Figure 11.6: Bright-Field TEM Images (a) and SADP (b) in Acetone

particles and the other was aggregation of welded ligament unclear nanoparticles. It was realized that many of welded ligament nanoparticles were caused by aggregation of very small unclear particles due to lower polarity of ethanol. The particle size in TEM was not likely revealed with DLS result because the irradiated light in DLS counted mostly accumulated species. Atomic composition of nanoparticles in ethanol was analysed by using SADP as shown in Figure 11.5 (b). In ethanol, mainly copper oxide nanoparticles as well as those in distilled water were observed. But, well dispersion and narrow size distribution without agglomeration or welded ligament were observed in the case of acetone as shown in Figure 11.6 (a). Corresponding selected area diffraction pattern in Figure 11.6 (b) revealed that the first and second rings were 111 for both copper and copper oxide regarding their intensities were comparable with 2.08 and 2.45 Angstrom (JCPDFWIN, 01-1241 Copper and 78-0428 Copper Oxide). It was noticed that the second 111 ring had higher intensity than the first one; it meant most of the particles from that region were mostly copper. The third 200 and the fourth 220 were indexed as pure copper and the fifth 222 was copper oxide. The reason for a formation of different types of nanoparticles was yet to be understood, this was related to the difference atoms or molecules in species around the plasma plume (Tilaki *et al.*, 2006).

CONCLUSIONS

Nanoparticles were fabricated successfully by pulsed laser ablation at low laser energy and high repetition rate on the copper target immersed in distilled water, ethanol and acetone. Spherical shape nanoparticles were observed in both distilled water and acetone, but welded ligament and few spherical nanoparticles in ethanol. The colour of the colloidal copper nanoparticles in distilled water showed light-green and the maximum absorption peak about 620 nm. In ethanol, light-brown colour and its maximum absorption peak 590 nm were observed, whereas dark-yellow colour and maximum absorption peak 580 nm in acetone. Mainly copper oxide nanoparticles were observed in distilled water and ethanol. Regarding of DLS result, the average size of nanoparticles in distilled water and ethanol were 37 nm and 85 nm, respectively. Both copper and copper oxide nanoparticles with the mean size of 10 nm were obtained in the case of acetone. Nanoparticles in ethanol were precipitated after a day, whereas a week in distilled water. A stable colloidal suspension was obtained only in the case of acetone. Thus, this technique offered an alternative method for preparation of nanoparticles in various liquids.

ACKNOWLEDGMENTS

The authors would like to thank Metallurgy Research Department, Ministry of Science and Technology, the Republic of the Union of Myanmar, the Graduate School, Chiang Mai University, Thailand and the Thailand International Development Cooperation Agency (TICA) for financial support. The Electron Microscopy Research and Service Centre (EMRSc), Faculty of Science, Chiang Mai University is thanked for TEM facilities.

REFERENCES

1. Andrei, K. V., Michel, M., Christopher, K. and John, H. T. L. 2003. Fabrication and Characterization of Gold Nanoparticles by Femtosecond Laser Ablation in an Aqueous Solution of Cyclodextrins. *Phys. Chem.*, **B 107**: 4527–4531.

2. Amikura, K., Kimura, T., Hamada, M., Yokoyama, N., Miyazaki, J. and Yamada, Y. 2008. Copper Oxide Particles Produced by Laser Ablation in Water. *Appl. Surf. Sci.*, **254**: 6976–6982.

3. Bohren, C. F. and Huffman, D. R. 1983. Absorption and scattering of light by small particles. Wiley, New York.

4. Becker, M. F., Brock, J. R., Cai, H., Henneke, D. E., Keto, J. W., Lee, J., Nichols, W. T. and Glicksman, H. D. 1998. Metal Nanoparticles Generated by Laser Ablation. *Nanostruct. Mat.*, **10**: 853–863.

5. Ho, C. and Hung-Ting, S. 2008. Synthesis and Magnetic Properties of Ni Nanoparticles. *Rev. Adv. Mater. Sci.*, **18**: 667–675.

6. Kabashin, A. V. and Meunier, M. 2003. Synthesis of Colloidal Nanoparticles During Femtosecond Laser Ablation of Gold in Water. *Appl. Phys.*, **94**: 7941–7943.

7. Lin, J., Lim, S. F., Mahmood, S., Tan, T. L., Springham, S. V., Lee, P. and Rawat, R. S. 2006. Synthesis and Characterization of FeCo Nanoparticle Colloid by Pulsed Laser Ablation in Distilled Water. 33rd EPS Conference on Plasma Phys. Rome **30I**: 1–4.

8. Nawathey, R., Vispute, R. D., Chaudhari, S. M., Kanetkar, S. M., Ogale, S. B., Mitra, A. and Date, S. K. 1989. Pulsed Laser Induced Vaporization from the Surface of a Binary Oxide (Zinc Ferrite) and Its Implications for Synthesis of Thin Films. *Appl. Phys.*, **8**: 3197–3204.

9. Patil, P. P., Phase, D. M., Kulkarni, S. A., Ghaisas, S. V., Kulkarni, S. K., Kanetkar, S. M. and Ogale, S. B. 1987. Pulsed-Laser Induced Reactive Quenching at Liquid-solid Interface: Aqueous Oxidation of Iron. *Phys. Rev. Lett.*, **58**: 238–241.

10. Pyatenko, A., Shimokawa, K., Yamaguchi, M., Nishimura, O. and Suzuki, M. 2004. Synthesis of Silver Nanoparticles by Laser Ablation in Pure Water. *Appl. Phys.*, **A 79**: 803.

11. Simakin, A. V., Voronov, V. V., Kirichenko, N. A. and Shafeev, G. A. 2004. Nanoparticles Produced by Laser Ablation of Solids in Liquid Environment. *Appl. Phys.*, **A 79**: 1127–1132.

12. Semaltianos, N. G. 2010. Nanoparticles by Laser Ablation. Critical Reviews in Solid State and *Mat. Sci.*, **35**: 105–124.

13. Tarasenko, N. V., Butsen, A. V. and Nevar, E. A. 2005. Laser-induced Modification of Metal Nanoparticles Formed by Laser Ablation Technique in Liquid. *Appl. Surf. Sci.* **247**: 418–422.

14. Tarasenko, N. V., Butsen, A. V., Nevar, E. A. and Savastenko, N. A. 2006. Synthesis of Nanosized Particles During Laser Ablation of Gold in Water. *Appl. Surf. Sci.* **252**: 4439–4444.

15. Tilaki, R. M., Zad, A. I. and Mahdavi, S. M. 2006. Stability, Size and Optical Properties of Silver Nanoparticles Prepared by Laser Ablation in Different Carrier Media. *Appl. Phys.*, A **84**: 215–219.

16. Tilaki, R. M., Zad, A. I. and Mahdavi, S. M. 2007. The Effect of Liquid Environment on Size and Aggregation of Gold Nanoparticles Prepared by Pulsed Laser Ablation. *Nanop., Res.* **9**: 853–860.

17. Tilaki, R. M., Zad, A., I. and Mahdavi, S. M. 2007. Size, Composition and Optical Properties of Copper Nanoparticles Prepared by Laser Ablation in Liquids. *Appl. Phys.*, A **88**: 415–419.

18. Thareja, R. K. and Shukla, S. 2007. Synthesis and Characterization of Zinc Oxide Nanoparticles by Laser Ablation of Zinc in Liquid. *Appl. Surf. Sci.* **253**: 8889–8895.

19. Tarasenko, N. V., Burakov, V. S. and Butsen, A. V. 2007. Laser Ablation Plasmas in Liquids for Fabrication of Nanosized Particles. *Astron. Obs. Belgrade,* **82**: 201–2011.

20. Yang, G. W. 2007. Laser Ablation in Liquids: Applications in the Synthesis of Nanocrystals. Progrs. *Mat. Sci.,***52**: 648–698.

Chapter 12

Institutionalizing Nanotechnology in Nepal

Suresh Kumar Dhungel

Nepal Academy of Science and Technology
P.B. Box – 3323, Khumaltar, Lalitpur, Nepal
E-mail: skdhungel@hotmail.com

ABSTRACT

Nanotechnology is a relatively new branch of technology, which basically deals with the engineering, and observation of things at measurements of 100 nm or less. It is basically a multidisciplinary area of Science and Technology. Though Nepal has ever growing number of students enrolled in the disciplines of Science and Technology in Universities each year, it has not been able to develop marketable technology of its own in many areas. Nepal has no liberty to spend much time, energy, and money for the research on pure sciences. Out of uncountable areas of applied research, Nanotechnology seems to be not very old and it is likely that Nepalese researchers can catch up the current pace of its progress if world- class facilities for research are put in place. With the initiation of research in the emerging field like Nanotechnology Nepal can not only create opportunities for young researchers within the country but also reverse the growing trend of Brain-drain into Brain-gain. Nepal Academy of Science and Technology (NAST) has taken the lead to institutionalize the research and development of the Nanotechnology in Nepal due to which Government of Nepal has kept the establishment of National Research Centre on Nanotechnology on the top of its priority list for the latest annual plan. NAST has initiated synthesis of metal oxide nanomaterials such as titanium dioxide in the form of nanotubes and nanoparticles targeting their applications in energy conversion through Dye Sensitized Solar Cell (DSSC) and water purification through Photocatalysis. The research laboratories of the universities of Nepal are mainly focusing on the development of nanocomposite polymers as well as nanoparticles of metals such as silver for their diversified applications. By institutionalizing Nanotechnology in the country like Nepal, it can also boost its research in advanced materials and discover innovative applications of the materials already synthesized elsewhere.

Keywords: *Nanotechnology, Nepal, Dye sensitized solar cell, Titanium dioxide, Nanoparticles, Nanotubes, Photocatalysis.*

INTRODUCTION

On December 29, 1959, Professor Richard Feynman, a Nobel Prize winner in Physics in 1965, presented a lecture entitled "There's Plenty of Room at the Bottom" during the annual meeting of the American Physical Society at the California Institute of Technology where he was a Professor. He presented the idea of manipulating and controlling things on an extremely small scale by building and shaping matter one atom at a time especially at the time when scientists thought most of the big discoveries had been made and that science just wasn't that exciting anymore. In his lecture he had described how the 24 volumes of the Encyclopedia Britannica could be written on the head of a pin (Williams L. and Adams W., 2007). This theoretical explanation is considered to be the foundation of present day Nanotechnology.

Nanotechnology is simply understood as the ability to observe, measure, manipulate, and manufacture things at the nanometer scale. A nanometer (nm) is one-billionth of a meter and at this scale length becomes comparable to the size of atoms and molecules. The word "nanotechnology" was first introduced in the late 1970s. While many definitions for nanotechnology exist, most groups use the National Nanotechnology Initiative (NNI) definition. According to NNI standard something is referred to as "nanotechnology" only if research and technology development at the atomic, molecular, or macromolecular levels is in the length scale of approximately 1 to 100 nm range, it creates and uses structures, devices and systems that have novel properties and functions because of their small size and has ability to control or manipulate on the atomic scale (Mongillo, 2007). Nanotechnology offers cutting-edge applications that will revolutionize the way we detect and treat disease, monitor and protect the environment, produce and store energy, improve crop production and food quality, and build complex structures as small as an electronic circuit or as large as an airplane. Nanotechnology is attracting increasing investment from governments and industries around the world.

Having completed more than a century and a half since the beginning of the institutionalization of the modern Science and Technology, Nepal still seems to be struggling in its attempts to carryout research activities in emerging disciplines of Science and Technology of which Nanotechnology is also the one. Nepal's geographical location between two giant neighbours with huge economies has not been very productive in terms of developing industries within the country, which would create an appealing environment for research and development in Science and Technology. The growth in the number of Scientists and Technologists returning to country after completing their studies and research activities abroad has created conducing environment in Nepal to put organized efforts for institutionalizing research activities in some prominent areas. Realizing this fact, Government of Nepal had already set policy a few years ago to establish research centres in three areas, *viz.* Nuclear Technology, Biotechnology and Space Technology in which some preliminary works are still in progress. Due to constant efforts of Scientists and Academicians working in Nanoscience and Nanotechnology within the country the Government of Nepal has realized need of establishing a dedicated research centre for Nanotechnology within the country, which is also reflected in the budget of the current fiscal year. If everything goes as planned this can be a milestone to comply with the global trend of research on newly emerged area of Nanotechnology.

Initiatives for Nanotechnology in Nepal

Different organizations active in Nepal for strengthening research in Science and Technology are trying at present to put Nanotechnology in their area of top priority. The initiatives taken by three major actors, Ministry of Science, Technology and Environment of Government of Nepal, Nepal Academy of Science and Technology and the Universities are briefly described here.

Government of Nepal

Government of Nepal has decided to set up Nanotechnology research centre in the country with following major objectives:

1. To have a world class research facility in the latest areas of Nanotechnology
2. To create environment for the Nepalese researchers to stay in Nepal and those working abroad to come back (Brain-Gain) and get involved in research activities within the country
3. To enhance the capacity of national institutions to collaborate in research activities with international counterpart
4. To exploit the full potential of the Nepalese scientists, technologists, and young researchers in different disciplines of S&T to develop native Nanotechnology in the country
5. To promote a multidisciplinary research hub for a holistic approach for the sustainable development of the country
6. To facilitate international collaboration for funding and research activities
7. To publish potential works in reputed international journals that shows our presence in broader scientific communities
8. To generate patents out of the inventions made during the research on technology
9. To have a paradigm shift from the culture of teaching science through 'Chalk and Talk' to 'learning by doing'
10. To build national capacity to carryout research activities in Nanotechnology for Masters as well as Doctoral degrees
11. To ensure Nepalese Scientists/Technologists carry out research activities as par with developed countries of the world

12. To attract industries to invest in Research and Development (R&D) and also initiate venture company in public-private partnership

13. To establish the priority of learning applied S&T over pure science in the country

14. To make the country capable or advancing and adopting modern technology

15. To prove that the country can make a quantum jump in improving the quality of lives of its people only by developing innovative technologies.

At Nepal Academy of Science and Technology (NAST)

Under the Materials Science and Devices Technology Laboratory of NAST, nanotechnology related research activities have been initiated. The laboratory has set four steps to carry out the activities: synthesis of nanomaterials in the form of nanoparticles, nanotubes or nanorods; characterization of synthesized materials; application of the synthesized materials for the fabrication of some sort of devices or processes; and finally measurement of the performance parameters of fabricated devices or processes.

Synthesis and Characterization of TiO_2 nanoparticles for Dye Sensitized Solar Cell application

With the emergence of nanotechnology, TiO_2 nanoparticles have been recognized as a significant candidate for multiple applications. It has also opened possibilities for developing cost competitive solar cells. Photoelectrochemical solar cells consist of a mesoporous dye coated metal oxide semiconductor such as TiO_2 to act as photoelectrode, a redox electrolyte and a counter electrode. TiO_2 has good stability under irradiation in solution but cannot absorb visible light because of its wide band gap of ~ 3.2 eV. Most of the commonly used DSSCs have TiO_2 films as photoelectrodes, which act as mediator for the transport of electrons. The photoelectrode is sensitized by the injection of electron from the dye, a metal-organic complex, used as sensitizer in the cell. Monolayer of dye adsorbed in the nanoporous surface of TiO_2 film absorbs light and goes to excited state where it injects electrons to the conduction band of TiO_2 while making transition to ground state. Significant improvements in the performance of DSSC have been made possible primarily due to the development of the high-performance nanoporous TiO_2 thin film electrodes that have a large surface area capable of adsorbing a large amount of photosensitizer in the form of monolayer.

One of the crucial factors determining the performance of the solar cells is the quality of the TiO_2 film on fluorine doped tin oxide (FTO) coated glass surface, which is prepared either by doctor blading or screen printing the paste of TiO_2 nanoparticles followed by sintering at a suitable temperature. The quality of the TiO_2 film depends on the type of material and method used for film deposition and subsequent sintering procedure. The properties of the films such as surface area, roughness, and pore size and film thickness determine its surface and electronic properties. Many effects related to the size of the nanoparticles of TiO_2 in the photoelectrode are yet to be understood.

Size and the type of the TiO_2 nanoparticles control the properties that lead to their potential application in different devices such as Dye Sensitized Solar Cell. The size of TiO_2 particles in the photoelectrode film can influence the solar cell performance in both ways. Films with larger particles have larger contact points between sintered colloidal particles or at the interface between the particles and the underlying substrate, allowing for easier dye access and better dye assembly whereas smaller particles have a larger surface area and have a greater number of contact points between sintered colloidal particles or at the interface between the particles and the underlying substrate, allowing for greater dye adsorption [Chou, 2007]. However, films consisting of larger particles have a smaller surface area for dye adsorption, which ultimately reduces the amount of light absorbed resulting in low photocurrent from the cell and the films consisting of smaller particles exhibit a larger number of grain boundaries to be overcome by the electrons injected by excited dye molecules, which results in a higher probability of electron trapping [Gracia *et al.*, 2004]. The comparative results of the solar cell electrodes consisting of TiO_2 nanoparticle films with varying particle sizes are presented elsewhere [Chou, 2007].

The synthesized nanoparticles must have good dispersion and high crystallinity. Anatase phase of TiO_2 has already established itself as a better candidate than rutile and brookite phases for the conversion of solar energy.

For this study, three types of TiO_2 nanoparticles were synthesized by hydrothermal process in acidic medium, the experimental details of which can be found elsewhere [Wu, 2002]. The powders of nanocrystalline TiO_2 particles of all the three types were subjected to X-ray diffraction (XRD) to characterize their phases and estimate the sizes of crystallites. Figure 12.1 show the comparison of the X-ray diffraction patterns of three different samples of TiO_2 nanocrystalline powders synthesized by the same process but in different lots where X-axis represents twice of the diffraction angle (2) in degrees and Y-axis represents the intensity in arbitrary unit (a.u.).

Synthesis of Self-organized TiO_2 Nanotubes and their Photocatalytic Application

The number of industries and the basic needs for human beings are increasing day by day, which is creating serious problem on the management of ever increasing environmental pollution. Most of the rural people have been suffering from water-born diseases due to the lack of access to the safe drinking water, especially in Nepal and similar least developed countries. Consequently, the environmental problems associated with toxic organic pollutants in water are the current issues to be solved for the development of a healthy environment. Water pollution is caused mainly from the effluents of factories, power plants, and mines situated either close to water source or away from sources. The sources of water pollution may be divided into two categories, *viz.* (i) Point-source pollution, in which contaminants are discharged from a discrete location. Sewage outfalls and oil spills are examples of point-source pollution. (ii) Non-point-source or diffuse pollution, referring to all of the other discharges that deliver contaminants to water bodies. Acid rain and unconfined run -off from agricultural or urban areas fall under this category.

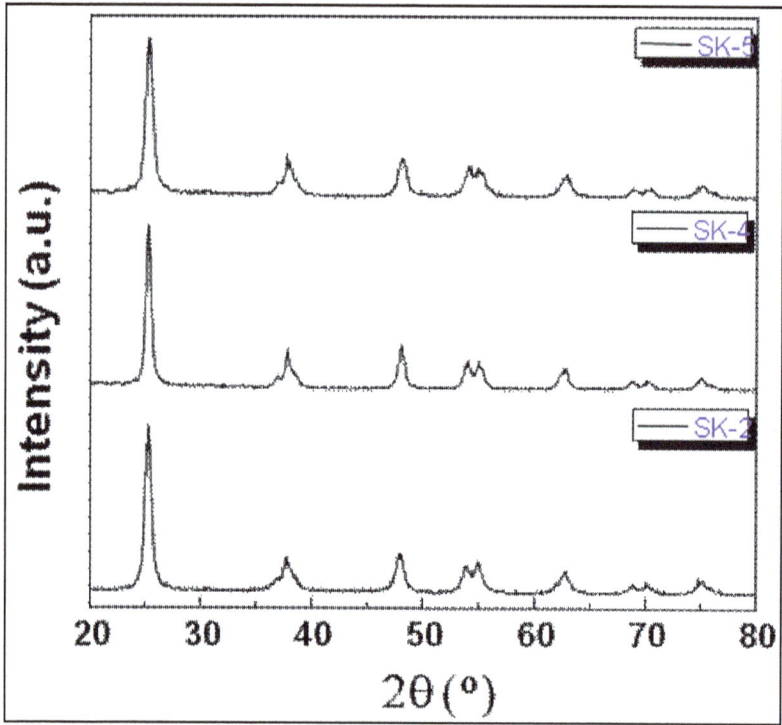

Figure 12.1: Comparison of X-ray Diffraction Patterns of Titanium Dioxide Nanoparticles Synthesized for the Fabrication of Dye Sensitized Solar Cells

In fact, all water pollutants are hazardous to humans. For example, sodium is implicated in cardiovascular disease, nitrates in blood disorders, mercury and lead can cause nervous disorders. Water pollution is due to many contamination in it such as particulates (silt and debris), microorganisms (*e.g.* endotoxins, pyrogens, DNA and RNA, cellular fragments and bacterial by-products, etc.), dissolved inorganic elements (*e.g.* phosphates, nitrates, calcium, magnesium, silicates, iron, chloride, fluoride, etc.), any other natural or man-made chemicals resulting from exposure to the environment, other heavy metals and their isotopes, dissolved organic elements (*e.g.* Pesticides, plant and animal remains or fragments, etc.). For a healthy environment and scientific applications require elimination of various types of contaminants. There are number of methods commonly used to purify water. Their effectiveness is linked to the type of contaminant being treated and the type of application the water will be used for. Some of the general methods of water purification are filtration, distillation, activated carbon adsorption, deionization, ultraviolet radiation and photocatalysis.

As the photocatalytic technique for water purification is an economical, simple and clean technology and hence the process can be very promising for the developing countries like Nepal. For the photocatalysis process, semiconductors are essential and for this TiO_2 especially the anatase form is the first choice because TiO_2 is relatively cheap, non-toxic, insoluble in water and very resistant to most chemicals. It also shows the highest photostability and resistance to so-called anodic photocorrosion. For this, TiO_2 nanoparticles are often used for the degradation of organic compounds (*e.g.* chlorinated alkenes and benzenes, dioxins, furans, PCB, etc.) and reduction of toxic metal ions [*e.g.*, Cr (V I), Ag (I) and Pt (II)] into less toxic corresponding metals in aqueous solutions under the illumination ultraviolet (UV) light. TiO_2 nanotubes are preferred for photocatalysis rather than TiO_2 nanoparticles (P25-commercially available TiO_2 nano-particles). Because of their (P25) extremely small size, it is hard to filter these particles from water after photocatalysis and these particles are also hydrophilic in nature. TiO_2 nanotubes provide a high surface area and high electron mobility as the carriers are free to move throughout the length of the nanotubes, which reduces e^--h^+ recombination rate and thus increases the efficiency of the system. A mechanism of the photocatalytic action of TiO_2 is the absorption of photons of energy equal or greater than its band gap energy which causes the formation of an electron and a hole on the surface or near it. The electron jumps from valence band to conduction band leaving behind a hole in the valence band. When this hole comes in contact with moisture, hydroxyl radical (OH^-) is formed, which has a high oxidation potential (2.8 V) and this oxidation potential is higher than other oxidising agent like ozone (2.07 V). These hydroxyl radicals (OH^-) break the bond between components of organic pollutant to yield the final product of CO_2, H_2O and inorganic ion of other elements present in the organic molecules instead of forming any organic toxic pollutant. The illuminated surface of TiO_2 is an excellent catalyst for the initiation of the oxidation of organic compounds.

The band gap of TiO_2 is 3.2 eV for anatase and 3.0 eV for rutile, which indicate that the light with wavelength in the UV range is required to excite the electron from the valence band. In the solar spectrum, the majority of the solar radiation lies in the visible light region while only about 4 per cent of the solar radiation lies in the UV region.

Therefore, in order to utilize solar radiation effectively, a new kind of photocatalysis which can absorb the majority of the solar radiation is desirable. One of the promising ways to activate TiO_2 in the visible light is the band gap engineering of TiO_2. There are various ways to scale down the band gap of TiO_2. Among them, deposition of secondary materials with narrow band gap is one of the techniques to create a suitable energy cascading system which can narrow down the band gap of the overall system and separate photogenerated e^--h^+ pairs. Silver phosphate is a semiconductor with narrow band gap of 2.4 eV and it has been recently investigated specially its photocatalytic activities by only very few research groups. The research group at NAST synthesized TiO_2 nanotubes through anodization and silver phosphate nanocrystals were deposited into TiO_2 nanotubes (TNTs) and the system was investigated for the visible light induced photocatalysis. The experimental details of which can be found elsewhere (Niraula *et al.*, 2014). Figures 12.2 and 12.3 show the SEM micrograph of the self assembled TiO_2 nanotubes synthesized by anodization and the nanotubes after deposition of silver phosphaste, respectively.

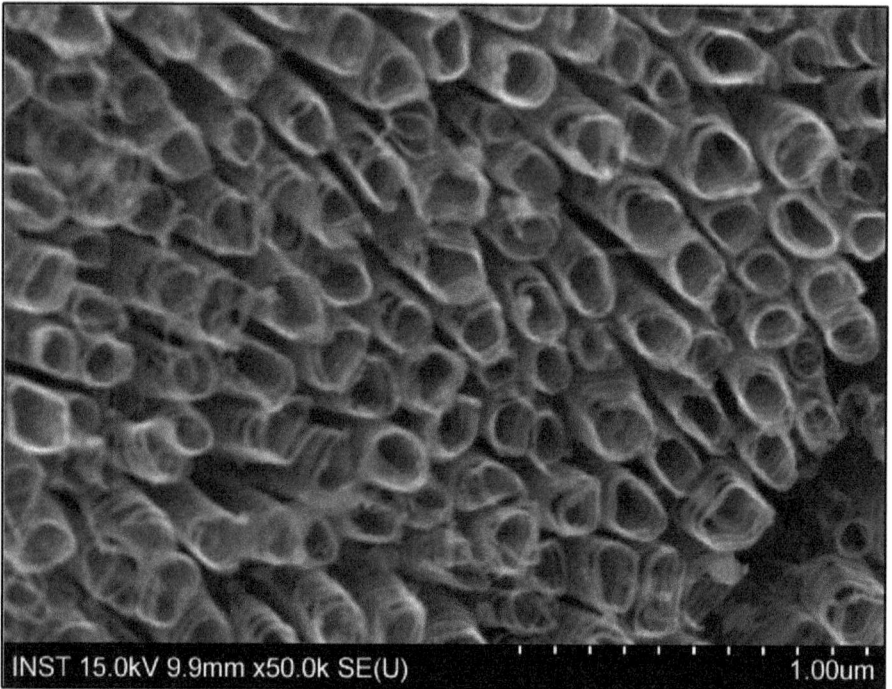

INST 15.0kV 9.9mm x50.0k SE(U)　　　　　　　1.00um

Figure 12.2: SEM Micrograph of Self-Assembled Titanium Dioxide Nanotubes Synthesized for their Possible Application in Water Purification through Photocatalysis after Band Gap Modification

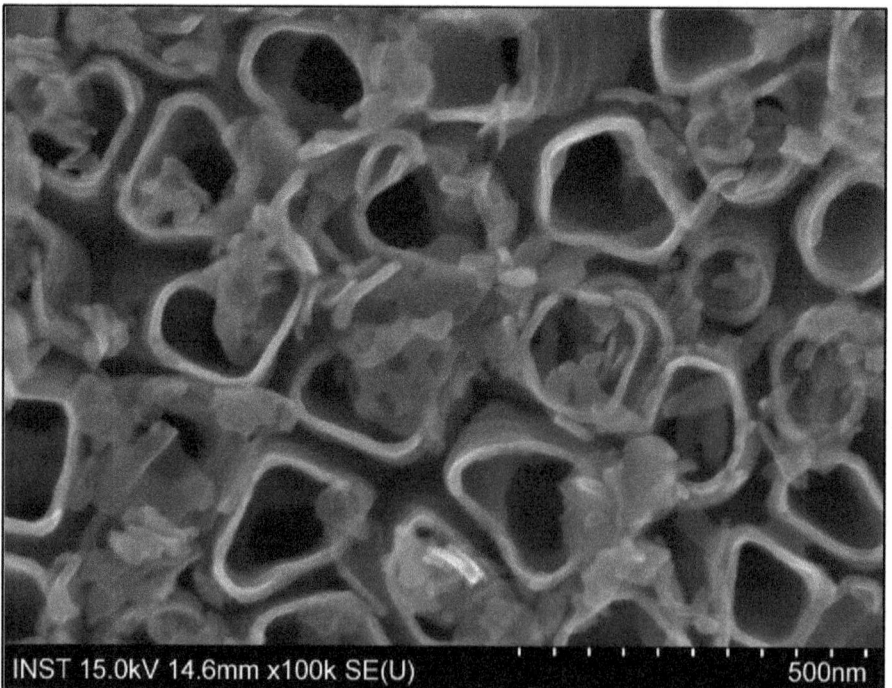

INST 15.0kV 14.6mm x100k SE(U)　　　　　　500nm

Figure 12.3: Titanium dioxide nanotubes after silver phosphate deposition

At Universities

Due to requirements of poor economy of country and need for huge investment to have facilities for research on globally emerging field of Nanotechnology, not even a single academic institution has been able to set up a laboratory dedicated for Nanotechnology in Nepal. However, some professors in the universities have initiated works related to nanomaterials synthesis on individual basis. The major areas covered by such research activities in the universities of Nepal are synthesis of nanocomposite polymers, nanostructures on silicon as well as metal surfaces through chemical routes, preparation of nanocrystalline films of metal oxide nanoparticles on different substrates and synthesis of metal nanoparticles for their diversified applications. Almost all of such works are being carried out in the laboratories of chemistry as they mostly follow the chemical routes that are relatively less cost intensive. Realizing the need of concerted effort to set up some facilities dedicated for research activities, especially for characterization of nanomaterials synthesized in different research laboratories of the country including that at the Universities as well as NAST, Materials Science and Devices Technology Laboratory of NAST has started installing world class instruments. X-ray Diffractometer was the first one among the instruments installed whereas NAST is aggressively involved for further strengthening of the laboratory to make the laboratory fully equipped for Nanotechnology applications.

FUTURE PROSPECTS

Despite the fact that Nepal is one of the least developed countries of the world and it has many priority areas other than research in the emerging field such as Nanotechnology, Government of Nepal seems to be quite positive to enhance the research on Nanotechnology. The positive environment has been created to raise the awareness level of the politicians, bureaucrats due to frequent use of terminology "Nanotechnology" in the national as well as international media and continuous efforts of the Scientists and Technologists of the sector. With this realizing from the Government of Nepal and due to constant feedback on the issue from NAST, it can be expected that Nepal is moving towards establishing at least a research centre dedicated for research and development of Nanotechnology in Nepal, which will a milestone towards institutionalizing Nanotechnology in the country.

CONCLUSIONS

Nepal has ever growing number of students enrolled in the disciplines of Science and Technology in Universities each year. It has not been able to develop marketable technology of its own in many areas due to resource constraint. Out of uncountable areas of applied research, Nanotechnology seems to be new and it is likely to have good impact on society if given a change with world class research facilities in place for research activities. The positive gesture of the Government of Nepal, determination of the Professors at the Universities and lead role played by the Scientists of NAST have been reflected in the latest decision taken by Ministry of Science, Technology and Environment. With the initiation of research in the emerging field like Nanotechnology Nepal can not only create opportunities for young researchers within the country but also reverse the growing trend of Brain-drain into Brain-gain.

ACKNOWLEDGEMENTS

The author would like to acknowledge Dr. Nabeen Kumar Shrestha and Mr. Subash Adhikari for their work related to the application of titanium dioxide nanotubes for photocatalysis at Materials Science and Devices Technology Laboratory of Nepal Academy of Science and Technology.

REFERENCES

1. Williams L., Adams W. (2007). Nanotechnology Demystified, McGraw – Hill Publication, United States of America.

2. Mongillo J. F.(2007). Nanotechnology 101, Greenwood Press, United States of America.

3. Chou T.M., Zhang Q., Russo B., Fryxell G.E., Cao G.(2007). Titania Particle Size Effect on the Overall Performance of Dye-Sensitized Solar Cells. *J Phys Chem C* 111: 6296-6302.

4. Gracia F, Holgado JP, Gonza´lez-Elipe AR (2004). Photoefficiency and Optical, Microstructural, and Structural Properties of TiO_2 Thin Films Used as Photoanodes, *Langmuir* 20: 1688-1697.

5. Hagfeldt A, Boschloo G, Lindstrom H, Figgemeier E, Holmberg A, Aranyos V, Magnusson E, Malmqvist L (2004). A system approach to molecular solar cells, *Coord Chem Rev*, 248:1501-1509.

6. Gregg BA (2004). Interfacial processes in the dye-sensitized solar cell, *Coord Chem Rev*, 248: 1215-1224.

7. Wu M., Lin G., Chen D., Wang G., He D., Feng S., Xu R. (2002). Sol-Hydrothermal Synthesis and Hydrothermally Structured Evolution of Nanocrystal Titanium Dioxide, *Chem. Mater.*, 14: 1974-1980.

8. Niraula M., Adhikari S., Lee D. Y., Kim E. K., Yoon S.J., Dhungel S.K., Lee W., Shrestha N.K., Han S. H.(2014). Titania nanotube-silver phosphate hybrid heterostructure for improved visible light induced photocatalysis, *Chemical Physics Letters*, 593: 193-197.

Chapter 13

Production of Nano Precipitated Calcium Carbonate from some Characterised Nigeria Limestone Deposits

O.E. Ojo, O.J. Omowumi, P.S.A. Irabor and G.N. Elemo

Department of Engineering,
Federal Institute of Industrial Research, Oshodi, Ikeja, Lagos, Nigeria
E-mail: isolyet@yahoo.com, sola_omowumi@yahoo.com,
iraborpsa@yahoo.com, gloria.elemo@fiiro.gov.ng

ABSTRACT

The chemical and physical properties of some Nigerian Limestone deposits were investigated. The samples were tested for various constitents, such as CaO, MgO, Fe_2O_3, Al_2O_3, SiO_2 and loss on ignition; average particle size, specific gravity and whiteness were also tested to determine the suitability for the production of Nano Precipitated Calcium Carbonate. The Yandev, Calabar, Jakura and Ukpilla limestone deposits are high calcium Limestone having CaO contents of 52.87 per cent, 54.10 per cent, 54.10 per cent and 51.16 per cent while the nano precipitated calcium carbonate got from each of them has 97.98 per cent, 98.86 per cent, 98.82 per cent, and 98.01 purity respectively which makes them suitable for Nano Precipitated Calcium Carbonate production. Also their quicklime and hydrated lime indicated high calcium lime products. The limestone deposits are of economic interest and therefore recommended for the production Nano Precipitated Calcium Carbonate for different uses.

Keywords: Calcination, Hydration, Precipitation, Carbonation, Lime and Nano Precipitated Calcium Carbonate.

INTRODUCTION

Limestone is a natural occurring mineral that consists principally of calcium carbonate but may also contain magnesium carbonate as a secondary component. It is 4 per cent of the earth crust.

It is found in many forms and is classified in terms of its origin, chemical composition, structure geological formation (Carr 1975; Barbara, 1990). Chemically, it is composed primarily of calcium carbonate, $CaCO_3$ and secondarily of magnesium carbonate $MgCO_3$, with varying percentage of impurities (Searle,1935). Although these carbonates occur in many other rocks, ores, and soils, in its broadest definition limestone is distinguished by a content of more than 50 per cent total carbonate; more restrictive interpretations demand at least 75 per cent or even 90 per cent (Kirk, 1981). In addition to showing varying degree of chemical purity, limestone assumed a bewildering number of widely divergent physical forms, including marble, travertine, chalk, calcareous marl, coral, shell, stalagmites, and stalactites. All these materials are essentially carbonate rocks of the same approximate chemical composition as conventional limestone (Driscoll, 1988; Boynton, 1980). The chemical composition and properties of limes and limestone depend on the nature of the impurities and the degree of contamination of original stone (Gilson, 1960; Knibbs, 1924). The reversible reaction involved in the calcination and recarbonation of lime-limestone is one of the simplest, and most fundamentals of all chemical reactions. Lime burning can be quiet complex and many empirical modifications are often necessary for efficient performance. There are three essential factors in the thermal decomposition of limestone:

1. The stone must be heated to the dissociation temperature of the carbonate
2. The minimum temperature must be maintained for certain duration
3. The carbondioxide involved must be removed rapidly.

At calcination temperature of 925–1340°C, dissociation of the limestone proceed gradually from the outer surface of the stone particle inward. If the dissociation of the particle is incomplete, there remains in the center of the particle a core of uncalcined carbonate stone that dissipate the concentration of the available lime (Oates, 1998). On the other hand, if the stone is calcined under severed calcining conditions (*i.e.* high temperature and long retention), the lime may become hard –burned or even dead-burned at sintering temperatures. Under these conditions the stone shrinks by 25 - 50 per cent of its original size.

The main use of calcium carbonate is in industrial applications like construction; for purification of iron from iron ore in a blast furnace; as extender in paint; as filler in plastic among others. In other to make it more usefulness, nanotechnology; which is the creation and use of materials or devices at extremely small scale is adopted.

Nanotechnology can equally be used for production of Nano precipitated calcium carbonate which makes it more useful than ordinary ground calcium carbonate. Calcium carbonate produced in precipitated form is also known as refined or synthetic calcium carbonate.

There are two reasons why precipitated calcium carbonate is produced; because there are several points in the production process where calcium carbonate can be purified, removing much of the rock from the deposit that is not calcium carbonate, impurities like fieldspar, heavy metals, silicaceous minerals e.t.c. The second reason is that the process allows the scientists to grow crystals of different shapes. The particles size is dictated by the control of reaction time, temperature, agitation pressure and rate of CO_2 addition.

The Nano calcium carbonate produced has outstanding performance in many applications where ground calcium carbonate does not perform maximally. For example, the Nano precipitated calcium carbonate gives better impact resistance in plastics than with ground calcium carbonate (Zhang *et al.,* 2002).

A substantial number of large limestone and dolomites deposits in Nigeria have been reported by space (Aliyu, 1996) and shown on Table 13.1. Limestone product is sold or used as crushed or broken stone, most of the description of limestone extraction concentrate on this use (Figure 13.1).

Table 13.1: Limestone Deposits in Nigeria

Location	State	Estimated Reserve in Million Tonnes
Igunmale	Benue	20.00
Ogbolokuta	Benue	10.16
Yandev	Benue	67.06
Itobe	Benue	Not yet quantified
Ubo	Kogi	20.00
Jakura	Kogi	68.00
Elebu	Kogi	Not yet quantified
Kwakuti	Niger	Not yet quantified
Bulum	FCT	Not yet quantified
Kalambaina	Sokoto	101.60
Gombe	Gombe	Not yet quantified
Muman	Adamawa	Not yet quantified
Nkalagu	Enugu	720.00
Odomoke	Enugu	200.00
Ukpilla	Edo	Not yet quantified
Siluko	Edo	Not yet quantified
Ewekoro	Ogun	7,135.00
Shagamu	Ogun	Not yet quantified
Ibeshe	Ogun	Not yet quantified
Mfamosing	Cross River	26.00

* Aliyu (1996)

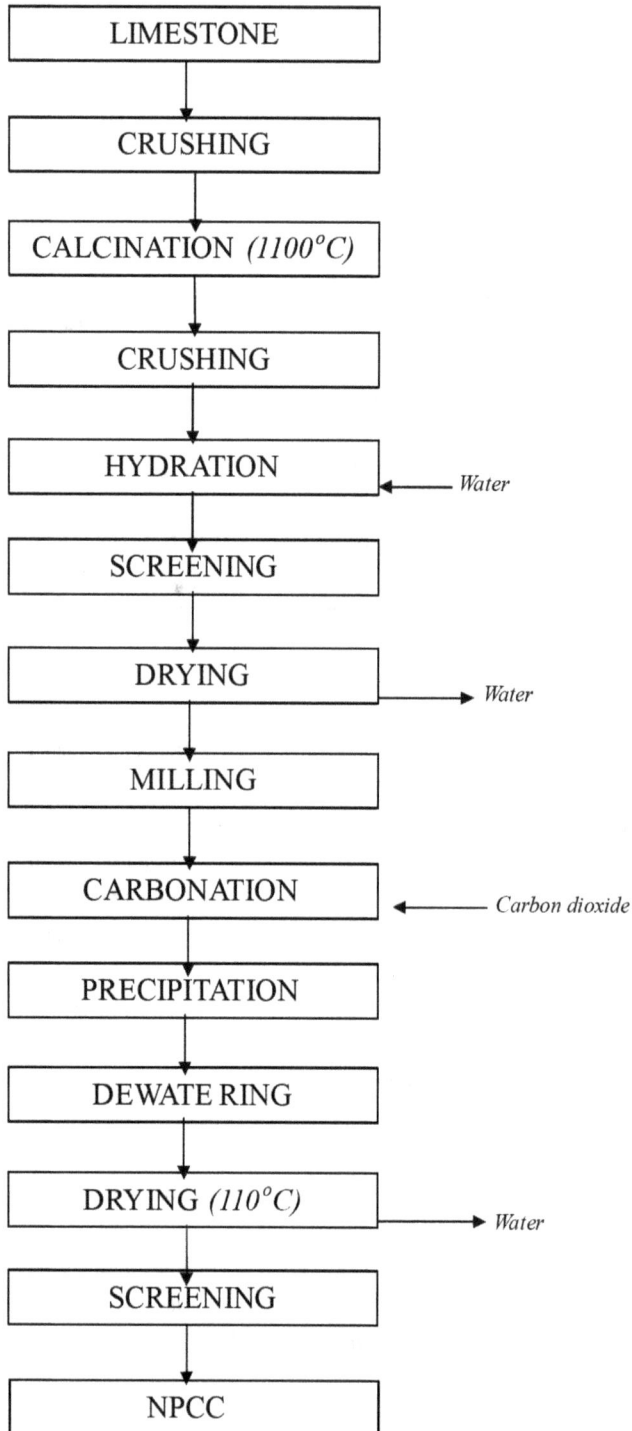

Figure 13.1: Flow Diagram for Production of Nano Precipitated Calcium Carbonate

MATERIALS AND METHODS

The samples were collected from six different deposits in Nigeria, Yandev, in Benue State; Calabar, in Cross River State; Ukpillar in Edo State; Jakura in Kogi State; Igbetti in Oyo State and Elebu in Kogi State.

The following equipment were used; Hammer, mill, Ball mill, Nerberthern Kiln, Stainless Steel dehydrator and Sieves.

Sampling Method

The sampling, inspection and rejection of the samples were conducted in accordance with the standard methods of sampling (ASTM C50; C75, 2003).

The Limestone lumps were first crushed with a hammer mill to reduce the size.

Calcination

The crushed samples were transferred into the kiln and calcined at 1100°C for 90 minutes to obtain an active Calcium Oxide (CaO).

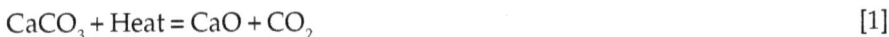

$$CaCO_3 + Heat = CaO + CO_2 \qquad [1]$$

where,

$CaCO_3$ - Limestone, CaO - Calcium Oxide, CO_2 - Carbondioxide

Milling

The calcined material was cooled and crushed with hammer mill to small pebbles (2-5 cm).

Hydration

20kg of the crushed materials was added to 50 litres of water then mixed rapidly for 10-15 minutes in a 100 litre capacity slaker.

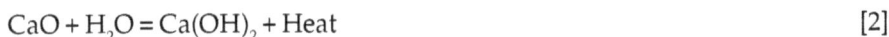

$$CaO + H_2O = Ca(OH)_2 + Heat \qquad [2]$$

where,

$Ca(OH)_2$ – Hydrated lime, H_2O- Water

The slaker was provided with a paddle flat headed agitator which was operated at a speed of 120 revolution per minute to obtain a 20 per cent weight by volume slurry. The reaction was found to be exothermic with maximum rise in temperature of about 70°C.

The Slurry was continuously agitated for an hour so as to achieve maximum conversion of Calcium Oxide to Calcium Hydroxide.

Carbonation

The resulting slurry was subjected to carbonation by passing a carbon dioxide-air mixture through the slurry at a gas velocity of about 10cm/sec. The Carbonation temperature was maintained in the range 25 to 40 degree Celsius. The Carbonation was completed within 80 minutes.

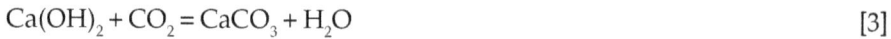

$$Ca(OH)_2 + CO_2 = CaCO_3 + H_2O \qquad [3]$$

where,

$CaCO_3$ –Nano Precipitated Calcium Carbonate, H_2O – Water

Chemical Analysis

The chemical analysis of limestone, lime and hydrated lime were carried out using (ASTM C25, 2003) method. The percentage compositions of the various constituent are recorded in Tables 13.2–13.4.

RESULTS

Properties percentage compositions of the various constituent are recorded in Tables 13.2–13.4.

Table 13.2: Chemical Analysis of Limestone Samples

Sample Locations	CaO	MgO	SiO_2	Al_2O_3	Fe_2O_3	LOI
Yandev	52.87	0.64	2.30	1.0	0.50	42.39
Calabar	54.20	0.57	–	–	–	42.62
Ukpilla	51.16	1.16	2.84	2.76	0.14	41.72
Jakura	54.01	0.58	1.88	0.35	0	42.69
*Limestone	54.54	0.59	0.70	0.68	0.08	42.90

Source: Kirk, 1981.

Table 13.3: Chemical Analysis of Quicklime

Sample Locations	CaO	MgO	SiO_2	Al_2O_3	Fe_2O_3	LOI
Yandev	95.14	0.32	1.08	0.40	0.24	0.38
Calabar	96.78	0.40	–	–	–	0.21
Ukpilla	93.27	0.60	1.12	0.3	0.1	0.42
Jakura	96.78	0.9	0.65	0.5	0.31	0.61
*Quicklime	93–98	0.3–2.5	0.2–2.5	0.1–0.5	0.1–0.4	–

Source: Kirk, 1981.

Table 13.4: Chemical Analysis of Hydrated Lime

Sample Locations	CaO	MgO	SiO_2	Al_2O_3	Fe_2O_3	LOI
Yandev	79.74	0.24	0.18	0.20	0.11	19.20
Calabar	86.14	0.61	–	–	–	0.21
Ukpilla	73.01	0.60	0.2	0.18	0.1	21.40
Jakura	79.74	0.61	0.52	0.12	0.12	25.45
*Hydrated Lime	71–74	0.5–2	0.2–0.5	0.1–0.2	0.1–0.2	24–25

Source: Kirk, 1981.

The properties of NPCC given below were carried out using (ASTM C97/C97M, 2003) method.

Table 13.5: Chemical Analysis of Hydrated Lime

Sample Locations	Average Particle Size (Microns)	Specific Gravity (g/cm³)	Bulk Density (g/cm³)	Whiteness (per cent)
Yandev	0.04 – 0.09	2.71	0.77	91
Calabar	0.04 – 0.08	2.58	0.60	93
Ukpilla	0.04 – 0.08	2.57	0.75	93
Jakura	0.04 – 0.08	2,55	0.75	92

DISCUSSION

Calcium Oxide

The calcium oxide content of 52.87 per cent, 54.10 per cent,51.16 per cent and 54.1 per cent for Yandev, Calabar, Ukpilla and Jakura respectively are within the acceptable range for high calcium limestone as reported by (Boynton, 1980). But the calcium oxide content of 36.72 per cent and 26.4 per cent for Igbetti and Elebu respectively samples indicate that the samples are dolomitic limestone. Chemical analysis on the quicklime and the hydrated lime also indicate this. (ASTM C911, 1947).

Magnesium Oxide

The magnesium oxide content of all the samples are within the internationally accepted value of 0.59 per cent for high calcium limestone and 20.45 per cent for dolomitic limestone according to (Boynton, 1980). The values obtained for hydrated lime also indicated a high calcium lime for all the samples, 71 – 74 per cent for high calcium and 41 – 45 per cent for dolomitic as reported by (Ames, 1975).

Silicon Dioxide

The silicon dioxide for all the samples is within the recommended value for quicklime 0.2 – 2.5 per cent. The silicon dioxide content of Igbetti samples is a bit higher than others' because of the primary impurities associated with the deposit. Also the values for hydrated lime are within the recommended value for high calcium hydrated lime

Aluminium Oxide

The aluminium content of all the samples are within are within the range 0.1 – 0.5 per cent for quicklime of high calcium content and 0.1 – 1.5 per cent for dolomitic type of quicklime. The values for hydrated lime are within the acceptable range of 0.1 – 0.2 per cent. High percentage of aluminium oxide is an indication of presence of impurities.

Iron III Oxide

The values for all fall within the standard value of 0.1 – 0.4 per cent for high calcium and 0.1 – 0.2 per cent for dolomitic quicklime except for Yandev, also 0.1 – 0.2 per cent for high calcium hydrated lime and dolomitic type for all the samples (ASTM C911, 1947).

Loss on Ignition

The percentage of LOI of hydrated lime at 1000°C for Jakura fall within the acceptable range of 24 – 25 per cent for high calcium hydrated lime as reported by Barbara (1990) while a lower values of LOI was observed for Ukpilla and Yandev.

CONCLUSIONS

The investigation on the chemical properties of the samples showed that not all the limestone deposit samples in Nigeria are good for the production of Nano Precipitated Calcium Carbonate their values compare favourably with known deposits. Deposits in Yandev, Calabar, Jakura and Ukpilla can be classified as high calcium limestone and high economical values. While the deposits in Igbetti and Elebu are dolomitic which make them not suitable for Nano Precipitated Calcium Carbonate High calcium Limestone could find very useful applications in almost every sector of the economy. These include pharmaceutical, agriculture, food and environmental sectors.

REFERENCES

1. Aliyu, A. (1996): potentials of the Solids Minerals Industry in Nigeria Raw Materials Research and Development Council pp.101.

2. Ames, G. (1975):Cement Raw Materials. Industrial Mineral rocks 4th edition. Pp. 140-150.

3. ASTM (C25, 1947): Methods of Chemical Analysis of Limestone, Quicklime and Hydrated Lime.

4. ASTM (C50, 1947): Sampling, Inspecting, Packaging, Marketing of Lime and Limestone Products.

5. ASTM (C75, 1947): Methods for Sampling Aggregates.

6. ASTM (C911, 1947): Specification for Quicklime, hydrated Lime and Limestone for chemical use.

7. Barbara, E. Stephen H, Gail, S, (1990): Ullman's Encyclopaedia of Industrial Chemistry, Fifth Completely Revised Edition Vol. A15 pp. 318 - 344.

8. Boynton, R. S. (1980): Chemistry and Technology of Lime and Limestone, John Wiley and Sons Inc. New York.

9. Carr, D. D. and Rooney, L. F. (1975): Limestone And Dolomite in Industrial Mineral Rocks Fourth Edition AIME, pp. 757 – 700.

10. Chemical Lime Fact (1975): National Lime Association.

11. Gilson, J. (1960): Carbonate Rocks Industrial Mineral and Rocks. American Institute of Mining and Metallurgical Engineers, New York pp. 125 – 130.

12. Kirk, O. (1981): Encyclopaedia of Chemical Technology. Third Edition Volume 14 pp. 350 – 368.

13. Knibbs, N. (1924): Lime and Magnesia E. Benn Ltd. London pp. 69.

14. O'Driscoll, M. (1988): Industrial Minerals pp. 42 – 50.

15. Searle, A. O. (1935): Limestone and its products. E. Benn Ltd. London.

Chapter 14
Barriers to Nanotechnology Transfer towards Business Perspectives

Odedele, Timothy Oladele[1], Sebastian Chukwuemezie Obasi[2] and Azikwe Peter Onwualu[3]

Raw Materials Research and Development Council (RMRDC)
(Federal Ministry Of Science And Technology)
Abuja
E-mail: [1]odedelermrdc@yahoo.com; [2]sebemobasi@gmail.com;
[3]ponwualu@yahoo.com

ABSTRACT

The term "nanotechnology" covers processes associated with the creation and utilization of structures in the 1.0 nanometer (nm) to 100 nm range. Nanofabrication involves engineering at the atomic length scale. It no doubt, offers substantial economic and societal benefits than any technology and holds the promise of both incremental improvements of existing products and the potential for revolutionary changes that could transform entire industries and create entirely new ones. The technology is already touching upon many aspects of medicine, including drug delivery, diagnostic imaging, clinical diagnostics, nanomedicines, and the use of nanomaterials in medical devices. To enable Nigeria become a major player in the nanotechnology within 5 years the Federal Government established Nigeria Nanotechnology Initiatives (NNI). The paper highlights the objectives of the NNI to assist in developing Nigerian efforts towards actualizing the gains of Nanotechnology. The scope of the activities cover areas that are relevant to Nigerian and global needs. Such areas include Medicine (disease detection and treatment), Agriculture (drought and treatment), Energy (solar cells and light emitting devices), Agriculture (drought resistant seeds and food preservation and genomics), Water purification and testing (nano- porous filters and bio – oxidants). The developed nations particularly U.S has invested considerably in nanotechnology research but nevertheless, transferring nanotechnology concept towards business perspectives is presently slow paced due to many identified barriers. Such barriers, both existing and potential that impede the transfer may limit the ability to capture the full benefits of nanotechnology, including economic growth, wealth and job creation, and improvements in the standard of living and quality of life of the people. These barriers may include capital issues, market readiness, regulatory uncertainties, health and safety, workforce readiness, public attitudes and perceptions, infrastructure, standards, nomenclature, and manufacturability. This paper therefore highlights causes and analysis of barriers to assist policymakers, so that government at all levels can help unleash the full potentials of nanotechnology for human and economic development.

Keywords: *Nanotechnology, Nanomaterials, Research, Development, Standardization, Workforce, Legislation, Market, Startup.*

INTRODUCTION

The term "nanotechnology" covers processes associated with the creation and utilization of structures in the 1 nanometer (nm) to 100 nm range. (John F. Sargent Jr.(2011)) Nanofabrication involves engineering at the atomic length scale. Engineering at this scale makes it feasible to create, atom by atom, fibers which are very small in diameter but extremely strong (John, 2011). In the health care domain, nanofabrication can be utilized to fabricate extremely minute probes that can detect disease by examining individual strands of DNA. Nanofabrication makes it possible to manufacture capillary systems for providing nutrients to man-made replacement organs (Theresa, 2007). The nanofabrication process has been used for creation of new chemical and biological substance detectors incorporating structures holding molecules that change their electrical conducting properties in the presence of the substances being detected. The development of a new class of nanoscale transistors, and molecular electronics, has also been made possible by the utilization of nonotechnology (Theresa, 2007).

Nanotechnology Applications and Business Opportunities

Nanotechnology is capable of producing products, materials and devices that impact a wide spectrum of industries and consumer products. Therefore, it is appropriate to view Nanotechnology as a "platform technology" with applications in a number of industrial sectors, and with potential for producing a variety of products. The list of current and potential nanotechnology applications continues to grow. However, it would be appropriate to consider the following areas of nanotechnology application as the most promising beneficiaries (not ranked in any manner):

- ✰ Electronics and Semiconductors
- ✰ Information Technology (Computing and Telecommunication)
- ✰ Aerospace and Automotive Industries
- ✰ Chemical Processes and Engineering
- ✰ Agriculture

☆ Energy

☆ Disease Diagnosis

☆ Health Monitoring

☆ Drug Delivery

☆ Food Processing and Storage

☆ Water Treatment and Air Pollution Control

According to Bradford(2003), the National Science Foundation, U.S, estimates the market for materials and devices engineered on a very tiny scale, the nano scale, will be $1 trillion by 2015.

Nano Business Alliance (2001) made an estimate of EUR 54 billion world market in nanotechnology especially in the following areas:

☆ Nanoparticles and composites(23 per cent)

☆ Ultra-thin laers(44 per cent)

☆ Measuring and analyzing nanostructures(24 per cent)

☆ Lateral nanostructures(3 per cent)

Other data (LuxCapital Report (2003)) showed that:

The number of nanotechnology patents has been growing significantly; many large corporations *e.g.* IBM and Samsung are among the most active patentees.

☆ More than 700 companies are involved in Nanotechnology

Nanotechnology Funding

The funding of nanotechnology in some countries are as shown in Table 14.1.

Table 14.1: Funding of Nanotechnology

Country	Current Funding for Nanoscience and Nanotechnologies
Europe	Nanotechnology R&D is about 1 billion euros, two-thirds of which comes from national and regional programmes.
Japan	Funding rose from $400M in 2001 to $800M in 2003 and is expected to rise by a further 20 per cent in 2015.
USA	The USA's 21st Century Nanotechnology Research and Development Act (passed in 2003) allocated nearly $3.7 billion to nanotechnology from 2005 to 2008 (which excludes a substantial defence-related expenditure). This compares with $750M in 2003.
UK	With the launch of its nanotechnology strategy in 2003, the UK Government pledged £45M per year from 2003 to 2009.

Source: US National Science Foundation (2003)

Nanotechnology Business Forecast

The report also showed that U.S. nanomaterials demand would reach $35 bil. in 2020. After a decade-long buildup, nanotechnology is beginning to see its first

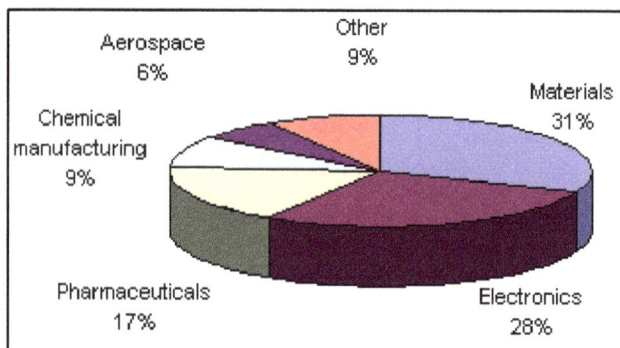

Figure 14.1: Estimates of the Nanotechnology Markets (2010-2015)
USD: 1.1 Trillion
Source: **US National Science Foundation (2003)**

commercial successes. The development of nanoscale materials is a key step in the eventual production of more sophisticated nanomachines, nanoelectronics and nanomedical devices. In fact, the move toward nanotechnology is a continuation of ongoing miniaturization efforts in many industrial sectors. Research in nanotechnology has focussed on reducing the size of existing manufacturing materials such as metal oxides through the use of new production technologies, and developing entirely new materials such as nanotubes and buckyballs that are intrinsically nanosized.

Table 14.2: Nanomaterials Demand (million dollars)

Item	2002	2007	2012	Per cent Annual Growth 2002-2020
Minerals	140	675	2,100	28
Metals	45	150	500	26
Polymers and chemicals	5	175	1,400	58
New Materials	10	100	500	41
Nanomaterials Demand	200	1,100	4,500	33

Source: U.S. Freedonia Group Inc. (2000)

The U.S. market for nanomaterials (which totaled only $125 million. in 2000) is expected to reach $35 billion by 2020 (Table 14.2). This growth will come from numerous applications that span the entire U.S. manufacturing sector. These include wafer polishing abrasives and high-density data storage media for the electronics industry; improved diagnostic aids for the medical community; transparent sunscreens, stain-resistant paints and wear-resistant flooring for consumers; cost-cutting equipment coatings for the defense industry; fuel-saving components for the auto industry; and better paper and ink for the printing industry. In the long run, however, the best opportunities are expected in health care and electronics, which together are expected to comprise nearly two-thirds of the market by 2020.

Nigerian Nanotechnology Initiatives (NNI)

The objective of the NNI is to develop Nigerian effort that will enable Nigeria to become a major player in the nano technology within 5 years. The scope of the activities will cover areas that are relevant to Nigerian and global needs in which Nigeria has real needs that can be met by developing strong capabilities in nanotechnology. These include:

- ☆ Medicine (disease detection and treatment)
- ☆ Agriculture (drought and treatment)
- ☆ Energy (solar cells and light emitting devices)
- ☆ Agriculture (drought resistant seeds and food preservation and genomics)
- ☆ Water purification and testing (nano- porous filters and bio-oxidants)

Consequently, the proposed Research Areas for Application in Nigeria are:

- ☆ Nanomedicine Nanoparticle synthesis and ligand conjugation
- ☆ Electronics Organic Solar fabrication and OLED fabrication and packaging
- ☆ Agriculture Seed coating with drought resistant layer and nanogenomically modified field cow for tropical milk production
- ☆ Water filtration Fabrication of nanoporous clays with nanoscale bio-oxidants
- ☆ Fabrication of nanoparticles using nano-precipitation methods (Gold, magnetite and gold/magnetite nano particles)
- ☆ Ligand conjugation of targets (that attach specifically to cancer, maleria – infected cells and FIV/HIV infected cells) to nanoparticles.
- ☆ Ligand conjugation of chemotherapy, malaria and HIV drugs to nanopartcles
- ☆ *In-vitro* (cell experiments) and *in vivo* (animal experiments) using ligand conjugated nanoparticles.
- ☆ Modeling and experiments to test for the detection and treatment of selected diseases.
- ☆ Faabricate solar cells and light emitting devices amorphous/ nanocrystalline silicon, organics.
- ☆ Developing stamping methods for pattern transfer and cold welding in non clean room environs
- ☆ Developing packaging and lamination techniques and their effects on device performance
- ☆ Study interface science and the influence of interfaces on charge transport
- ☆ Developing polymer coating methods for the fabrication of drought resistant seeds
- ☆ Testing seeds in green houses with well controlled soils and environments that stimulate

Common Strategies for Nano-Technology Transfer Towards Business Perspectives

A number of strategies can be adopted in transferring nanotechnology results into business enterprise. Some of these include:

Nanotechnology Business Start Up

Licensing IP

In some industries, patents are not critical to business success – firms focus more on swift execution than on intellectual property (IP) protection. This is not the case for nanotech firms. IP has been a central issue to every nanotech startup. The inception of a company is synonymous with the acquisition of the company's initial IP. Most commercialization efforts start with taking steps to protect IP through the filing of patents. Most patents in the area of nanotech are generated by either large companies or by universities or by government labs. Many startups in nanotechnology get at least their initial IP from universities or government labs. In the US for instance, some of the California based government labs/agencies that license IP in the area of nanotech are NASA, Lawrence Livermore National Laboratories, and Lawrence Berkeley Labs. Likewise, universities have offices that focus on the commercialization of their locally generated IP.

Spin-Outs

The nanotechnology startup companies can also be formed by a parent company spinning-out a business unit. In the recent IPO market environment, these spin-outs have not gone public, but are typically held as subsidiaries. A recent small-tech example is the MEMS CAD company Coventor, who spun out their RF MEMS unit to create WiSpry. Previously Coventor had spun-out another business unit into a new company to focus on optical MEMS. The parent company has a number of advantages in doing this. First, the net value of the two separate companies can potentially be higher, especially if the parent is a large company. Secondly, by spinning out a division, the parent allows for other sources of capital to fund the operation.

Independent Entrepreneur

The nanotechnology business start-ups can also be formed through the independent entrepreneur who generates the IP. This case is not always the practice because the complexity and expense required to develop a new nanotechnology and file the appropriate IP is considerable, and this is easily affordable by most independent entrepreneurs. The development phase is expensive for a number of reasons. Nanotechnologies are based on physical science. Therefore the capital costs to setup a laboratory to do research and development tends to be high. For instance, one commonly used piece of equipment in nanotechnology, an atomic force microscope (AFM), costs about $100,000 for the least expensive model. And there are many more pieces of equipment that are typically required. At the far extreme, many nano companies plan to use semiconductor-like manufacturing facilities. It is widely known that a state of the art semi-laboratory today costs billions of dollars. This is opposed to a software company where the only capital costs are those of computers and inexpensive software development tools.

Funding

There are many sources of funding. The ones typically considered for a nanotech startup are: friends and family, Venture Capitals, government, and corporate partners. We can consider friends and family as a single category. Usually this category can only fund the writing of the business plan and perhaps for licensing some IP from university or other sources. As stated before, nanotech companies usually have significant capital requirements to make real progress. But because of the potential viability of nanotechnology, it is possible to find high net-worth venture capital that will put in significant funds. An example of this is MagiQ Technologies. This company's last round of funding of $6.9M was done entirely by angels which included Jeff Bezos, the founder of Amazon.com (Aragon, 2004). The government is another source of potential funding.

Growth

Partnering with a larger corporation is one of the strategies commonly used by nanosetup executives to facilitate the growth of their companies. This approach gives access to manufacturing and sales avenues which are very expensive to develop for a startup company. For instance, Thinfilm Electronics and Intel corporation. Thinfilm is developing a new type of non-volatile memory technology in which Intel has invested. If Thinfilm technology succeeds, easy access to a large market through Intel's existing market position is possible. Another strategy for growth is to spin off technologies from a common underlying technology. Without loss of focus, it could be a good approach for a company that has developed a platform technology which can make impact in many application areas.

Barriers to Nanotechnology Transfer Towards Business Enterprise in Nigeria

Environmental, Health and Safety Issues

The unique properties of these nanotechnology materials are a double edged sword because they can be tailored for beneficial properties and at the same time may also have unknown innocuous consequences, such as new toxicological and environmental effects. The following examples illustrate how the same nanotechnology material may be both potentially beneficial and potentially harmful to human health and environment (John, 2011).

☆ Nanoscale silver is highly effective as an antibacterial agent in wound dressings, clothing, and washing machines, but there are general concerns that widespread dispersion of nanoscale silver in the environment could kill microbes that are vital to waste water treatment plants and to ecosystems. (John, 2011) Some beneficial bacteria, for example, break down organic matter, remove nitrogen from water, aid in animal digestion, protect against fungal infestations, and even aid some animals in defense against predators.

☆ Due to size of nanoscale particles they may have the potential to penetrate the blood-brain barrier, a structure that protects the brain from harmful substances in the blood but they may affect the delivery of therapeutic agents (John, 2011). The characteristics of certain nanoscale materials may assist the development of pharmaceuticals to purposefully and beneficially cross this barrier and deliver medicine directly to the brain to treat, for example, a brain tumor. The harmful aspect, however, is the possibility of nanoscale particles to unintentionally pass through the blood-brain barrier causing harm to humans and animals (John, 2011).

☆ It is also generally believed that certain nanoscale materials are highly chemically reactive due to their high surface-to-volume ratio. This is a property which can be positively applied in catalysis, treatment of groundwater contamination, and site remediation. This property which is also being explored for use in protective masks and clothing as a defense against chemical and biological agents can potentially result to cell damage in animals (John, 2011).

☆ Carbon nanotubes (CNTs) despite their potential uses in a wide range of applications (*e.g.*, materials, batteries, memory devices, electronic displays, transparent conductors, sensors, medical imaging),CNTs can exhibit properties similar to asbestos fibers and might become lodged in organs (*e.g.*, lungs, kidneys, livers), harming humans and animals (John, 2011).

Considering the Environmental, Health and Safety (EHS) issues, nanomaterials play decisive roles in their distribution through environment, ecosystem and human body. Due to their biological activities/or unique properties they may gain access into human body through the main ports of entry such as the skin, lungs, gastrointestinal tract. Several toxicological studies have reported that nonomaterials can be cytotoxic, neurotoxic, genotoxic and ecotoxic (Agnieszka *et al.*, 2012.)

These apprehensions of the potential EHS effects of nanomaterials constitute serious barrier to nanotechnology transfer to business enterprises.

Research and Development

Research and Development is the first and most important process link in the long chain of different parallel processes leading directly and indirectly towards achieving the objectives of nanotechnology transfer towards business perspectives. Though university laboratories may lead to IP rights and patents but using such R&D as the basis for carrying out the required engineering and experiment with prototypes suitable for transfer to business may be a barrier. The gap from science research and development to product manufacturing and markets is presently wide. The involvement of government in fostering R&D is minimal in Nigeria and there is a missing link between university and government laboratories and companies to know what R&D are available and the potential benefits which companies may receive if they invest in these R&D projects. Generally R&D infrastructures and facilities are expensive and may not be affordable by small nanotechnology companies.

Investment

In developing countries, it is difficult to get venture capitalists who are interested in a transformational nanotechnology program that will take more than three (3) years to pay out.

Funding agencies seem to focus more on larger companies leaving small companies in precarious funding situations. Their model does not fit into today's research because of the time of research. It takes many years to come to production stage. Earlier investment will require higher funding. The venture capitalists have moved away from entrepreneurs and small companies to larger companies. Leadership should therefore come from State and Federal governments to support innovation because research may take between 3-4 years or up to 10 years to complete. Funding must be earmarked for risks and marshalling resources. The federal government in Nigeria is not adequately involved in endeavors such as bringing together academia, businesses, researchers, local and state government and investors.

The main barrier is that there is usually a long gestation period from research to development. Even though small businesses get federal grants, others get funding from private investors. But there is problem of transiting from government research to commercial ventures and the connection facilitating relationship between public/private funding and government information is also not adequate. A venture capital fund is usually planned to operate for ten years, with investments made in small companies during the first four years. Presently there are some nanotech investment opportunities but they do not seem to have promising high returns to satisfy fund investors' desires and objectives. Before ten years, the invested small companies with valuable technology need to find and be acquired by established large companies to bring financial returns to the venture capital firm. But venture capital firms do not know how to locate a large company that needs the invested small company and the search could take an additional four years or more. There should be a more efficient way for a large company to find external funding sources like venture capital firms that would have possible interest in advanced research projects.

Intellectual Property (IP)

In some cases, there is increasing problem due to increasing number of patents conflicting and serve to limit their operations. There is need to enter into more cross licensing so that companies can operate their business with less possibility of conflicts and litigation. After obtaining patents, the problem of using the rights in order to gain some benefits is still common. Usually, in other technologies, it is possible for venture portfolio companies with valuable intellectual property which appear to be a competitive threat to negotiate the most desirable terms for their acquisition by larger companies. Nanotechnology is different from some other technologies because it is a platform technology with applications in diverse industrial sectors and very different products. The small nanotech company could choose to use its intellectual property rights in many of these sectors with different arrangements to expand its opportunities to enter new markets and exploit income sources. The problem from a large company perspective is that too many problems arise when attempting to use nanotechnology intellectual property as a platform to pursue commercialization in diverse fields, rather than concentrating on a particular product.

Workforce Development and Education

There exists a major education gap between needed skills and the current workforce. Better curriculum is needed at all levels of education that stresses science, biology, physics, mathematics, chemistry and in the area of nanotechnology. The nation must start to think of drastic measures in considering many years for research and development to commercialization. Having the right people with the right training is critical to transfer of nanotechnology towards business enterprises. A gap exists but could be fixed with the proper tertiary education especially M.Sc., Ph.D. in areas relevant to nanotechnology.

Government Budget

Funding for basic research is essential and needs to be increased. Additionally, in Nigeria for instance, the science research findings that emerge from the laboratories are usually dumped before evolving into application that has commercial viability due to inadequate funding for early proto-typing and early stage development. Federal, state, and regional governments should consider providing more technical assistance to the private sector. Federal funding cutbacks were considered a barrier to important research projects, especially at the national science and technology institutions. There must be a leverage of federal and state funds with private sector funding. Government funding is vital to help finance nanotechnology infrastructure that requires higher investments and costs for multidisciplinary ventures, and risk research of the environment and human health.

Nanotechnology Standards

Measurement of nano standards must be established. The government agencies in Nigeria lack excellent equipment and research information that start-ups could work with and potential users have problems getting through the bureaucracy. Measurement of nano materials is a major issue. Some concerns for the future of nanotechnology will be manufacturing the right equipment and tools. Many of the needed support systems do not exist. The real production capability and industry that exists in the real sense may need assistance from the government for their infrastructural needs. There are many potential issues that may require regulation.

Global Barriers

There is global barrier considering the potential environmental applications and implications of nanotechnology. An international risk research network and coordination for public safety and health is lacking. Every debate over harmonization is about national differences in beliefs about workers, the environment, competitiveness, etc. A common database for nanomaterials risk data, standardization, characterization and nomenclature is also still not available (Ronald *et al.*, 2007) Such database is to facilitate comprehensive risk analysis and characterization of nanomaterials classes (*e.g.* carbon nanotube, metal and metal oxide). Global concern is growing since about 75 per cent of known nanotechnology

R&D investment worldwide is done by foreign nations, and even more unknown amounts by private industry, thus making environment, health, and safety all international issues (Ronald *et al.*, 2007).

Instrumentation and Metrology

Adequate instrumentation and metrology which are considered vital to the development of the basic terminology and comprehensive nomenclature of nanomaterials are still lacking. Metrology, the science of measurement, underpins all other nanoscience and nanotechnologies not only because it allows the characterization of materials in terms of dimensions but also in terms of attributes such as electrical properties and mass. Advanced instrumentation and sophisticated metrology needed to be developed to characterize properties of nanomaterials and products are not available in Nigeria. Greater precision in metrology will assist the development of nanoscience and nanotechnologies. Presently there are inadequate characterization and measurement tools and capabilities to enable monitoring and processing control based on nanoscale features.

Public Perception

Nanotechnology acceptance by the public is still at its low ebb considering the types of issues affecting public health and safety. The public impression generally is that risks from nanotechnology would outweigh the benefits derived. For example, fear that cell phone use caused brain cancer forced the some agencies in U.S to perform a short-term study (Ronald *et al.*, 2007).The evidence did not support the hypothesis or perception that cell phone usage was related to brain cancer. Most problematic in this "public perception and media exposure" was that the scientific community was not prepared to answer that question on issues such as dealing with nano particle soot and pollution that will need to be addressed. Some in the public and members of the press don't understand nanotechnology and are afraid of the consequences, side effects, waste product, toxic clouds etc. Concerns have been expressed that the very properties of nanoscale particles being exploited in certain applications (such as high surface reactivity and the ability to cross through cell membranes) might also have negative health and environmental impacts (John, 2011). There is immediate need to focus efforts on the types of nanoparticles already being used by industry, as these pose the most immediate exposure threat to humans and the environment.

Risk Management

There is serious challenge in evaluating risk associated with the manufacture and use of nanomaterials. The diversity and complexity of the types of materials available and being developed, as well as the seemingly limitless potential uses of these materials are not presently well managed. As an integral part of the innovation and design process of products and materials containing nanoparticles or nanotubes, toxicological information on the risk of release of these components throughout the life cycle of the product should be made available to the relevant regulatory authorities (Agnieska *et al.*, 2012). The similarity between carbon nanotubes and asbestos fibers has been highlighted by the toxicology community and is an issue of potential concern. Carbon nanotubes exhibit some characteristics that are similar to asbestos fibers with regards to shape, size and bio-persistency (Agnieska *et al.*, 2012). Whether this indicates a similar toxicity is not known at present and an integrated research is insufficient despite the current responsible attitude adopted for their handling in the wider scientific community.

An integrated risk research framework by government is low to manage nanotechnology environmental, health and safety issues by coordinating agencies in Nigeria.

Nanotechnology Materials

Developing and validating methods to evaluate the toxicity of engineered nanomaterials is required, but not adequately available in Nigeria. Much of nanoscience and many nanotechnologies are concerned with producing new or enhanced materials without thorough evaluation of toxicity level.

CONCLUSIONS AND RECOMMENDATIONS

Despite the aforementioned barriers to the transfer of nanotechnology concept to business enterprise in Nigeria, the interesting development is the establishment of Nigeria Nanotechnology Initiative (NNI) by the Federal Government as the starting point for the development of nanotechnology. It is also our hope that with time NNI will address the identified barriers. Significant barriers to nanotechnology transfer to business perspectives can be substantially reduced, if not completely eliminated, if the following recommendations are adopted:

Environmental, Health and Safety Issues (EHS)

It is quite obvious that the current body of knowledge of how nanoscale materials might affect humans and the environment is insufficient to assess, address, and manage the potential risks. While there is agreement on the need for more EHS research, there are differing views on the level of funding required, how it should be managed, and related issues. To accomplish this, there is need to develop sensitive analytical methodologies, tools and an acceptable protocol for screening, characterization and monitoring of nanomaterials in the work place, laboratory, homes and environment. Therefore, considering the EHS issues there is serious need to develop and design predictive models for nanomaterials toxicity using computational intelligent systems(Artificial neural network, neuro-fuzzy systems, hybrid support vector machines and fuzzy inference systems). The objective is to develop computational/ predictive model used to establish knowledge domains, risk modeling and nano-informatics capabilities to reliably assist decision making

Therefore, the following are recommended:

☆ Development of computational intelligent predictive models for nanomaterials toxicity

☆ Development of standardized methods, risk evaluation, risk assessment and management protocol

☆ Information sharing, common database for research that uses standard protocols to generate knowledge.

Investment/Government Budget

Funding for basic research is essential and needs to be increased. Additionally, the critical stage is when science emerges from the laboratories and evolves into commercial applications. There is need to provide adequate funding for early proto-typing and early stage development. Federal, state, and regional governments should consider providing more technical funding to the private sector. There is a need for medium/long term funding to help out groups that may have a five to ten year cycle research issue. A national fund may be set up for universities to teach people how to be entrepreneurs, to fund more research and patent protection, and for infrastructure improvements (laboratories, clean rooms, equipment and nanotechnology tools).

More Sophisticated and Early Market Research

It is needed to bridge the science culture-to-commercialization gap. Markets and future products must be identified early in the R&D stage, followed by periodic impartial reviews as innovations are transformed into prototypes that are placed into production and finally offered for sale.

New Laws and Regulations

There is need to establish new federal and state laws and regulations that encourage and offer tax incentives to encourage safer environment by business; make and promote public purchases of desirable nanotechnology products and services; amend existing regulations to favour certain industrial conduct and outcomes for good public policy; and support more education and training of researchers and workers.

The laws also need to encourage nanotechnology small and medium business growth, the expansion and novel financing of more multidisciplinary R&D, better intellectual property protection, and development of larger, more sophisticated nanotechnology corporations and venture capital funds.

Research and Development

Small companies would prefer to obtain university R&D that is developed to the latest stage when it is just about ready for production, without having to pay for prior R&D. The small start-up companies or small businesses need more access to federal and university labs. Government policy should consider financial assistance to new nanotechnology ventures that require special needs for infrastructure and facilities. The university infrastructure is essential and should not be available only for the largest firms. Genuine partnerships should be established between small businesses and these groups since not all of the start-up businesses can afford the research equipment needed for their work University laboratory scientific results may lead to intellectual property rights and basic patents. Nanotechnology is a multidisciplinary field. Advances in the area will require the expertise of chemists, physicists, materials scientists, biochemists, molecular biologists, engineers, toxicologists and medical scientists working together. Chemistry and physics are central to most nanotechnologies. R&D.Infrastructure availability is lacking, yet crucial to assist businesses, especially small companies that cannot afford the cost of nanotechnology instrumentation, equipment and facilities. Nanotechnology virtually demands university and industry cooperation due to basic science innovations, expensive laboratories, and need for highly trained workers. Federal, state and local government support is needed to encourage more networking, strategic alliances and joint ventures for expanding international collaboration involving universities, R&D laboratories, investors, manufacturers and product distributors.

ACKNOLEDGEMENTS

The authors wish to thank Dr. M.A. Jolaoso, Dr. A. Assanga, Mr. O. Adewole, Dr. M.L. Buga, Mrs. I.O. Ejuya, Engr. J.O. Adekunle, Mrs. Rachael Kotso and Mr. Felix Adigwe for their support and inputs into this paper. Your ideas have been very valuable and contributed immensely to the success of this paper.

REFERENCES

1. Adams, L. (2003, October). Video is Versatile. *Quality Magazine*, 32.Ahlgren,Martin, and Franchi, Helena Jonsonn., Policy for a New Industrial Revolution- A Study of Nanotechnology in the USA. Swedish Institute forGrowth Policy Studies.

2. Aitken, R., Butz, T., Colvin, V., Maynard, A., *et al.*, November 2006. Safe Handling of Nanotechnology. Nature Publishing Group. Vol. 444. No. 16. pp. 267-269.

3. Anderson, P., and Tushman, M. L. (1990). Technological Discontinuities and Dominant Designs: A Cyclical Model of Technological Change. *Administrative Science Quarterly*, 35, 604-633.

4. Aragon, L. (2004, July 1, 2004). Nano-Bubble Ahead? *Venture Capital Journal*, July 1, 2004,

5. Agnieszka Gajewicz a, Bakhtiyor Rasulev b, Tandabany C. Dinadayalane b, Piotr Urbaszek a, Tomasz Puzyn a,Danuta Leszczynska c, Jerzy Leszczynski (2012) Advancing risk assessment of engineered nanomaterials: Application of computational approaches.

6. Anthony Waitz and Wasig Bothare: Nanotechnology Commercialization Best Practices http://www.quantronainsight.com/paper/030915.commerciali-zation.pdf

7. Bergman, B. (2005, April 1). License to Grow: An Explosion of Patent Filings Brings With it an Increase in Litigation Cases. What Can a Savvy Investor Do? *Venture Capital Journal*.

8. Braunschweig, C. (2003, January 1). Nano Nonsense: Venture capitalists are searching for the next big thing in the smallest of technologies. But even with the most powerful electron microscope, they will find it very difficult to detect a profit. *Venture Capital Journal*, 1.

9. Braunschweig, C. (2004, May 31). Nanotech Company Raises $45M Recap. *Private Equity Week*, 11(21), 2.

10. Brookstein, Darrell. (2005). *Nanotech Fortunes- Make Yours in the Boom*. San Diego: The Nanotech Company.

11. Bruns, B., 2001, Open Sourcing Nanotechnology Research and Development: Issues and Opportunities, IOP Electronic Journals, Vol. 12, (3), pp.198-210.*Chemical Week* 167, no. 42 (Dec. 14, 2005): p. 22-23.

12. Christopher, A. (2000, October 1). The IT Hot List: Leading VCs Say Where the Smart Money is Headed. *Venture Capital Journal*.

13. Conner, J. (2005). *Foresight Ideas and Other Nano Media*. Retrieved December 2, 2005, from www.foresight.org

14. Coopers and Lybrand (1996). Three Keys to Obtaining Venture Capital.

15. Darby, M., Zucker, L., 2003 Grilichesian Breakthroughs: Inventions of Methods of Inventing and Firm Entry in Nanotechnology, National Bureau of Economic Research.

16. Davies, J. C. (2006, January 11). Stricter Nanotechnology Laws Are Urged. The *Washington Times*, A02.

17. Davey, Michael E. 2006. Manipulating Molecules: Federal Support for Nanotechnology Research. CRS Report for Congress. Department of Health and Human Services. 2007. Progress Toward Safe Nanotechnology in the Workplace: A Report from the NIOSH

18. Foley, Edward T. and Hersam, Mark C., 2006. Assessing the Need for Nanotechnology Education Reform in the United States. Nanotechnology Law and Business. Vol. 3. No. 4. pp.467-484.

19. John F. Sargent Jr.(2011). Nanotechnology and Environmental, Health,and Safety: Issues for Consideration

20. Michael Darby, and Lynne Zucker(July 2003): Grilichesian Breakth Troughs, Inventions of methods of Inventing and firm entry in Nanotechnology, National Bureau of Economic Research.

21. Nanosysterm: Molecular Machinery, Manufacturing and Computation (http://www.e drexler.com/d/06/00/nanosysterms. toc.html, 2006 ISBNO-471-57518-6.

22. Ronald D.Mc Neil, Jung Lowe J D,Ted M, Joseph Cronin, Dyanne Ferk (September 2007). Barriers to Nanotechnology Commercialization. Report prepared for U.S. Department of Commence, Technology Administration

23. Theresa Deitz (2007). Mitigation of Barriers to Commercialization of Nanotechnology: An Overview of Two Successful University-Based Initiatives

Chapter 15

Synthesis of Fe Doped SnO_2-TiO_2 Nanocatalysts via Sol-gel Method and their Structural and Catalytic Activities against Pollutants

*Fozia Iram and Muhammad Akhyar Farrukh**

Department of Chemistry,
GC University Lahore, Lahore 54000, Pakistan
**E-mail: akhyar100@gmail.com*

ABSTRACT

Here we report novel and facile synthesis of iron doped tin oxide-titanium oxide nanocatalysts with varying molar concentrations of SDS by sol gel method. The techniques used for the characterization of nanoparticles, Fourier Transform Infrared Spectroscopy (FTIR), Thermal Gravimetric Analysis (TGA), Powder X-Ray Diffraction (XRD), Transmission Electron Microscopy Analysis (TEM), Scanning Electron Microscope (SEM) and Energy Dispersive X-Ray Microanalysis (EDX) confirm successful synthesis of nanocatalysts. The prepared nanoparticles were applied to degrade methylene blue dye. Results suggest that these nanocatalysts may be envisaged for the treatment of waste waters in textile industries.

Keywords: Nanocatalysts, Sol-gel method, Doping, Morphology, Degradation, Methylene blue.

INTRODUCTION

A number of technological systems have been developed for the removal of organic pollutants such as dyes to meet the strict International environmental standards in this technological era (ISO 14001, March 2013). The commonly used scientific methods to remove dyes and other organic waste are adsorption (Dejohn and Hutchins, 1976), biological methods (biodegradation) (Patil and Shinde, 1988; More, 1989) and ozonation (Slokar and Le Marechal, 1998).

There is about 15 per cent loss of the total world production of dyes during the dying process and it is released in the textile effluents (Zolinger, 1991). The ecosystem is highly disturbed with the release of these colored waste waters and it is frightful source of pollution in the aquatic life (Akpan and Hameed, 2009). The release of several hazardous dyes from textile industries in waste water poses a serious threat to human health and aquatic medium due to toxic and carcinogenic effect of these dyes (Borker and Salker, 2006).

The important scientific mechanisms for removal of these toxic dyes from waste water are adsorption on high surface area supports, chemical precipitation, sedimentation, biological membranes and ion- exchange processes. The problems with these methods are that they are slow, require expensive equipment and may lead to the transfer of primary pollutants into secondary pollutants which in turn demands further removal (Gaya and Abdullah, 2008).

The Heterogeneous Catalysis is newly developed technique and it is considered as emerging destructive technology amongst newly developed oxidation processes since it leads to total mineralization of many organic pollutants (Herrmann, 1999; Schiavello, 1988; Guillard, 1993; Al-Ekabi and Ollis, 1993; Legrini, 1993). The TiO_2, Fe_2O_3 and ZnO nanoparticles have been used for degradation of methylene blue up to present time (Ahmed, 2013; Ai-Dong *et al.*, 2010; Farrukh, 2012).

In the present work, we make an attempt to synthesize iron doped tin oxide-titanium oxide nanoparticles by sol gel method with different concentrations of SDS. The prepared samples are investigated using developed techniques as FTIR, XRD, SEM, EDX, TGA and TEM. Moreover, the catalytic performance of the samples in degrading methylene blue dye in dark, in sunlight and under UV radiation was estimated using UV-Visible spectrophotometer.

MATERIALS AND METHODS

The chemical reagents used were titanium (IV) tetraisopropoxide $Ti(OCH(CH_3)_2)_4$ from Daejung, tin (IV) chloride pentahydrate $(SnCl_4.5H_2O)$ from Sigma Aldrich, sodium dodecyl surfactant (SDS) from Merck, NaOH pellets from Panreac, iron chloride hexahydrate $FeCl_3.6H_2O$ from Merck. All reagents were of analytical grade and were used without further purification. Distill water from purification system (favorit W4L). Methylene blue was supplied by a textile firm and used as received.

Degradation of methylene blue was monitored using spectrophotometer UV-1700 Shimadzu. The functional groups of nanoparticles were analyzed by FTIR MEDAC M2000 spectrophotometer. The thermogravimetric measurements carried out on a TA series SDT Q600 TGA-DSC instrument. The transmission electron micrographs obtained by Philips CM12, 80 kV TEM. The surface morphology and percentages of elements present in the samples investigated using Hitachi S3400 SEM/EDX. The structure of the material was determined by X'Pert PRO PANalytical XRD Powder with Cu Ka1 source of wavelength 1.540598 Å and Ka2 of wavelength 1.544426 Å.

Synthesis of Nanoparticles

To prepare tin oxide-titanium oxide nanocomposite by sol-gel method, titanium (IV) tetraisopropoxide (0.1 M) and tin (IV) chloride pentahydrate (0.1 M) were added to 50 mL distilled water in a flask and stirred for 5 minutes then NaOH (0.8 M) was added in the flask. The synthesis was carried out using NaOH with the reactants and the ratio of NaOH to reactants was 8:1. The 0.004, 0.006, 0.008, 0.010 and 0.012 M SDS concentrations were used to prepare five samples. After 4 hours of stirring the resulting product was centrifuged at 5000 rpm for 15 minutes each time during washing and at first it was washed three times with distilled water, then three times with ethanol, and once again three or more times with distilled water until the pH of the solution became 7. After drying at 150 °C for six hours, the product was calcined at 600 °C for three hours.

Doping of Nanoparticles

To dope the nanoparticles, 100 mL of iron chloride hexahydrate $FeCl_3.6H_2O$ ($4.2×10^{-3}$ M) solution was prepared and approximately 1.00 g of above prepared tin oxide-titanium oxide nanocomposite (catalyst) was dispersed in solution and stirred for 2 hours. The suspension was centrifuged at 5000 rpm for 15 minutes each time during washing and washed three times with distilled water then three times with ethanol and again three times with distilled water until pH of the solution became 7. After drying at 150 °C for six hours, the product was calcined at 600 °C for three hours. Figure 15.1 shows five samples of prepared nanoparticles with varying SDS concentration.

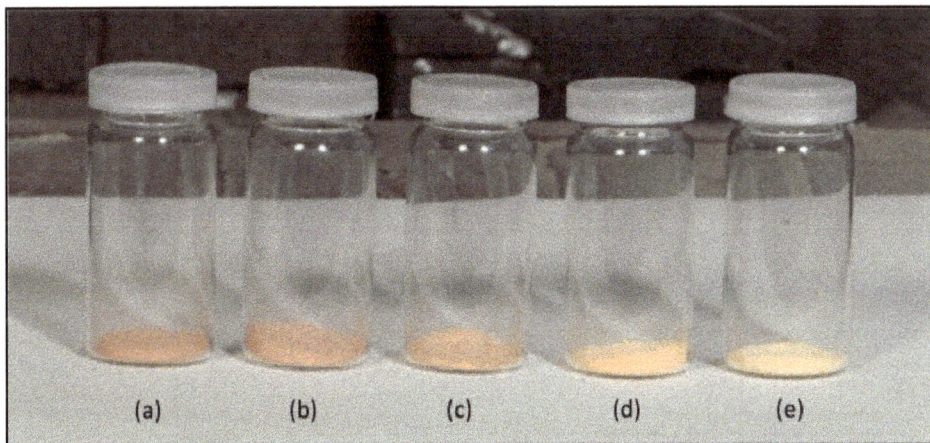

Figure 15.1: (a) tinti-4 (SDS Conc. 0.004 M) (b) tinti-6 (SDS Conc. 0.006 M) (c) tinti-8 (SDS Conc. 0.008 M) (d) tinti-10 (SDS Conc. 0.010 M) (e) tinti-12 (SDS Conc. 0.012 M)

Catalytic Reaction

A mixture of 5 mg iron doped tin oxide-titanium oxide nanocatalyst and 10 ppm solution of methylene blue in water was added into a cuvette at room temperature. The catalytic activity was determined using UV-Vis spectrophotometer (UV-1700 Shimadzu) by measuring the change in absorbance at 664 nm. The catalytical activity of prepared nanocatalysts was studied in dark, in sunlight and under UV lamp for the time one minute, half hour and one hour each. All the solutions were freshly prepared in water.

RESULTS AND DISCUSSION

FTIR spectrums of samples with different SDS concentrations are shown in Figure 15.2. The peaks from 3294 to 3394 cm^{-1} are attributed to O-H bending and stretching vibrations of absorbed water at the surface of Ti^{+4} and Sn^{+4} cations (Ivanda, 1998). The vibration bands from 2326 to 2341 cm^{-1} are due to CO_2 adsorbed on the cations Ti^{+4} and Sn^{+4} surfaces. In samples tinti-6 (0.006 M SDS concentration) and tinti-10 (0.010 M SDS concentration) the peaks at 2337 cm^{-1} and 2341 cm^{-1} respectively are more sharp as there is more absorption of CO_2 during calcination (Scaranto, 2005) and air. The vibration peaks from 1651 to 1674 cm^{-1} are because of bending vibrations of water molecules trapped in prepared samples (Adnan, 2010). The peaks from 1404 to 1496 cm^{-1} are attributed to C-H bending vibrations while peaks from 1353 to 1369 cm^{-1} are due to C-H rocking vibrations (Martin, 1996). The absorption peaks from 1130 to 1153 cm^{-1} are assigned to O-H defomative mode (Mazloom, 2013). The vibration bands from 501 to 609 cm^{-1} are attributed to Sn-O stretching vibrations (Farrukh,

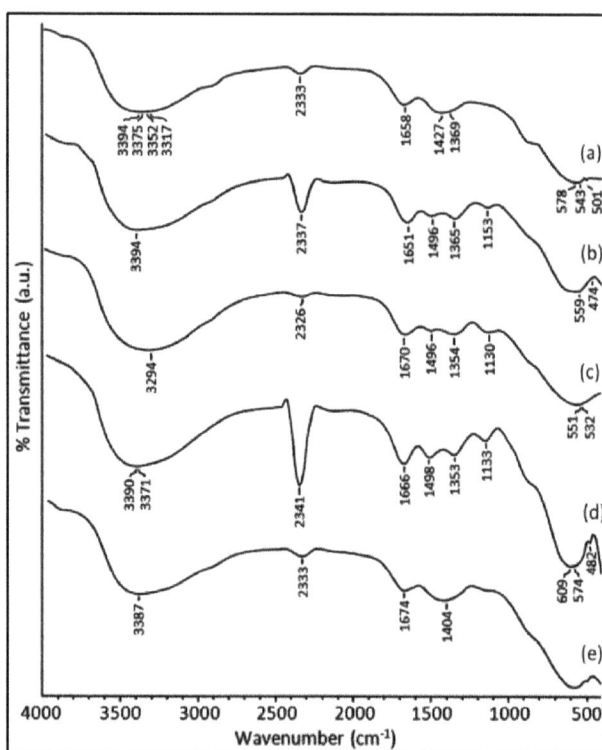

Figure 15.2: FTIR of Samples (a) tinti-4 (SDS Conc. 0.004 M)
(b) tinti-6 (SDS Conc. 0.006 M) (c) tinti-8 (SDS Conc. 0.008 M)
(d) tinti-10 (SDS Conc. 0.010 M) (e) tinti-12 (SDS Conc. 0.012 M)

2010). The absorption bands at 428 and 474 cm^{-1} are assinged to TiO$_2$ stretching vibrations (Nagaveni, 2004).

To study the thermal stability of nanoparticles they were subjected to TGA analysis between room temperature to 1000°C (Figure 15.3). As it can be noted from this figure, a total weight loss during the whole temperature range is 13.5 per cent. The weight loss happened in six stages. The first stage is from room temperature to 150°C, where 4 per cent weight loss is caused by atmospheric moisture adsorbed. The second stage is from 150 to 260°C, in which 1.5 per cent weight loss is caused by loss of physically absorbed moisture on the surface of the sample. The third stage is from 260 to 500°C and 2 per cent weight loss is happened by degradation of organic groups contained in the sample. The fourth stage is from 500 to 710°C and it showed 1 per cent weight loss due to degradation of iron. The fifth stage is from 710 to 840°C with 2.5 per cent weight loss because of the degradation of tin dioxide. The sixth stage is from 840 to 1000°C, and it further caused 2.5 per cent weight loss due to degradation of titanium dioxide.

The SEM images of the samples tinti-4 (SDS concentration 0.004 M) and tinti-8 (SDS concentration 0.008 M) shown in Figures 15.4 (a) and (b) respectively both

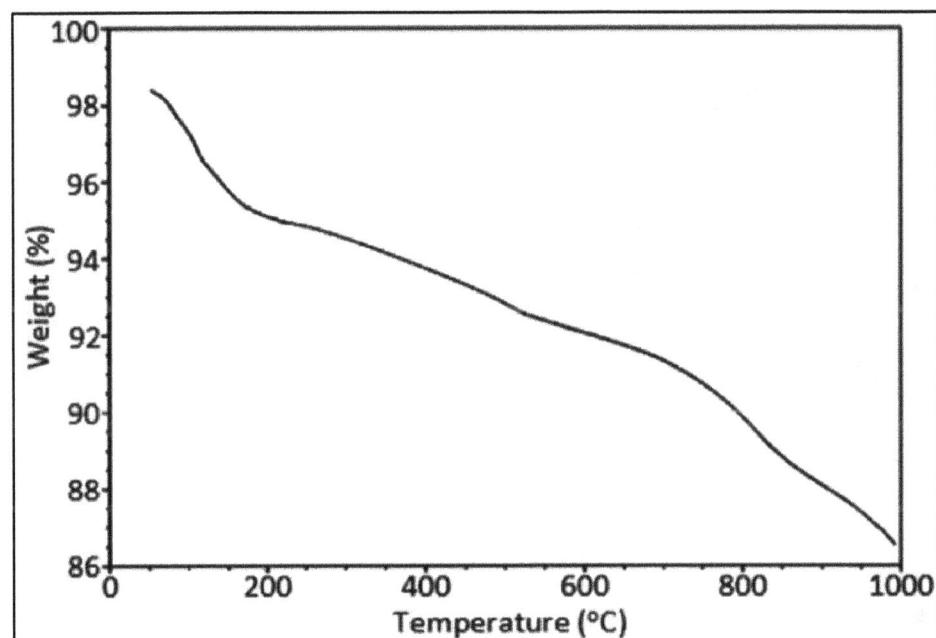

Figure 15.3: TGA of Prepared Samples

display rod like morphology while porous rock like morphology revealed in Figure 15.4 (c) shown by sample tinti-12 (0.012 M SDS concentration).

The EDX analysis of prepared nanoparticles is carried out to check the purity of the product and to know the elements present in the sample and their percentages. In

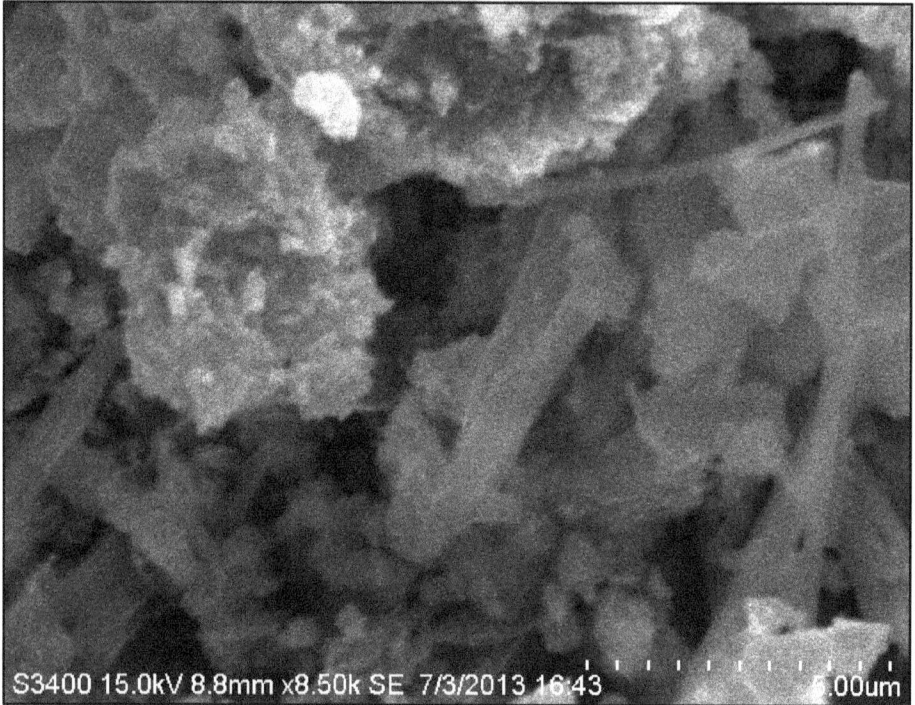

Figure 15.4(a): SEM Image of tinti-4 (SDS Conc. 0.004 M) at 5 µm

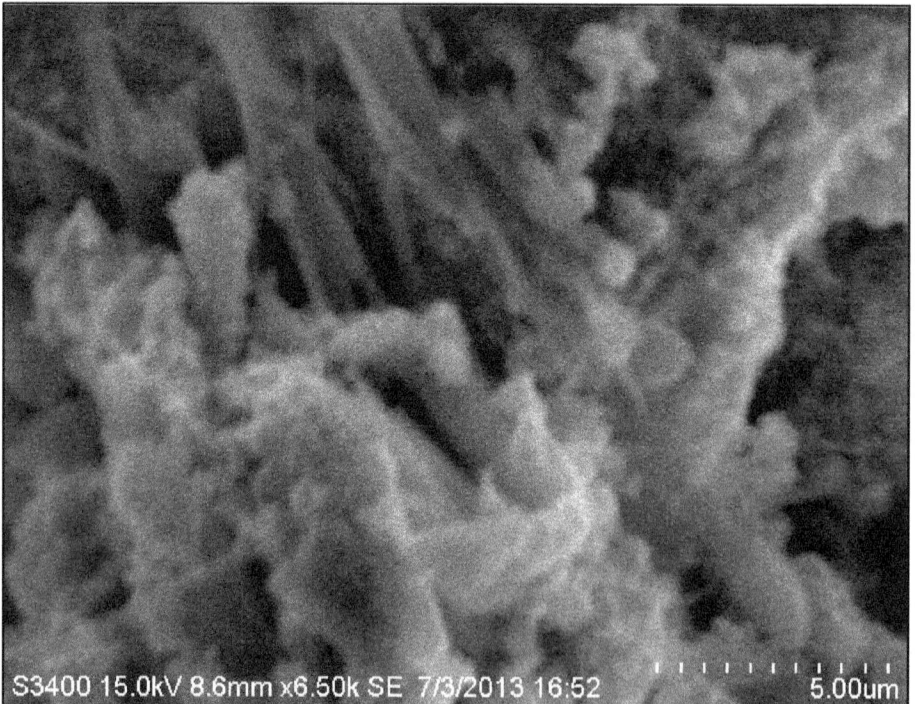

Figure 15.4(b): SEM Image of tinti-8 (SDS Conc. 0.008 M) at 5 µm

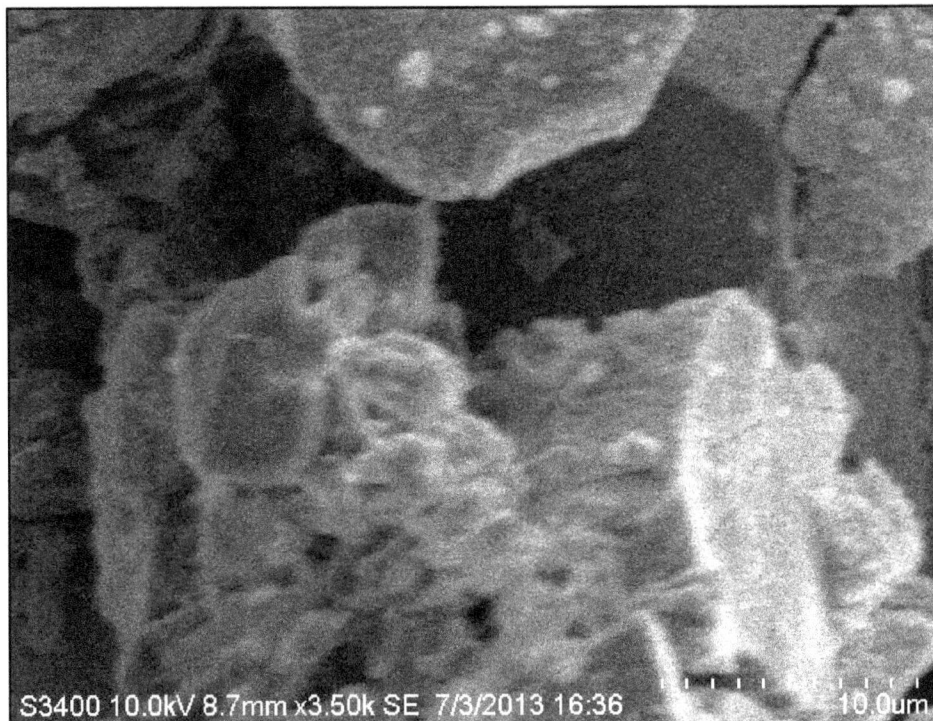

Figure 15.4(c): SEM Image of tinti-12 (SDS Conc. 0.004 M) at 10 μm

Figure 15.5(a) EDX of tinti-4 (0.004 M SDS concentration) the elements oxygen, titanium, iron and tin have weight percentages 27.49, 35.4, 5.33, 31.78 and atomic percentages 60.24, 26.66, 3.44 and 9.66 respectively. Figure 15.5 (b) EDX of tinti-8 (0.008 M SDS concentration) shows that the elements oxygen, titanium, iron and tin have weight percentages 50.86, 28.69, 5.54, 14.91 and atomic percentages 6979, 17.92, 2.18, 10.11 respectively. The elements oxygen, titanium, iron and tin have weight percentages 6.44, 52.06, 25.81, 15.69 and atomic percentages 11.07, 67.24, 14.2 and 7.49 respectively as shown in Figure 15.5 (c) EDX of tinti-12 (0.012 M SDS concentration). The results of EDX analysis confirm that the prepared samples are pure with desired chemical stoichiometry as no peak of any other element can be seen.

Figure 15.6 presents XRD spectrum of nanocatalysts with different SDS concentrations their 2θ values were compared with the ICDD database to identify the phase purity and composition formed. The h k l values and diffraction peaks are explained as under. The diffraction peaks at 2θ values of 26.57° corresponded to the 110 reflection planes of tetragonal SnO₂ (PDF#770448). The diffraction peaks at 27.0°, 27.29°, 27.33°, 35.13°, 35.64°, 35.85°, 53.79° and 54.22° corresponded to the 110, 110, 110, 101, 101, 101, 211 and 211 reflection planes of triclinic TiO₂ respectively (PDF#896975). The diffraction peaks at 35.23°, 48.41°, 52.92°, 52.99°°and 53.06° corresponded to the 110, 024, 11-6, 11-6 and 11-6 reflection planes of trigonal

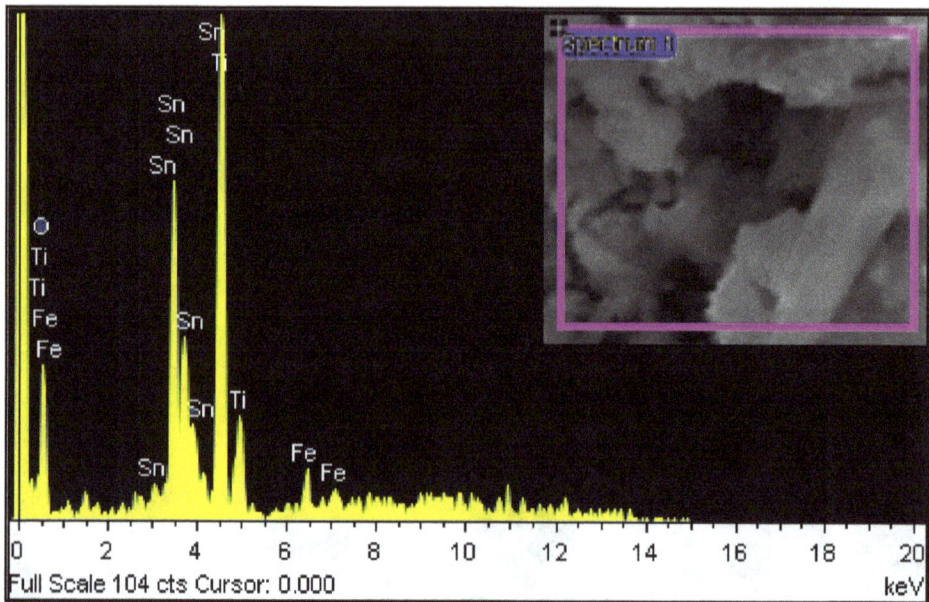

Figure 15.5(a):. EDX of tinti-4 (0.004 M SDS Conc.)

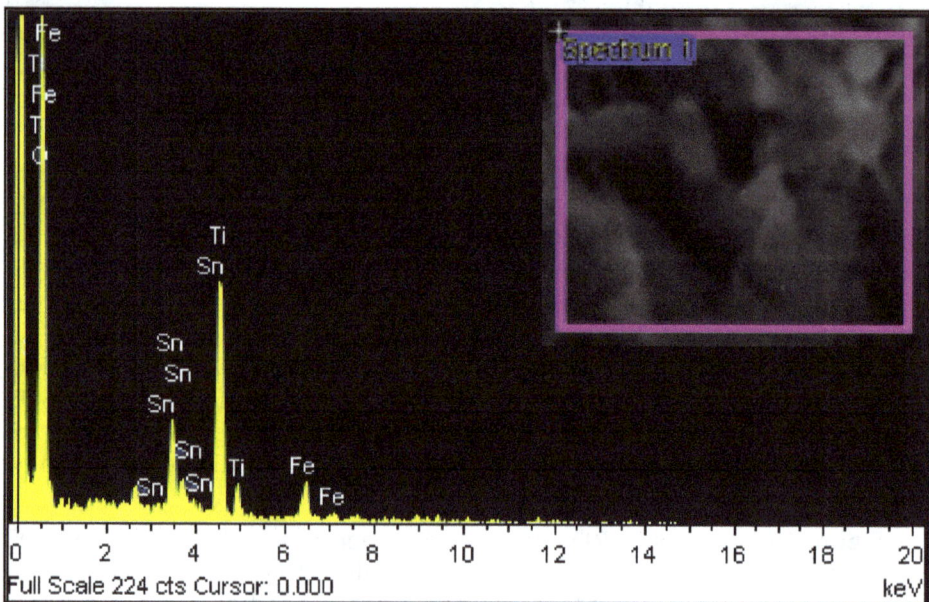

Figure 15.5(b): EDX of tinti-8 (0.008 M SDS Conc.)

(rhombohedral) lattice of Fe-TiO$_3$ respectively (PDF#892811). The diffraction peaks at 61.99° corresponded to 440 planes of cubic lattice of Fe-SnO$_2$ (PDF#710693). The diffraction peaks at 44.13° and 44.35° corresponded to the 110 and 110 reflection planes of cubic lattice of iron respectively (PDF#851410). The average crystallite size

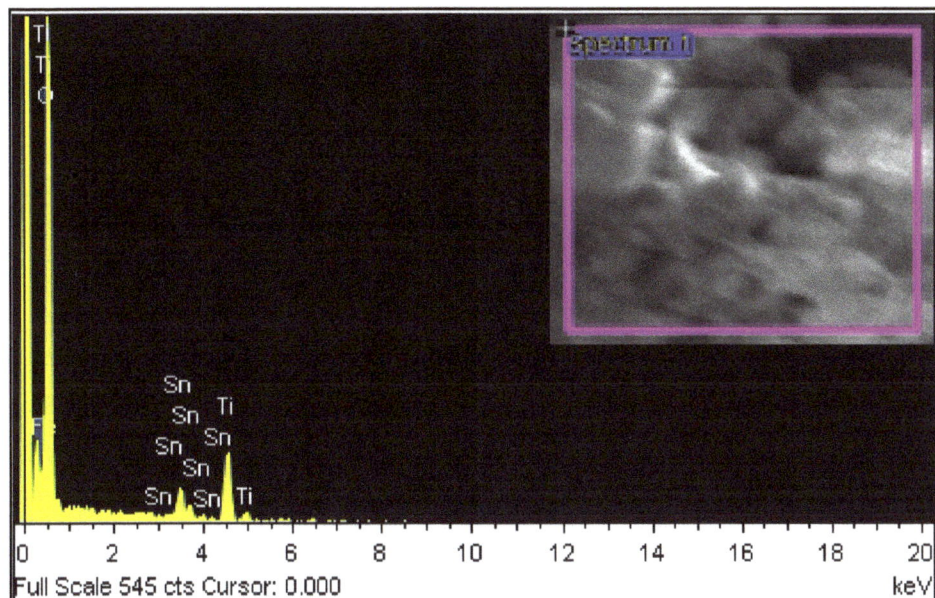

Figure 15.5(c): EDX of tinti-12 (0.012 M SDS Conc.)

(1.99 nm) was determined from the broadenings of corresponding peaks by using Scherrer's equation:

$$D = \frac{k\lambda}{\beta(\cos\theta)}$$

where,

D is the mean crystallite size, k is the grain shape dependent constant 0.89, λ is the wavelength of the incident beam in nm, 5 is the Bragg reflection angle, and 5 is the line broadening at half the maximum intensity in radians.

Catalytic Degradation of Methylene Blue

Methylene blue degradation in the presence of nanocatalysts prepared with varying molar concentrations of SDS was studied in dark, in sunlight and under UV irradiations for the reaction time one minute, half hour and one hour each.

Nanocatalysts; tinti-4 (SDS concentration 0.004 M), tinti-6 (SDS concentration 0.006 M), tinti-8 (SDS concentration 0.008 M), tinti-10 (SDS concentration 0.010 M), tinti-12 (SDS concentration 0.012 M) were used to degrade methylene blue by one minute stirring in dark, their rate constant (k) values were found to be 0.33, 0.25, 0.3, 0.45, 0.39 min^{-1} and percentage degradation 1.97, 2.20, 2.56, 2.69, 3.91 per cent respectively.

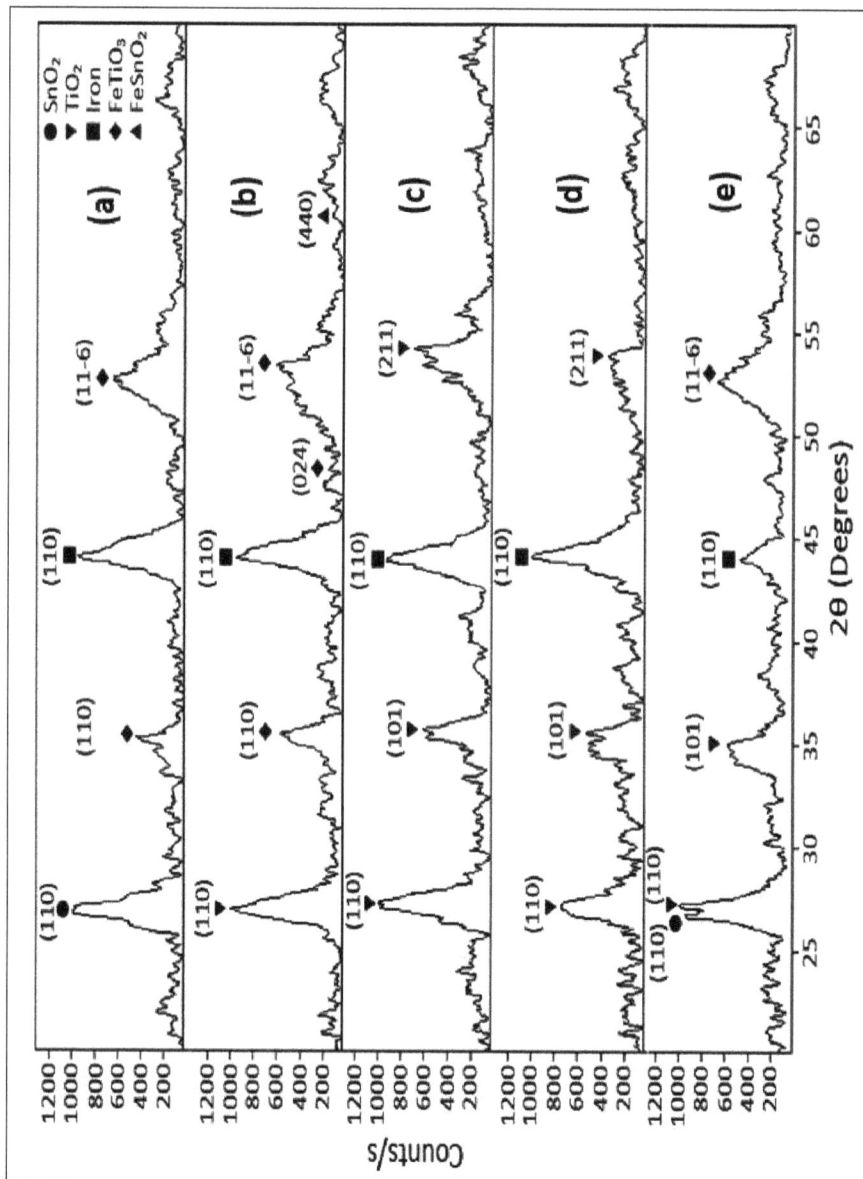

Figure 15.6: XRD of (a) tinti-4 (SDS Conc. 0.004 M) (b) tinti-6 (SDS Conc. 0.006 M) (c) tinti-8 (SDS Conc. 0.008 M) (d) tinti-10 (SDS Conc. 0.010 M) (e) tinti-12 (SDS Conc. 0.012 M)

Table 15.1: In Dark, the Degradation of Methylene Blue by One Minute Stirring

Sample Code	k Value min^{-1}	Per cent Degradation	SDS Conc.
tinti-4	0.33	1.97 per cent	0.004 M
tinti-6	0.25	2.20 per cent	0.006 M
tinti-8	0.3	2.56 per cent	0.008 M
tinti-10	0.45	2.69 per cent	0.010 M
tinti-12	0.39	3.91 per cent	0.012 M

Nanocatalysts; tinti-4 (SDS concentration 0.004 M), tinti-6 (SDS concentration 0.006 M), tinti-8 (SDS concentration 0.008 M), tinti-10 (SDS concentration 0.010 M), tinti-12 (SDS concentration 0.012 M) were used to degrade methylene blue by half hour stirring in dark, their rate constant (k) values were found to be 0.4, 0.51, 0.34, 0.35, 0.18 min^{-1} and percentage degradation 1.58, 1.68, 1.79, 1.81, 2.21 per cent respectively.

Table 15.2: In Dark, the Degradation of Methylene Blue by Half Four Stirring

Sample Code	k Value min^{-1}	Per cent Degradation	SDS Conc.
tinti-4	0.4	1.58 per cent	0.004 M
tinti-6	0.51	1.68 per cent	0.006 M
tinti-8	0.34	1.79 per cent	0.008 M
tinti-10	0.35	1.81 per cent	0.010 M
tinti-12	0.18	2.21 per cent	0.012 M

Nanocatalysts; tinti-4 (SDS concentration 0.004 M), tinti-6 (SDS concentration 0.006 M), tinti-8 (SDS concentration 0.008 M), tinti-10 (SDS concentration 0.010 M), tinti-12 (SDS concentration 0.012 M) were used to degrade methylene blue by one hour stirring in dark, their rate constant (k) values were found to be 0.5, 0.42, 0.41, 0.29, 0.51 min^{-1} and percentage degradation 0.95, 1.39, 1.48, 1.54, 1.60 per cent respectively.

Table 15.3: In Dark, the Degradation of Methylene Blue by One Hour Stirring

Sample Code	k Value min^{-1}	Per cent Degradation	SDS Conc.
tinti-4	0.5	0.95 per cent	0.004 M
tinti-6	0.42	1.39 per cent	0.006 M
tinti-8	0.41	1.48 per cent	0.008 M
tinti-10	0.29	1.54 per cent	0.010 M
tinti-12	0.51	1.60 per cent	0.012 M

Nanocatalysts; tinti-4 (SDS concentration 0.004 M), tinti-6 (SDS concentration 0.006 M), tinti-8 (SDS concentration 0.008 M), tinti-10 (SDS concentration 0.010 M), tinti-12 (SDS concentration 0.012 M) were used to degrade methylene blue by one

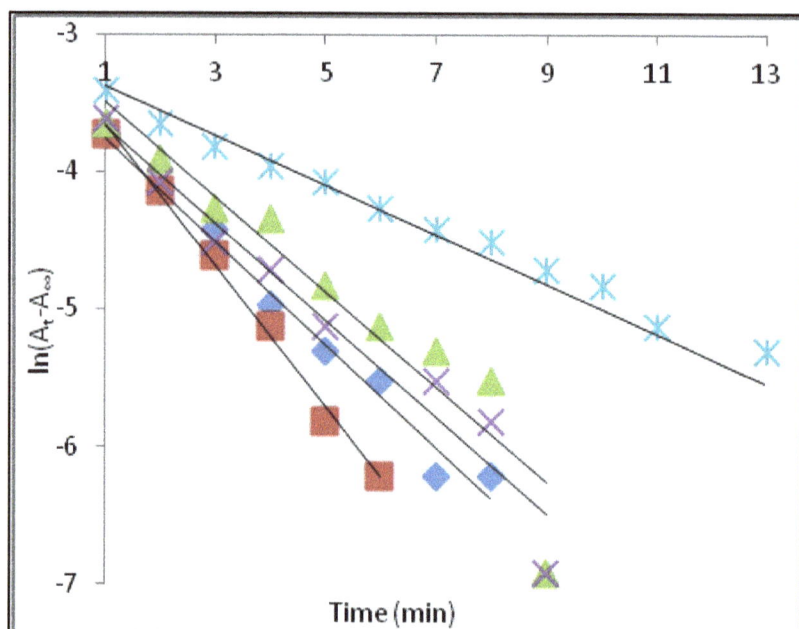

Figure 15.7: Catalytic Degradation of Methylene Blue in Dark by Half Hour Stirring. Plot of $\ln(A_t-A_\infty)$ versus time show first order reaction

◆ tinti-4 (SDS Conc. 0.004 M) ■ tinti-6 (SDS Conc. 0.006 M) ▲ tinti-8 (SDS Conc. 0.008 M) ✕ tinti-10 (SDS Conc. 0.010 M) ✳ tinti-12 (SDS Conc. 0.012 M)

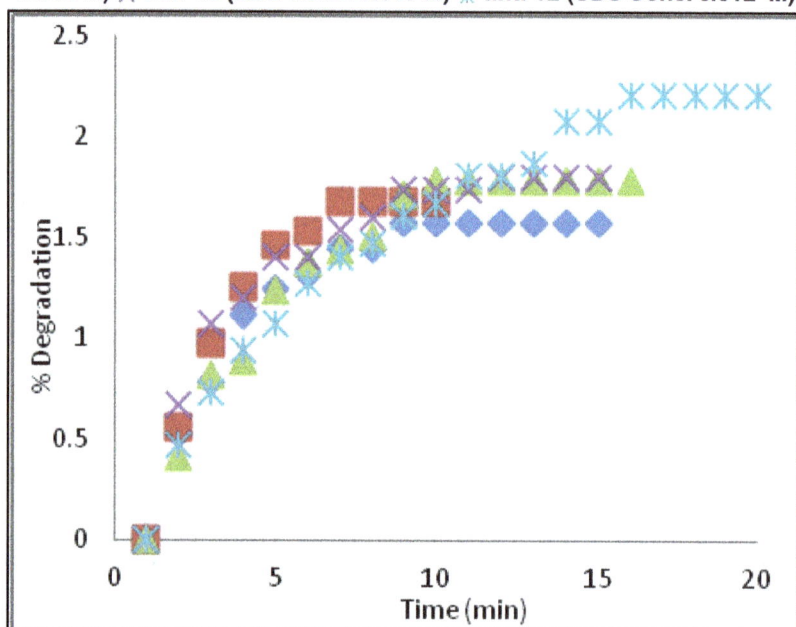

Figure 15.8: Catalytic Degradation of Methylene Blue in Dark by Half Hour Stirring. Plot of per cent degradation versus time

◆ tinti-4 (SDS Conc. 0.004 M) ■ tinti-6 (SDS Conc. 0.006 M) ▲ tinti-8 (SDS Conc. 0.008 M) ✕ tinti-10 (SDS Conc. 0.010 M) ✳ tinti-12 (SDS Conc. 0.012 M)

minute stirring in sunlight, their rate constant (k) values were found to be 0.54, 0.29, 0.42, 0.33, 0.35 min⁻¹ and percentage degradation 2.73, 3.02, 3.54, 3.63, 4.83 per cent respectively.

Table 15.4: In Sunlight, the Degradation of Methylene Blue by One Minute Stirring

Sample Code	k Value min⁻¹	Per cent Degradation	SDS Conc.
tinti-4	0.54	2.73 per cent	0.004 M
tinti-6	0.29	3.02 per cent	0.006 M
tinti-8	0.42	3.54 per cent	0.008 M
tinti-10	0.33	3.63 per cent	0.010 M
tinti-12	0.35	4.83 per cent	0.012 M

Nanocatalysts; tinti-4 (SDS concentration 0.004 M), tinti-6 (SDS concentration 0.006 M), tinti-8 (SDS concentration 0.008 M), tinti-10 (SDS concentration 0.010 M), tinti-12 (SDS concentration 0.012 M) were used to degrade methylene blue by half hour stirring in sunlight, their rate constant (k) values were found to be 0.35, 0.35, 0.35, 0.38, 0.31 min⁻¹ and percentage degradation 3.40, 3.69, 4.23, 4.33, 4.95 per cent respectively.

Table 15.5: In Sunlight, the Degradation of Methylene Blue by Half Hour Stirring

Sample Code	k Value min⁻¹	Per cent Degradation	SDS Conc.
tinti-4	0.35	3.40 per cent	0.004 M
tinti-6	0.35	3.69 per cent	0.006 M
tinti-8	0.35	4.23 per cent	0.008 M
tinti-10	0.38	4.33 per cent	0.010 M
tinti-12	0.31	4.95 per cent	0.012 M

Nanocatalysts; tinti-4 (SDS concentration 0.004 M), tinti-6 (SDS concentration 0.006 M), tinti-8 (SDS concentration 0.008 M), tinti-10 (SDS concentration 0.010 M), tinti-12 (SDS concentration 0.012 M) were used to degrade methylene blue by one hour stirring in sunlight, their rate constant (k) values were found to be 0.32, 0.39, 0.33, 0.33, 0.38 min⁻¹ and percentage degradation 3.76, 4.12, 4.14, 4.18, 4.97 per cent respectively.

Table 15.6: In Sunlight, the Degradation of Methylene Blue by One Hour Stirring

Sample Code	k Value min⁻¹	Per cent Degradation	SDS Conc.
tinti-4	0.32	3.76 per cent	0.004 M
tinti-6	0.39	4.12 per cent	0.006 M
tinti-8	0.33	4.14 per cent	0.008 M
tinti-10	0.33	4.18 per cent	0.010 M
tinti-12	0.38	4.97 per cent	0.012 M

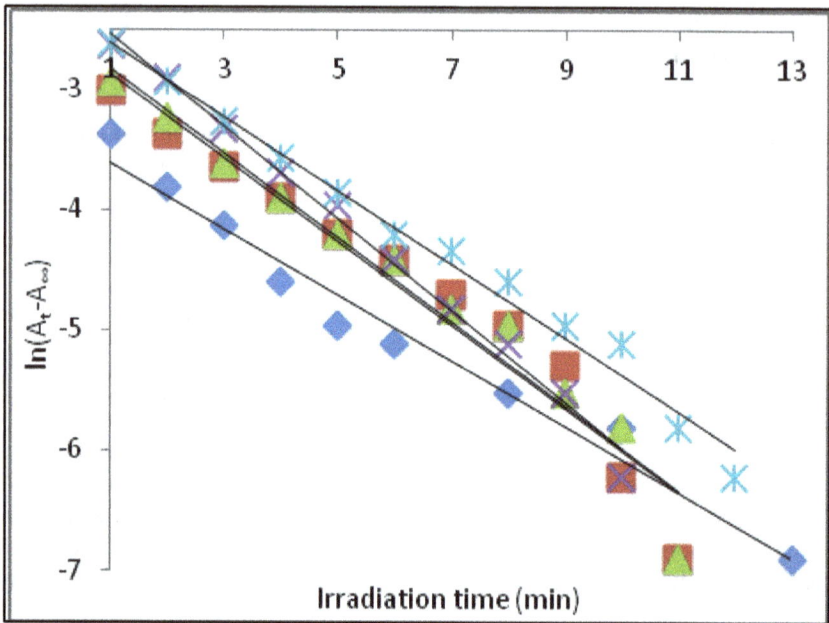

Figure 15.9: Catalytic Degradation of Methylene Blue in Sunlight by Half Hour Stirring. Plot of $ln(A_t-A_\infty)$ versus time show first order reaction

◆ tinti-4 (SDS Conc. 0.004 M) ■ tinti-6 (SDS Conc. 0.006 M) ▲ tinti-8 (SDS Conc. 0.008 M) × tinti-10 (SDS Conc. 0.010 M) ✳ tinti-12 (SDS Conc. 0.012 M)

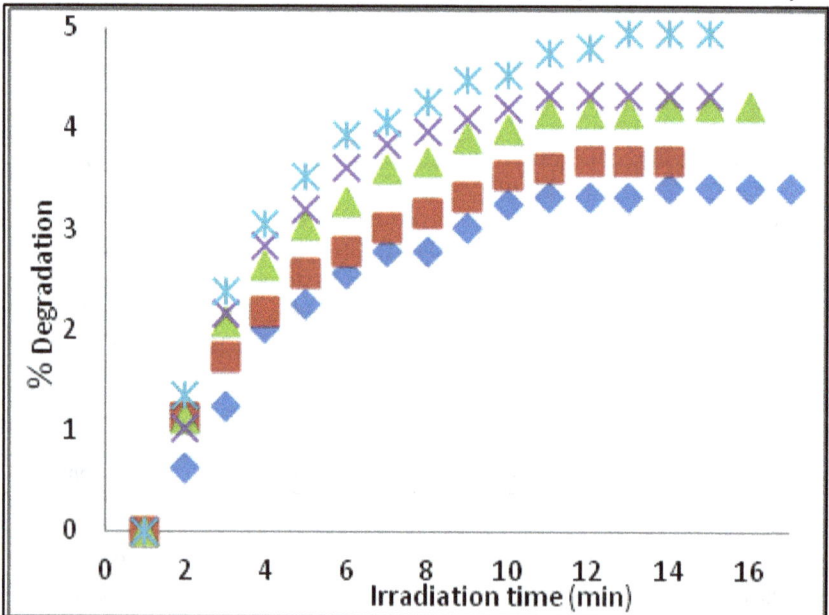

Figure 15.10: Catalytic Degradation of Methylene Blue in Sunlight by Half Hour Stirring. Plot of per cent degradation versus time

◆ tinti-4 (SDS Conc. 0.004 M) ■ tinti-6 (SDS Conc. 0.006 M) ▲ tinti-8 (SDS Conc. 0.008 M) × tinti-10 (SDS Conc. 0.010 M) ✳ tinti-12 (SDS Conc. 0.012 M)

Nanocatalysts; tinti-4 (SDS concentration 0.004 M), tinti-6 (SDS concentration 0.006 M), tinti-8 (SDS concentration 0.008 M), tinti-10 (SDS concentration 0.010 M), tinti-12 (SDS concentration 0.012 M) were used to degrade methylene blue by one minute stirring in UV light, their rate constant (k) values were found to be 0.51, 0.31, 0.38, 0.39, 0.36 min^{-1} and percentage degradation 3.58, 3.85, 4.15, 4.55, 4.62 per cent respectively.

Table 15.7: In UV Light, the degradation of Methylene Blue by One Minute Stirring

Sample Code	k Value min⁻¹	Per cent Degradation	SDS Conc.
tinti-4	0.51	3.58 per cent	0.004 M
tinti-6	0.31	3.85 per cent	0.006 M
tinti-8	0.38	4.15 per cent	0.008 M
tinti-10	0.39	4.55 per cent	0.010 M
tinti-12	0.36	4.62 per cent	0.012 M

Nanocatalysts; tinti-4 (SDS concentration 0.004 M), tinti-6 (SDS concentration 0.006 M), tinti-8 (SDS concentration 0.008 M), tinti-10 (SDS concentration 0.010 M), tinti-12 (SDS concentration 0.012 M) were used to degrade methylene blue by half hour stirring in UV light, their rate constant (k) values were found to be 0.27, 0.35, 0.36, 0.36, 0.27 min^{-1} and percentage degradation 2.32, 2.80, 4.04, 4.13, 5.75 per cent respectively.

Table 15.8: In UV Light, the Degradation of Methylene Blue by Half Hour Stirring

Sample Code	k Value min⁻¹	Per cent Degradation	SDS Conc.
tinti-4	0.27	2.32 per cent	0.004 M
tinti-6	0.35	2.80 per cent	0.006 M
tinti-8	0.36	4.04 per cent	0.008 M
tinti-10	0.36	4.13 per cent	0.010 M
tinti-12	0.27	5.75 per cent	0.012 M

Nanocatalysts; tinti-4 (SDS concentration 0.004 M), tinti-6 (SDS concentration 0.006 M), tinti-8 (SDS concentration 0.008 M), tinti-10 (SDS concentration 0.010 M), tinti-12 (SDS concentration 0.012 M) were used to degrade methylene blue by one hour stirring in UV light, their rate constant (k) values were found to be 0.48, 0.38, 0.4, 0.46, 0.35 min^{-1} and percentage degradation 3.91, 4.15, 4.20, 4.22, 4.87 per cent respectively.

Table 15.9: In UV Light, the Degradation of Methylene Blue by One Hour Stirring

Sample Code	k Value min⁻¹	Per cent Degradation	SDS Conc.
tinti-4	0.48	3.91 per cent	0.004 M
tinti-6	0.38	4.15 per cent	0.006 M
tinti-8	0.4	4.20 per cent	0.008 M
tinti-10	0.46	4.22 per cent	0.010 M
tinti-12	0.35	4.87 per cent	0.012 M

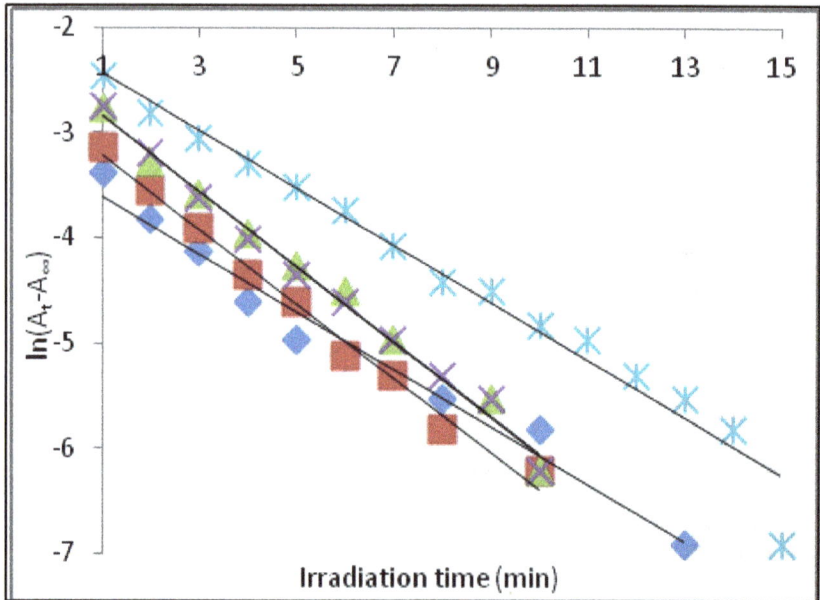

Figure 15.11: Catalytic Degradation of Methylene Blue Under UV Irradiation by Half Hour Stirring. Plot of $\ln(A_t-A_y)$ versus time show first order reaction

◆ tinti-4 (SDS Conc. 0.004 M) ■ tinti-6 (SDS Conc. 0.006 M) ▲ tinti-8 (SDS Conc. 0.008 M) ✕ tinti-10 (SDS Conc. 0.010 M) ✳ tinti-12 (SDS Conc. 0.012 M)

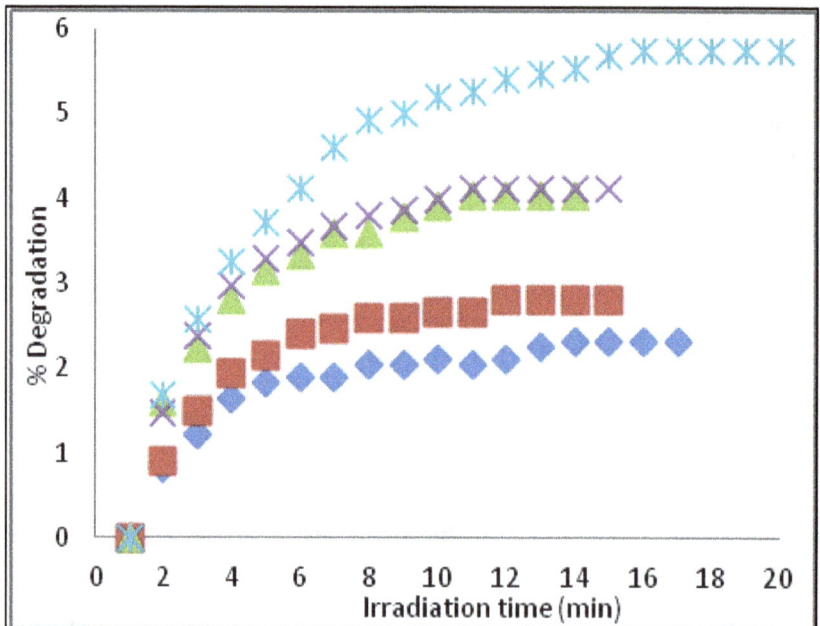

Figure 15.12: Catalytic Degradation of Methylene Blue Under UV Irradiation by Half Hour Stirring. Plot of per cent degradation versus time

◆ tinti-4 (SDS Conc. 0.004 M) ■ tinti-6 (SDS Conc. 0.006 M) ▲ tinti-8 (SDS Conc. 0.008 M) ✕ tinti-10 (SDS Conc. 0.010 M) ✳ tinti-12 (SDS Conc. 0.012 M)

Table 15.10: Total per cent Degradation of Methylene Blue in Dark, in Sunlight and in UV Light

Sample Code	Total Per cent Degrad. in Dark	Total Per cent Degrad. in Sunlight	Total per cent Degrad. in UV Light	SDS Conc.
tinti-4	4.5 per cent	9.89 per cent	9.81 per cent	0.004 M
tinti-6	5.27 per cent	10.83 per cent	10.8 per cent	0.006 M
tinti-8	5.83 per cent	11.91 per cent	12.39 per cent	0.008 M
tinti-10	6.04 per cent	12.14 per cent	12.9 per cent	0.010 M
tinti-12	7.72 per cent	14.75 per cent	15.24 per cent	0.012 M

In our previous work ZnO Nanoflakes degrade methylene blue 9.57 per cent under UV light (Farrukh, 2012). In comparison thereof, the Fe doped SnO_2-TiO_2 nanocatalysts in the present work degrade methylene blue 15.24 per cent under UV light. The above results show that as the concentration of SDS increases in the nanocatalysts the percentage degradation of methylene blue also increases because the surface area of nanocatalysts increases by increasing the concentration of surfactant (SDS); the SEM images also support the results. In all reaction conditions sample tinti-12 (SDS concentration 0.012 M) show greater degradation of methylene blue as compared to other samples as it has porous rock like morphology so its surface area is greater than other samples having simple rod like morphology.

CONCLUSIONS

An easy and simple process was used for large scale synthesis of iron doped tin oxide-titanium oxide nanocatalysts with different molar concentration of SDS. The sample tinti-4 (0.004 M SDS concentration) and tinti-8 (0.008 M SDS concentration) show rod like morphology while tinti-12 (0.012 M SDS concentration) display porous rock like morphology. The sample tinti-12 (0.012 M SDS concentration) show maximum degradation of methylene blue 15.24 per cent under ultra violet radiations because of increased surface area revealed from its porous morphology. Furthermore the prepared nanoparticles have the ability to degrade methylene blue even in dark so may be promising candidate for practical applications in the field of catalysis.

REFERENCES

1. Adnan, R., Razana, N.A., Rahman, A., and Farrukh, M.A., 2010. Synthesis and characterization of high surface area tin oxide nanoparticles via the sol gel method as a catalyst for the hydrogenation of styrene. *Journal of Chinese Chemical Society*, 57, pp. 222–229.

2. Ahmed, M.A., Emad, E., El-Katori., Zarha, and Gharni, H., 2013. Photocatalytic degradation of methylene blue dye using Fe_2O_3/TiO_2 nanoparticles prepared by sol–gel method. *Journal of Alloys and Compounds*, 553, pp. 19–29.

3. Ai-Dong, L., Kong, J. Z., Xiang, Y. L., Zhai, H. F., Zhang, W. Q., Gong, Y. P., Wu, D., 2010. Photo-degradation of methylene blue using Ta-doped ZnO nanoparticle. *Journal of Solid State Chemistry*, 183(6), pp. 1359–1364.

4. Akpan, U.G., and Hameed, B.H., 2009. Parameters affecting the photocatalytic degradation of dyes using TiO_2-based photocatalysts: A review. *Journal of Hazardous Materials*, 170(2–3), pp. 520–529.

5. Al-Ekabi, H.A., and Ollis, D., 1993. Photocatalytic Purification and Treatment of Water and Air, *In:* (Eds.), Elsevier, Amsterdam.

6. Borker, P., and Salker, A.V., 2006. Photocatalytic degradation of textile azo dye over $Ce_{1-x}Sn_xO_2$ series. *Materials Science and Engineering:* B, 133(1–3), pp. 55–60.

7. Dejohn, P.B., and Hutchins, R.A., 1976. Treatment of dye wastes with granular activated carbon. *Textile Chemist and Colorist*, 8, pp. 69.

8. Farrukh, M. A., Heng, B. T., and Adnan, R., 2010. Surfactant controlled aqueous synthesis of SnO_2 nanoparticles via the hydrothermal and conventional heating methods. *Turkish Journal of Chemistry*, 34, pp. 537–550.

9. Farrukh, M.A., Thong, C. K., Adnan, R., and Kamarulzaman, M. A., 2012a. Preparation and characterization of zinc oxide nanoflakes using anodization method and their photodegradation activity on methylene blue. *Russian Journal of Physical Chemistry* A, 86(13), pp. 2041–2048.

10. Gaya, U.I., and Abdullah, A.H., 2008. Heterogeneous photocatalytic degradation of organic contaminants over titanium dioxide: A review of fundamentals, progress and problems. *Journal of Photochemistry and Photobiology C: Photochemistry Reviews*, 9(1), pp. 1–12.

11. Guillard, C., Herrmann, J.M., and Pichat, P., 1993. Heterogeneous photocatalysis: an emerging technology for water treatment. *Catalysis Today*, 17(1–2), pp. 7.

12. Herrmann, J.M., 1999. Water Treatment by Heterogeneous Photocatalysis. *In:* F. Jansen, R.A. van Santen (Eds.), Environmental Catalysis, Catalytic Science Series, Vol. 1, Imperial College Press, London, Chapter 9, pp. 171–194.

13. Ivanda, M., Music, S., Popovic, S., and Gotic, M., 1998. XRD, Raman and FTIR spectroscopic observations of nanosized TiO_2 synthesized by sol gel method based on an esterification reaction. *Journal of Molecular Structure*, pp. 645–649.

14. Legrini, O., Oliveros, E., and Braun, A.M., 1993. Photochemical processes for water treatment. *Chemical Reviews*, 93(2), pp. 671–698.

15. Martin, C., Martin, I., Rives, V., Grzybowska, B., and Gressel, I., 1996. A FTIR spectroscopy study of isopropanol reactivity on alkali-metal-doped MoO_3/TiO_2 catalysts. *Spectrochimica Acta* Part A, 52, pp. 733–740.

16. Mazloom, J., Ghodsi, F. E. and Gholami, M., 2013. Fiber-like stripe ATO (SnO_2:Sb) nanostructured thin films grown by sol gel method. *Journal of Alloys and Compounds*, 579, pp. 384–393.

17. More, A.T., Vira, A., and Fogel, S., 1989. Biodegradation of trans-1, 2-dichloroethylene by methane-utilizing bacteria in an aquifer simulator. *Environmental Science and Technology*, 23(4), pp. 403–406.

18. Nagaveni, K., Hedge, M. S., Ravishankar, N., Subbanna, N., and Madras, G., 2004. Synthesis and structure of nanocrystalline TiO$_2$ with lower band gap showing high photocatalytic activity. *Langmuir*, 20, pp. 2900–2907.

19. Patil, S.S., and Shinde, V.M., 1988. Biodegradation studies of aniline and nitrobenzene in aniline plat waste water by gas chromatography. *Environmental Science and Technology*, 22(10), pp. 1160–1165.

20. Scaranto, J., Pietropolli, A., Charmet, Stoppa, P., and Giorgianni, S., 2005. Vinyl halides adsorbed on TiO$_2$ surface: FTIR spectroscopy studies and ab initio calculations. *Journal of Molecular Structure*, 741, pp. 213–219.

21. Schiavello, M., 1988. Photocatalysis and Environment. *In:* Trends and Applications, Kluwer Academic Publishers, Dordrecht.

22. Slokar, Y.M., and Le Marechal, A.M., 1998. Methods of decoloration of textile wastewaters. *Dyes and Pigments*, 37(4), pp. 335–356.

23. Zolinger, H., 1991. Color Chemistry. *In:* Synthesis, Properties and Applications of Organic Dyes and Pigments, VCH, Germany.

Chapter 16

Synthesis and Characterization of Few-layer Graphene from High Purity Sri Lankan Vein Graphite

Iresha R. M. Kottegoda[1]*, Liyanage D.C. Nayanajith[1],
Xuanwen Gao[2], Jun Wang[2], Jia-Zhao Wang[2],
Hua-Kun Liu[2] and Yosef Gofer[3]

[1]*Materials Technology Section of Industrial Technology Institute,*
No. 363, Bauddhaloka Mawatha, Colombo 07, Sri Lanka
[2]*Institute for Superconducting and Electronic Materials,*
University of Wollongong, NSW 2519, Australia
[3]*Department of Chemistry, Bar Ilan University,*
Ramat-Gan, 5290002, Israel
*E-mail: iresha@iti.lk

ABSTRACT

We report the synthesis of good quality few-layer graphene on a large scale using high purity natural graphite available in Sri Lanka. The properties of graphene depend on the graphite source used to synthesize it. Each graphite source exhibits characteristic properties resulting unique graphene suitable for diverse applications. The work focused on synthesis of graphene from Sri Lankan vein graphite with purity exceeding 98 per cent. Initially, graphite oxide was synthesized from graphite using modified Hummer method. Subsequently, graphene was synthesized from the intermediate graphite oxide by a thermal method in an inert atmosphere. The as prepared graphene was characterized by X-ray diffraction, Fourier transform infrared spectroscopy, Scanning electron microscopy, Raman etc. The results indicate that the graphene prepared in the present study is highly exfoliated and it has a Brunauer-Emmett-Teller specific surface area of 398 m^2 g^{-1}. The graphene, which exists in stacks of only a few layers, supposed to be less than 7 layers, would be promising for vast variety of applications.

Keywords: *Graphite, Graphite oxide, Graphene, Characterization, Vein graphite.*

INTRODUCTION

Graphene is a single atomic layer of graphite arranged in a two-dimensional honeycomb lattice (Novoselov, 2004). It has become the focus of research among almost the entire scientific community (Novoselov, 2004; Geim, 2007; Berger, 2006; Geim, 2009; Li, 2008). A vast variety of practical applications are emerging, including the creation of new materials and the manufacture of innovative electronics (Hong, 2010; Ansari, 2009; Yong, 2010; Liang, 2009; Kottegoda, 2011; Guo, 2010). The most attractive feature of graphene is the possibility that it can be synthesized from natural graphite. The latter is a well known low-cost natural resource abundant in some countries such as Sri Lanka, Malagasy, Mexico, West Germany, and North and South Korea. The properties of graphene obviously depend on the graphite source used to synthesize it. In Sri Lanka alone, different graphite sources exhibit different chemical and physical characteristics and have purity levels suitable for different applications. Sri Lankan vein graphite with purity exceeding 98 per cent was used for the present study.

The development of an economical and efficient method to synthesize high quality graphene from graphite for a particular application is really a challenge. Simple as well as advanced chemical and physical methods have been used to isolate graphene from graphite. These include exfoliation (either physical/mechanical or chemical) (Pan, 2009; Guo, 2009) and solution based direct and indirect methodologies (Li, 2008; Nethravathi, 2008; Park, 2009, Stankovich, 2007). The present work is aimed at the synthesis and characterization of few-layer graphene on large scale using a thermal reduction method. The method adapted was a modification for thermal reduction methods in literature (Zhao, 2011; Li, 2012). Agitation method, heating and the firing step of graphite oxide was modified which enabled synthesis of graphene with high surface area on large scale.

MATERIALS AND METHOD

Natural graphite was obtained from Kahatagaha Graphite Lanka (Ltd.) in Sri Lanka. All other chemicals are of analytical grade and were used without any further purification.

Preparation of Materials

Graphite oxide (GO) was synthesized by modified Hummers method (Hummers 1958) and it was used to synthesize graphene by the hydrothermal method in our previous study (Kottegoda, 2011; Xu, 2009)]. In contrast a simple and low cost thermal reduction method was introduced to prepare multilayer graphene in the present study. The GO was dispersed in water by agitation for one hour. The mixture was then dried in an oven at 80 °C for 2 h. The resulting GO was fired at 500 °C in argon for

30 min. The enhancement of the conductivity marked the conversion of insulating GO to conducting graphene.

Materials Characterization

The morphology of the samples was investigated using a JEOL JSM 6460A scanning electron microscope. XRD analysis was carried out using a Regaku Ultima IV X-Ray Diffractometer with Cu Ka radiation and a graphite monochromator. X-ray photoelectronic spectroscopy (XPS) analyses were performed with a Kratos AXIS-HS spectrometer, using monochromatized Al Ka source. Scans ran at 150 W and measurements were carried out at room temperature, under vacuum conditions. FTIR spectra were collected using a Brooker Tenser 27. BET specific surface area was measured using a Tri Star 3000 analyzer by N_2 adsorption at 77 K. Raman spectroscopy was carried out using a JOBIN YVON HR800 Confocal Raman system with 632.8 nm diode laser excitation on a 300 lines/mm grating at room temperature.

RESULTS AND DISCUSSION

Figure 16.1 shows the schematic diagram of graphite, graphite oxide and few layer graphene prepared from Kahatagaha Graphite. The color of the GO synthesized from graphite was brilliant brown, in contrast to the normal observation of dark brown GO produced by the typical Hummers Method.

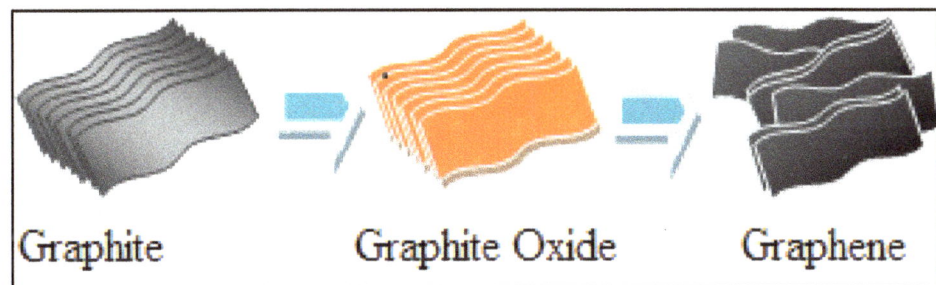

Figure 16.1: Schematic Diagram of Graphite, Graphite Oxide and Graphene

X-Ray Diffraction (XRD) Analysis

Figure 16.2 present the XRD spectra of graphene and graphite oxide (GO) synthesized from graphite. XRD spectrum of Graphite obtained from the Kahatagaha mines in Sri Lanka is also included as an inset. The sharp XRD peaks of graphite appeared at about 26° degrees indicate that the Graphite used to synthesized graphene and GO are highly crystalline. The disappearance of the characteristic 2q peak of graphite and the appearance of the GO peak at about 11° as in Figure 16.2(a), clearly shows that the graphite is completely converted to GO during the chemical oxidation. The GO is highly hydrophilic and well dispersed in water, in contrast to graphite. It retains its original laminar structure and shows sharp XRD peaks with considerable intensity. The corresponding *d*-spacing of the diffractions from the (002) plane for GO is about 0.85 nm and similar to the value obtained in our previous study (0.84 nm) (Kottegoda, 2011), The GO samples were reduced using thermal method in contrast to our previous work where hydrothermal reduction process was used. The

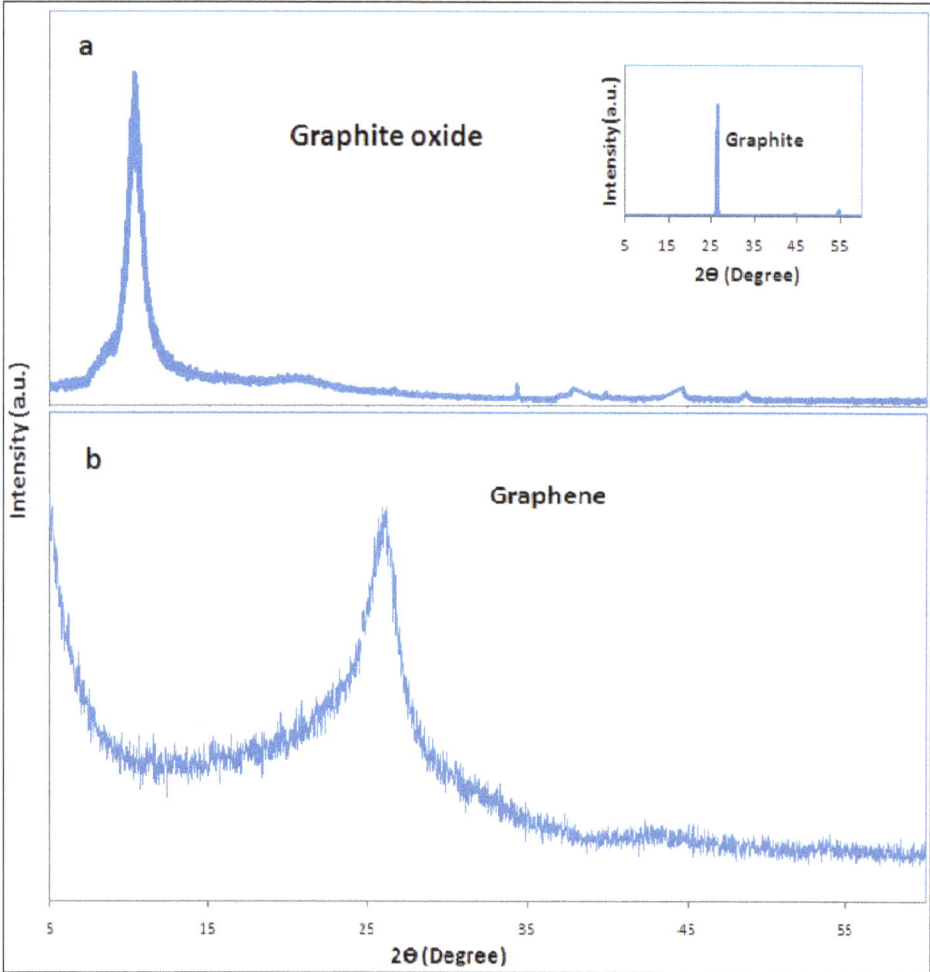

Figure 16.2: XRD Spectra of (a) Graphite Oxide,
(b) Few Layer Graphene, and Natural Graphite as an Inset of (a)

previous method was not efficient in terms of cost, time and yield therefore was not followed in the present study. The novel thermal reduction step introduced in the present study involves firing dried graphite oxide directly in argon flow which was effective in preparing graphene on a larger scale. Further purification (removal of oxygen functionalities) was achieved by further sintering in Argon for 1-2 hours depending on the sample purity.

The reduction of GO to graphene was noticeable with the disappearance of the corresponding XRD peak for GO. When the GO is reduced to graphene, there is a color change from brown to black (Figure 16.1), and the rigid graphite changes to flexible curly shape as shown in SEM images. The peak corresponding to graphite appears at about 2q = 26° in Figure 16.2 and is sharp and intense; whereas that of the few-layer graphene was broad and low in intensity. The peak for few-layer graphene is generally broader and less intense than the corresponding one for graphite, which is a common feature. The difference in broadness and sharpness is attributable to the presence of various functional groups such as C-OH, COOH, and COC in graphene. Most of the adsorbed OH groups and the other functional groups such as COOH are removed from the graphene structure on further reduction in argon. The crystalline size of graphene is about 1.2 nm, as derived from the Scherrer equation applied to the (002) plane. The smaller crystalline size of the graphene means that the surface area is high.

Field Emission Scanning Electron Microscopy (FE-SEM)

Graphene, when imaged via field emission scanning electron microscopy (FE-SEM), show disassembly of graphite stacks into large flexible graphene single sheets or stacks of several layers, which are oriented freely and appear similar to silky soft clothes (Figure 16.3). Graphene synthesized in this study seems to be stacked in few layers. The firing of graphite oxide in argon at high temperature resulted in rapid removal of oxygen and water in graphite oxide breaking the stacks in the original material similar to pop corn. In addition, the sintering in argon promotes further removal of oxygen and water remains in the structure and within graphene layers.

X-ray Photoelectronic Spectroscopy (XPS)

XPS analysis and FTIR analysis were conducted to identify the nature of oxygen functinalites present on graphene after being reduced from GO. C 1s XPS spectra of graphene and GO are compared in the Figure 16.4. The GO's carbon shows main unoxidized carbon (C-C) at 284.9 eV and large oxidized carbon at ca 286.2 eV. It has higher oxidation state carbon, at ca. 288.6 eV, which can be attributed to carboxyl and carboxylate groups. The presence of unoxidized carbon in GO indicates the presence of graphite stacks in the structure. The C 1s spectra of graphene also can be disintegrate into two main components as indicated in Figure 16.4 corresponding to different oxygen-containing functional groups. C-C (Graphene/graphite) at 284.9 eV and C-O at 286.2 eV.

The results reveal the existence of various oxidized carbon in graphene (after reduction from graphite oxide) as oxygen containing surface groups, like alcohols, ethers, carbonyls, quinons, and small amount of carboxylates (low intense peak at 288.7 eV). XPS analysis further reveals that graphene synthesized in this study still containing oxygen functionalities, though the percentage is low. However, further removal of these oxygen containing groups is necessary for further improvement of the conductivity and the other properties of graphene. Longer time firing under argon or high temperature firing (above 800°C) under argon would further remove the oxygen containing functional groups in the structure.

Fourier Transform Infrared Spectroscopy (FTIR)

FTIR analysis of graphene and GO are indicated in Figure 16.5 which also indicative the presence of various functional groups on graphene structure. Graphite loses its extended conjugated orbital system on oxidation with strong acids and attaches oxygen-containing functional groups such as COH and COC, acquiring

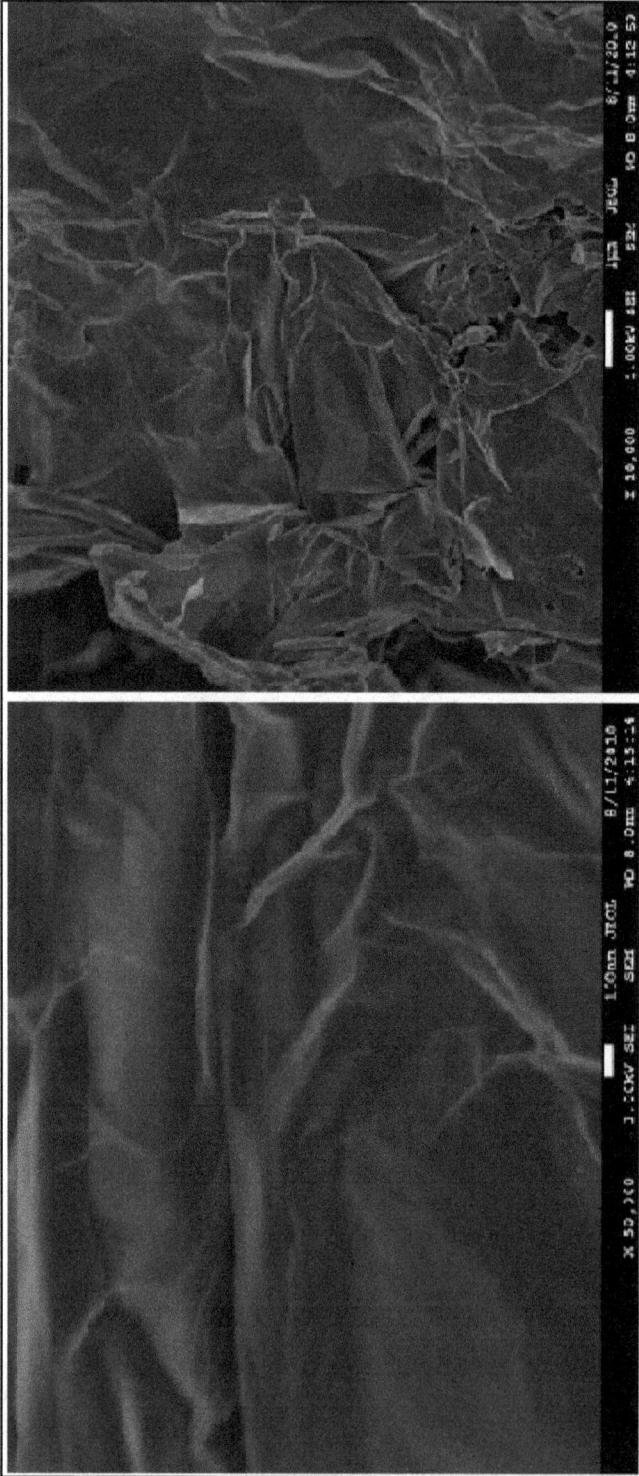

Figure 16.3: FE-SEM Images of Few Layer Graphene

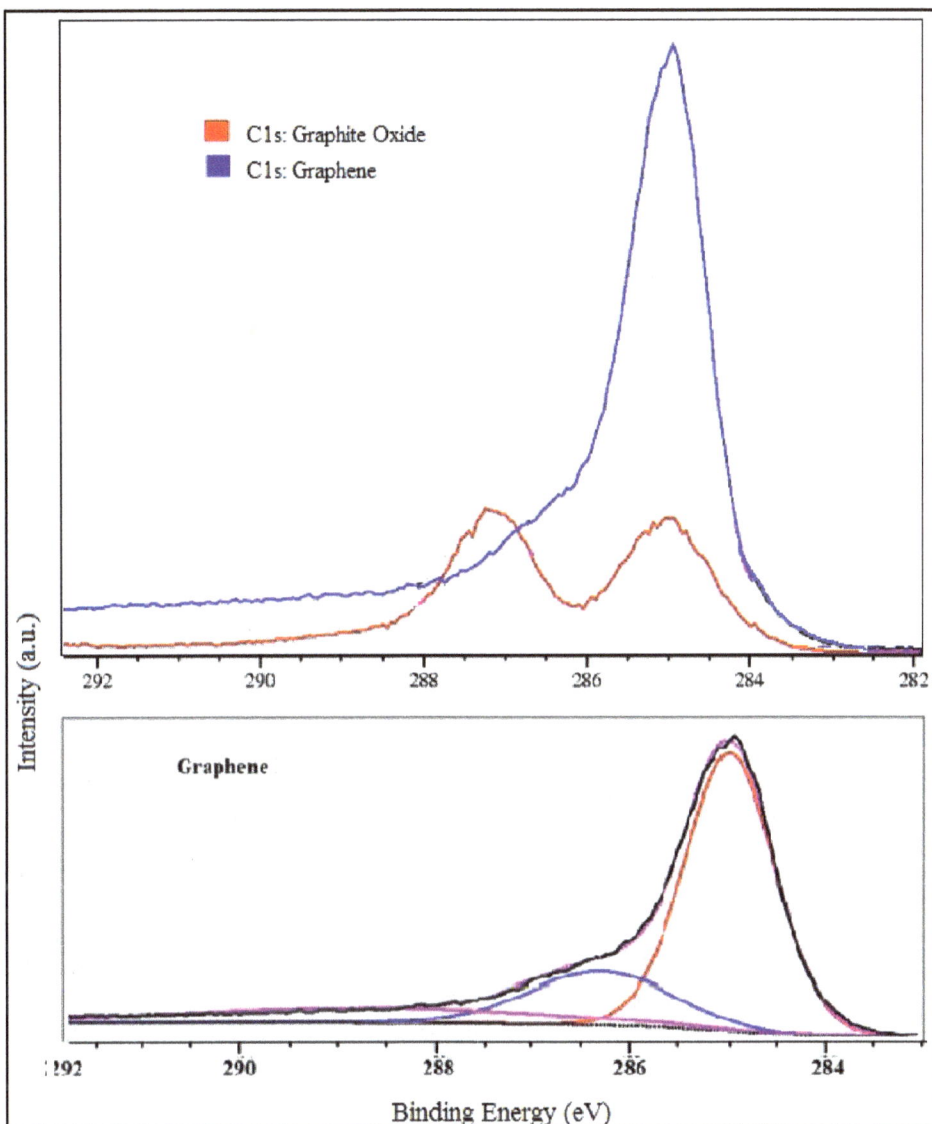

Figure 16.4: C 1s XPS Spectra of Graphite Oxide and Graphene

insulating properties. The formation of GO can be observed through the reduction of the conductivity of the original graphite and observation of the corresponding peaks for GO through FTIR (Szabo, 2005; Paek, 2009).

The broad peak ranging from 3800–2200 cm^{-1} is attributable to O–H stretching vibrations of absorbed water molecules and structural OH groups prominent for GO, indicating high inclusion and/or attachment of water to the GO structure. The peak in the low frequency region close to 1622 cm^{-1} in Graphite Oxide is attributable to O-H vibrations of water, which observed to be reduced on formation of graphene,

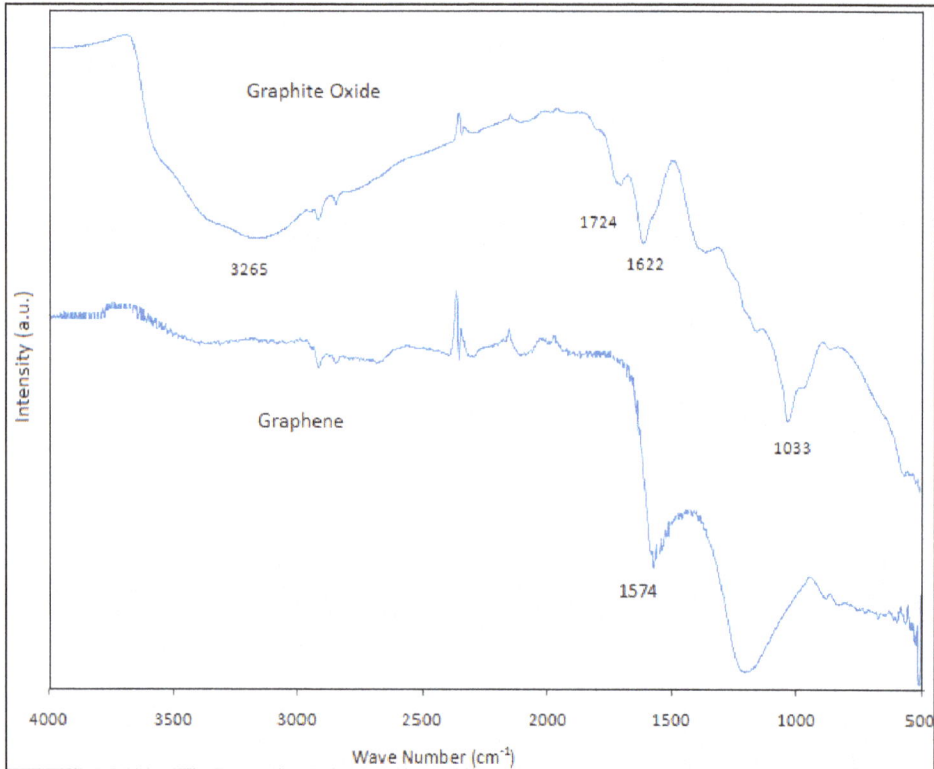

Figure 16.5: FTIR Spectra of Graphite Oxide and Graphene

since the samples are annealed at high temperature (Szabo, 2005). The slight difference in the peak position for the sample from literature believed to be due to the difference in hydrogen bonding and other interactions which are unique to the samples, although further experimental evidence and further investigation are required to support this argument. Relatively weak peaks for the functional groups, such as C=O ($1724\ cm^{-1}$ were observed after the reduction of GO, demonstrating that the amounts of most of the oxide groups attached to or included in the material have been reduced. The peak at $1622\ cm^{-1}$ was also reduced upon reduction of GO, indicating that they are mostly from H_2O. The band ranging from 3800–$2200\ cm^{-1}$ (O-H stretching vibration) is reduced, but not eliminated completely, even by firing at high temperature ($500\,°C$), which allows the remaining component to be assigned to structural OH groups of reduced GO. The adsorbed water is completely removed at that temperature. The appearance of a new peak at about $1574\ cm^{-1}$ reflects the skeletal vibration of graphene (C-C) (Szabo, 2005), which is further increased when the as-prepared graphene is further annealed under argon flow for a few hours. The adsorbed water and many of the other surface groups seems to be reduced in the structure. Therefore, FTIR spectral data also support the fact that the GO has been reduced to graphene, although groups such as C-OH are present to certain extent which should be further reduced or may even be beneficial to some applications.

The resistance of graphene was reduced from 5.00 kW to 0.01 kW after argon treatment longer, which also supports the argument that the reduction of surface functional groups such as C-OH, C-O-C, and C-OO occurs after the argon treatment which improves the conductivity. Highly conducting nature of graphene synthesized by the present method would be beneficial in application as anode in lithium ion batteries. The electrochemical performance study of graphene is in progress which would be published separately. There is a possibility even to replace the conductor used in anode fabrication partially using high conducting graphene which has high surface area as shown below.

BET Specific Surface Area Analysis

Since graphene is composed of a monolayer of carbon atoms packed into a dense honeycomb crystal structure, the inherent surface area of a sample with single graphene sheets can be as high as <"2630 m^2 g^{-1} (Paek 2009, Stoller 2008). Graphene synthesized by chemical methods, however, is always in the forms of stacks of several graphene layers. In the present study, the BET surface analysis revealed the specific surface areas of Graphene to be 398 m^2 g^{-1}, suggesting that the degree of exfoliation of graphite layers is high or sheet size of Graphene is small and therefore it is few layer graphene. The presence of extremely thin layers of graphene is also observed through FE-SEM suggesting extensive exfoliation. BET surface area analysis, however, is not a direct measurement of the degree of exfoliation of graphite; nevertheless, it can support the observation of exfoliation of graphite.

Raman Spectroscopy

The Raman spectra for graphene are shown in Figure 16.6. Raman spectroscopy is a powerful non-destructive technique to study carbonaceous materials such as graphene and also for examining the ordered and disordered crystal structures and distinguishing the single and multilayer characteristics of graphene layers (Guo, 2009; Stoller, 2008; Stankovich, 2006). In perfect graphite, the G band is highly intense (in-plane bond stretching motion of C sp^2 pairs), whereas the D band is generally active in the presence of high disorder in the graphene. Furthermore, G-band was observed at about 1581 cm^{-1} during the present study. It had been shown that the peak frequency of the G band of the single layer graphene at 1585 cm^{-1} shifts about 6 cm^{-1} into lower frequencies after stacking several graphene layers. For 2–6 layers of graphene G band have even shifts to 1579 cm^{-1}. Therefore G-band at 1581 cm^{-1} is attributable to mostly few layer (<6) graphene (Guo, 2009; Stoller, 2008; Stankovich, 2006).

Sri Lanka natural graphite had been shown high capacity and rate capability as an anode in Lithium ion batteries exceeding the theoretical capacity of graphite (Kottegoda, 2002; Kottegoda, 2005). The preliminary investigation revealed that the graphene synthesized in the present study also exhibits high capacity and rate capability as will be revealed in our future studies. In addition few layer graphene showed good conductivity as filler in conductive polymer which needs to be study further.

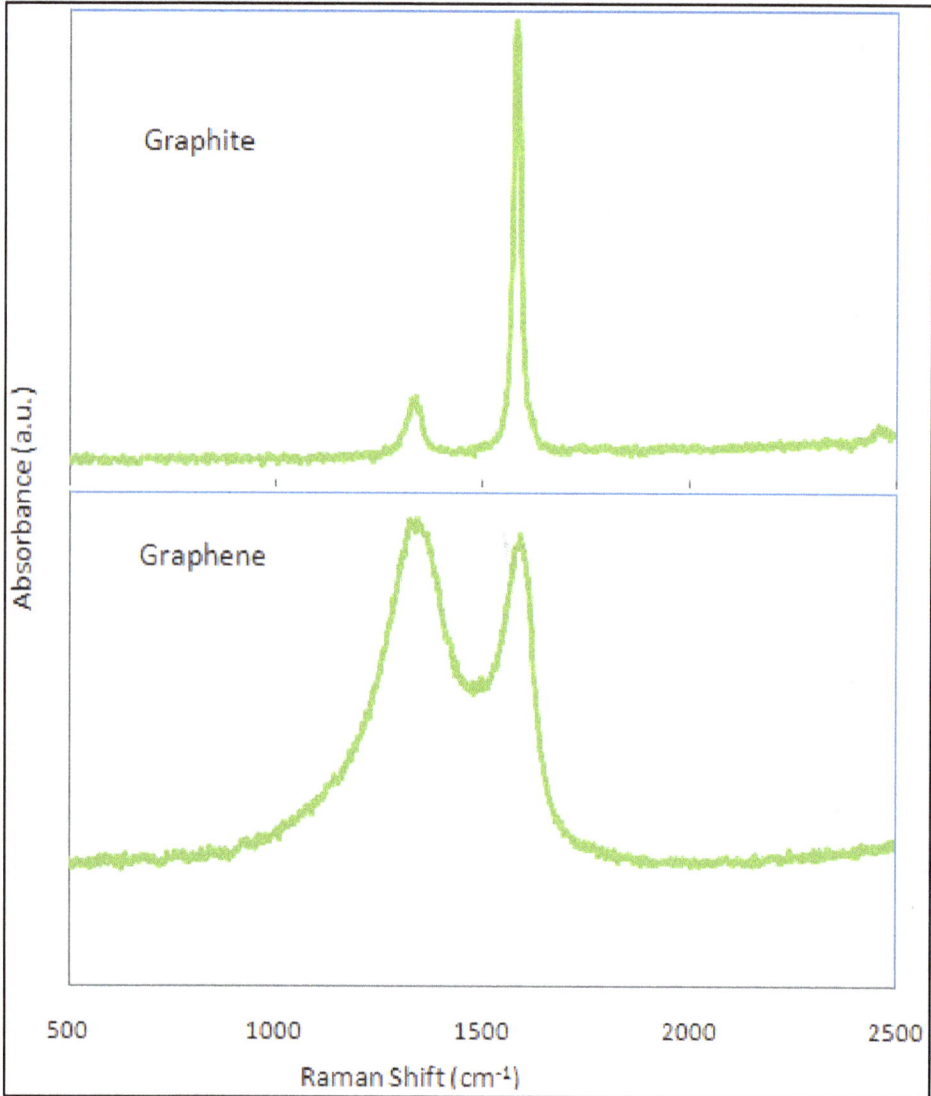

Figure 16.6: Raman Spectra of Graphite and Graphene

CONCLUSIONS

Few-layer graphene synthesized from high purity vein graphite from Sri Lanka showed high surface area. The thermal reduction method to prepare graphene from graphite oxide was found to be an effective method to prepare graphene on a large scale. The multilayer graphene synthesized from Sri Lankan graphite has the potential to be used in future electronic devices.

ACKNOWLEDGEMENTS

Financial support provided by Australian Research Council (ARC) and NRC/ Treasury Grant Sri Lanka. Authors thank Mr. Amila Jayasinghe from Sri Lanka and Dr. Feher Robert from Germany for their support in BET analysis.

REFERENCES

1. Ansari S, Giannelis EP (2009). *J Polym Sci* Pt B – Polym Phys 47(9): 888–897.

2. Berger C, Song ZM, Li XB, Wu XS, Brown N, Naud C, *et al.* (2006). *Science* 312: 1191-1196.

3. Geim AK (2009). *Science* 324: 1530-1534.

4. Geim AK, Novoselov KS (2007). *Nat Mater* 6: 183-191.

5. Guo SJ, Dong SJ, Wang EW (2010). *ACS Nano* 4(1): 547–555.

6. Guo HL, Wang XF, Qian QY, Wang FB, Xia XH (2009). *ACS Nano* 3: 2653-2659.

7. Hong WJ, Bai H, Xu YX, Yao ZY, Gu ZZ, Shi GQ (2010*). J Phys Chem C* 114(4): 1822–1826.

8. Hummers WS, Offeman RE (1958). *J Am Chem* Soc 80: 1339.

9. Liang MH, Zhi LJ (2009). *J Mater Chem* 19 (33): 5871–5878.

10. Li D Muller MB, Gilje S, Kaner RB, Wallace GG (2008). *Nat Nanotechnol* 3: 101-105.

11. Li T, Gao L (2012). *J Solid State Electrochem* 16: 557–561.

12. Li XL, Wang XR, Zhang L, Lee SW, Dai HJ (2008). *Science* 319: 1229-1232.

13. Nethravathi C, Rajamathi M (2008). *Carbon* 46: 1994-1998.

14. Novoselov KS, Geim AK, Morozov SV, Jiang D, Zhang Y, Dubonos SV, *et al.* (2004). *Science* 306: 666-669.

15. Pan D, Wang S, Zhao B Wu M, Zhang H, Wang Y, *et al.* (2009). *Chem Mater* 21:3136-3142.

16. Park S, Ruoff RS (2009). Nat Nanotechnol. 4: 217-224.

17. Kottegoda IRM, Idris NH, Lu L., Wang JZ, Liu HK (2011). *Electrochim Acta* 56: 5815-5822.

18. Kottegoda IRM, Kadoma Y, Ikuta H, Uchimoto Y, Wakihara M (2002). *Electrochem Solid-State Lett* 5(12): A275-A278.

19. Kottegoda IRM, Kadoma Y, Ikuta H, Uchimoto Y, Wakihara MJ (2005). *Electrochem Soc* 152 (8):A, 1595-99.

20. Paek SM, Yoo EJ, Honma I (2009). *Nano Lett* 9: 72-75.

21. Stoller MD, Park SJ, Zhu YW, An JH, Ruoff RS (2008). *Nano Lett* 8(10):3498-3492

22. Stankovich S, Dikin DA, Dommett G H B, Kohlhaas KM, Zimney E J, Stach EA, *et al.* (2006). *Nature* 442(7100): 282-6.

23. Stankovich S, Dikin DA, Piner RD, Kohlhaas KA, Kleinhammes A, Jia Y, *et al.* (2007). *Carbon* 45: 1558–1565.

24. Szabo T, Berkesi O, Dekany I (2005). *Carbon* 43(15): 3186-3189.

25. Xu C, Wang X, Yang L, Wu Y (2009). *J Solid State Chem* 182:2486-2490.

26. Yong V, Tour JM (2010). *Small* 6(2): 313–318.

27. Zhao X, C. Hayner M, Kung MC, Kung HH (2011). *Adv Energy Mater* 1: 1079–1084.

Chapter 17

Anacardic Acid Capped Metal Chalcogenide Nanoparticles

S. Mlowe[1,2], E.B. Mubofu[2], F.N. Ngassapa[2]
and N. Revaprasadu[1]*

[1]*Department of Chemistry, University of Zululand,
Private Bag X1001, Kwa-Dlangezwa, 3886, South Africa*
[2]*Department of Chemistry, University of Dares Salaam,
P.O. Box 35061, Dares Salaam, Tanzania*
*E-mail: ebmubofu@gmail.com

ABSTRACT

Nanotechnology is increasingly being exploited in almost all diverse fields and has led to scientific and another or next industrial revolution. Thus no country would like to be left behind in accruing the benefits of this promising field. In Tanzania, nanotechnology is in its infancy stage and few research groups exist and are involved in nanomaterials. The groups are mostly researching on the synthesis and application of nanomaterials as in water purification, catalysis, drug delivery and energy. This paper report results of some of the ongoing researches where a naturally occurring oil, anacardic acid is used as a capping agent in the synthesis of well dispersed metal chalcogenides. The low temperature synthesis of anacardic acid capped lead and cadmium chalcogenide nanoparticles is discussed. The potential of this work lies in the use of greener solvent (anacardic acid) in the synthesis of lead and cadmium chalcogenide nanoparticles at reasonably low temperature. The anacardic acid capped PbE (E=Se, Te and S) nanoparticles in the shape of spheres and cubes have been synthesized via a solution based reaction and thermolysis at 140 °C and 160 °C. Similarly, anacardic acid capped CdE (E = S, Se and Te) nanoparticles displayed sharp absorption bands and characteristic strong Stokes shifted emission peaks. These semiconductor nanoparticles capped by anacardic acid, an environmentally benign naturally occurring capping ligand were synthesized at relatively low temperature.

Keywords: *Anacardic acid, Metal chalcogenide, Nanoparticles, Optical properties, Electron microscopy.*

INTRODUCTION

Cadmium and lead chalcogenide (CdE and PbE where E = S, Se and Te) nanomaterials offer enormous interest in applications such as biomedical labeling reagents (Bruchez *et al.*, 1998: Chan and Nie, 1998), photovoltaic and optoelectronic devices (Greenham *et al.*, 1996: Mokari *et al.*, 2007: Wang *et al.*, 2005). The Bohr radii of PbE for example, show that these materials exhibit strong quantum confinement. The unique optical properties of these nanomaterials are dictated by their structure, shape and size, and rendering them tunable band gap, which are frequently used to emit wide range of wavelength.

Synthetic methodologies employing surface passivating agents such as amines and thiols are commonly used to control the particle size at the nanodimensional level so as to achieve quantum confinement. Various synthetic routes such as microwave irradiation (Zhu *et al.*, 2000), solvothermal (Gautham and Sheshadri, 2004; Xie *et al.*, 2000), chemical bath deposition (Raniero *et al.*, 2010), interfacial deposition, (Thomas *et al.*, 2013) are available/common for the synthesis of chalcogenide nanoparticles. Moreover, high temperature thermolysis has been used in the synthesis of cadmium chalcogenide nanoparticles wherein dimethyl cadmium was used as the cadmium source (Murray *et al.*, 1993) while tri-n-octylphosphine chalcogenide (TOPE) was the chalcogenide source. This method however is deemed not suitable for large scale production of nanomaterials due to the high reaction temperatures and the toxic nature of the metal alkyl. To overcome these drawbacks, three alternative methods have been proposed and developed. Firstly, the design of low temperature processing methods (He and Gu 2006), replacing $(CH_3)_2Cd$ as Cd-metal source by CdO (Boatman *et al.*, 2005) and other Cd metal salts (Maseko *et al.*, 2010: Mntungwa *et al.*, 2011) and lastly the use of safe, cheaper, natural and more air stable coordinating solvents (Akhtar *et al.*, 2010: He and Gu 2006: Sapra *et al.*, 2006). Recently, we reported the synthesis of lead chalcogenide nanoparticles capped by anacardic acid, a naturally occurring oil which is extracted from cashew nut shell liquid (CNSL) (Mlowe *et al.*, 2013). The potential of this work is in using the greener solvent (anacardic acid) in the synthesis of chalcogenide nanoparticles at relatively low temperature.

MATERIALS AND METHODS

Materials and Instruments

All chemicals used were of analytical grade and of highest purity available. Selenium powder, tellurium powder, sulfur powder, sodium borohydride (NaBH$_4$), lead and cadmium carbonates, deionized water, methanol, toluene and tri-*n*-octylphosphine (TOP) were purchased from Sigma-Aldrich. Anacardic acid was isolated from solvent extracted cashew nut shell liquid (CNSL) using the method described by Paramashivappa *et al.*, 2001, with slight modifications as reported by Lucio *et al.*, 2010. A Varian Cary 50 Conc UV-Visible spectrophotometer was used to carry out the optical measurements. Photoluminescence of the particles was done using a Perkin-Elmer LS 55 Luminescence spectrometer. The crystalline phase was identified by X-ray diffraction (XRD), employing a scanning rate of 0.05° min^{-1} in a 2θ range from 20 to 80°, using a Bruker AXS D8 diffractometer equipped with nickel filtered Co Kα radiation (λ = 1.5418 Å) at 40 kV, 40 mA and at room temperature. JEOL 1010 TEM with an accelerating voltage of 100 kV, Megaview III camera, and Soft Imaging Systems iTEM software was used to determine the morphology. HRTEM was done with a JEOL 2010 transmission electron microscope operated at an accelerating voltage of 200 kV.

Solvent Extraction of CNSL from cashew nut shells

Several pre-treatment processes were carried out on the cashew nut samples (*Anacardium occidentale*) prior to extraction process to ensure a high degree of purity. The processes include washing, drying, de-shelling as well as pulverizing in order to create a better surface area exposure of the shells to the solvent to improve extraction of the CNSL. In this method, solvents were used to extract the CNSL from the shells of the cashew nuts (Paramashivappa *et al.*, 2001). The shells were soaked in petroleum ether for 3 days to result into a brown oily product (CNSL) which contains a mixture of compounds. This was followed by solvent removal from the coloured liquid under reduced pressure using a rotary evaporator at about 40°C. Solvent extracted cashew nut shell liquid contains anacardic acid (60-65 per cent), cardanol (10 per cent), cardol (15-20 per cent) and traces of methylcardol (Figure 17.1).

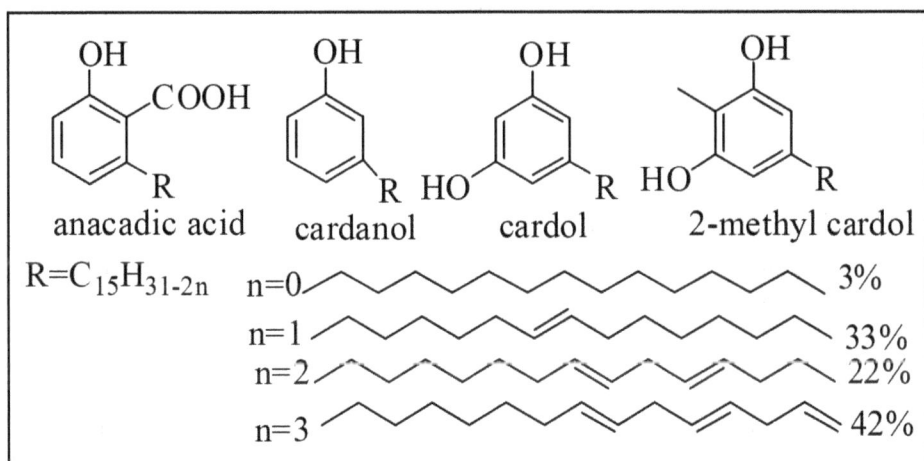

Figure 17.1: Components of Cashew Nut Shell Liquid

Isolation of Anacardic Acid from CNSL

The isolation of anacardic acid from CNSL was carried out using a procedure reported by Paramashivappa *et al.*, 2001, with slight modifications reported by Lucio *et al.*, 2010. Anacardic acid was selectively isolated as calcium anacardate. The isolation was carried out by dissolving the extracted CNSL (50 g) in 5 per cent aqueous methanol (300 mL) followed by addition of calcium hydroxide (25 g) with stirring. Then the reaction was left at room temperature for 24 h. Calcium anacardate precipitates were vacuum-filtered and washed thoroughly with 5 per cent aqueous methanol (200 mL). The crushed calcium anacardate cake was transferred into a flask contained a stirred mixture of 6.0 M HCl (200 mL) and 300 mL of ethyl acetate. The mixture was stirred for 1 h. The organic layer was washed twice with distilled water (100 mL), dried over anhydrous sodium sulphate and concentrated under reduced pressure using a rotary evaporator to yield anacardic acid (heterogeneous mixture of saturated, monoene, diene, and triene).

Synthesis of CdE and PbE Nanoparticles

The chalcogen powder was reduced to the corresponding ion by adding 0.32 mmol of chalcogen powder to 20.0 mL of deionized water in a three neck flask at room temperature. A 0.79 mmol solution of sodium borohydride was added to the flask contents and the flask was purged with nitrogen flow to create an inert atmosphere. The reduction reaction was carried out for 2 h with continuous stirring. A 0.32 mmol solution of the cadmium salt was added to the reduced ion solution and stirred for 5 min, followed by the addition of excess methanol to form the bulk CdE which was isolated by centrifugation and dispersed in 6.0 mL of TOP. The resultant CdE-TOP mixture was then injected into 6.0 g of anacardic acid, pre-heated to 140 °C. The reaction temperature was kept for between 1 hour and 2 hours. The reaction contents were then cooled to room temperature, followed by the addition of excess methanol to flocculate the nanoparticles. The anacardic acid capped CdE nanoparticles were isolated after centrifugation. The synthetic method of PbE (E = S, Se, Te) is similar to that of CdE and involved the reduction of sulfur, selenium or tellurium powder with sodium borohydride ($NaBH_4$) to produce sulfide, selenide or telluride ions. This was followed by the reaction with a lead salt where the as-formed lead chalcogenide was thermolysed in an anacardic acid (140°C or 160°C) to form the nanocrystalline materials.

RESULTS AND DISCUSSION

The coordinating solvent plays a crucial role in controlling the growth process, stabilizing the resulting nanoparticles dispersion, and electronically passivating the semiconductor surface (Murray *et al.*, 1993). Anacardic acid was chosen in this work as it is a naturally occurring oil solvent extracted from cashew nut shell liquid which is found in abundance in Tanzania. Furthermore, anarcadic acid has a bulky alkyl chain with a carboxylic functionality and boils at 179 °C. Overall this preparation route is environmentally friendly because it uses relatively lower reaction temperature and anarcadic acid is a naturally occurring solvent.

Optical Properties

Figures 17.2(a-c) show the absorption and photoluminescence spectra of anacardic acid capped CdS, CdSe and CdTe nanoparticles synthesized at 140°C. All three spectra show the effect of quantum confinement. CdS, CdSe and CdTe absorption peaks were at lower wavelength which indicates the blue shift with reference to that of their 515, 716 and 827 nm bulky band gaps respectively. The CdSe spectrum shows three distinct resolved electronic transitions, which could be assigned to the excitonic absorption features of a nanosized CdSe particle (Ithuria *et al.*, 2008). This has been theoretically predicted (Efros *et al.*, 1996) and experimentally shown for CdSe nanoparticles thermolysed via an organometallic route (Norris *et al.*, 1996). For

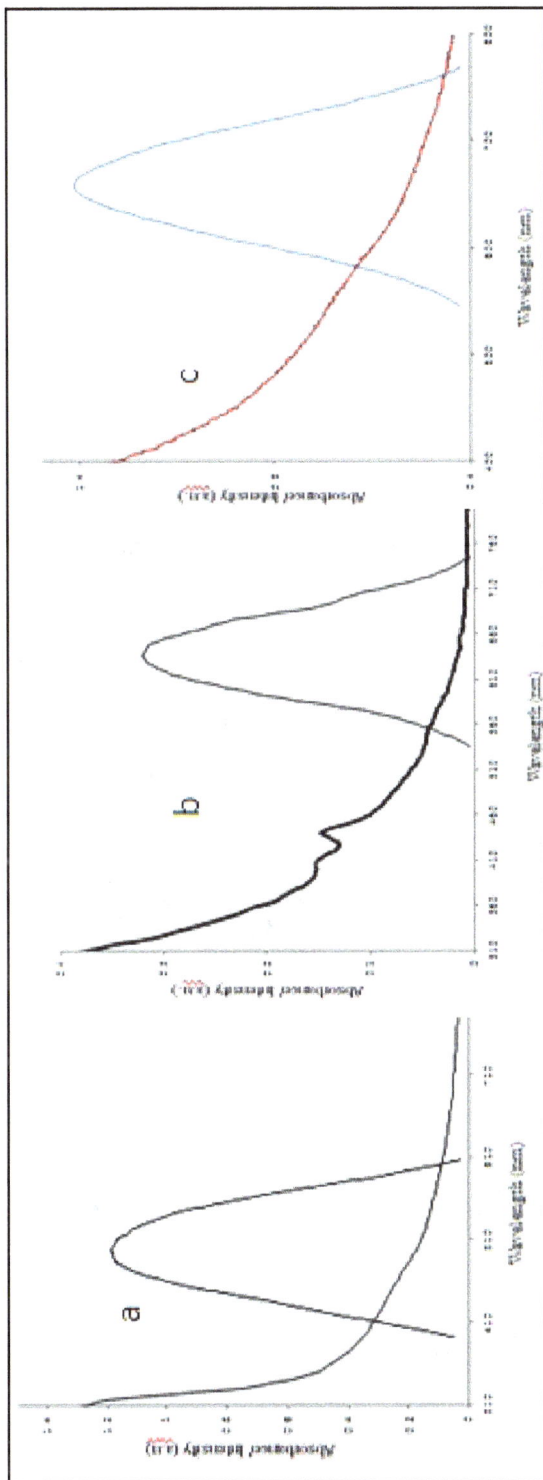

Figure 17.2(a-c): Absorption and Photoluminescence (PL) Spectra of Anacardic Acid Capped (a) CdS, (b) CdSe and (c) CdTe Nanoparticles respectively as Synthesised at 140 °C

CdSe, the emission peak is red shifted to that of absorption maximum, which can be attributed to a combination of relaxation into shallow trap states and the size distribution (Bawendi *et al.*, 1992). All three PL spectra justify highly monodispersed samples and narrow emission line widths indicating growth of nanoparticles with few electronic defect sites as a result of the efficiency of anacardic acid to electronically passivate the nanoparticles.

Structural Properties

Figure 17.3 shows the TEM and HRTEM images of anacardic acid capped PbSe synthesized at 140 °C. Both anacardic acid capped PbSe and PbS nanoparticles had/ have close to spherical shapes while those of PbTe were cubes. The observed shape of PbS particles is similar to the olive oil capped PbS nanoparticles earlier reported by other workers (Akhtar *et al.*, 2010). The PbSe nanoparticles formed were regular and predominantly spherical shaped particles. Some particles are joined together to form chain-like aggregate particles which are vivid in the TEM images in Figure 17.3. The average particle size of the spheres was 13.25 ± 3.35 nm. The corresponding HRTEM image shows that the particles are single crystals with observable distinct lattice fringes (Figure 17.3c). The lattice spacing of 3.22 Å was estimated from the HRTEM image which is assigned to the [200] plane of PbSe. The HRTEM images also provided

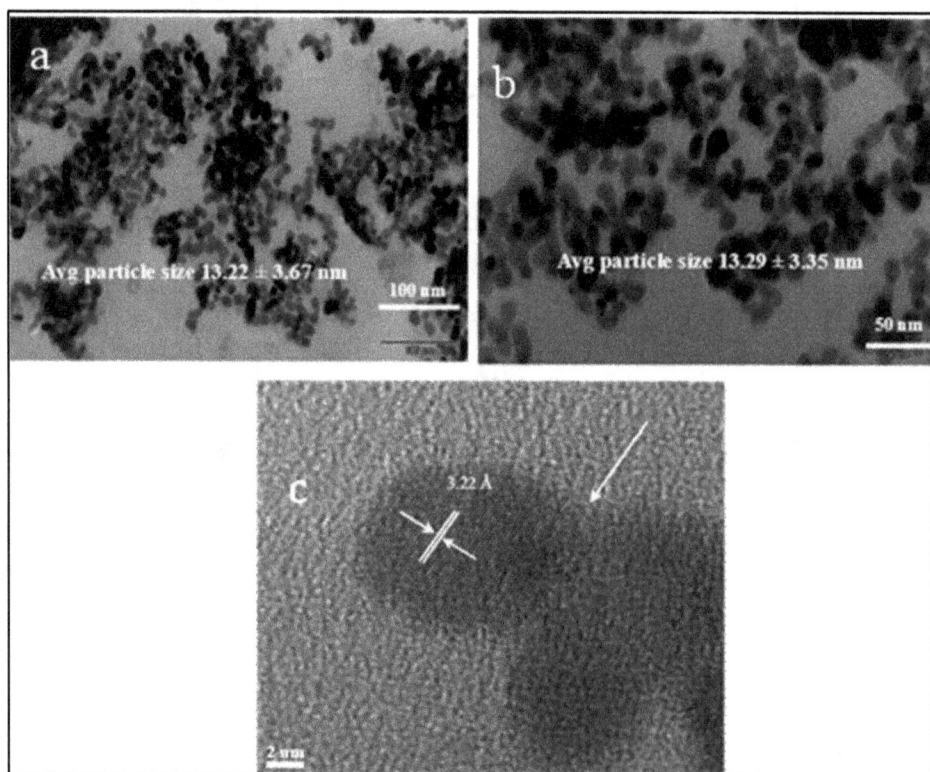

Figure 17.3: TEM and HRTEM Images of Anacardic Acid Capped PbSe Nanoparticles Synthesized at 140 °C when PbCl$_2$ was Used as Lead Source (1h)

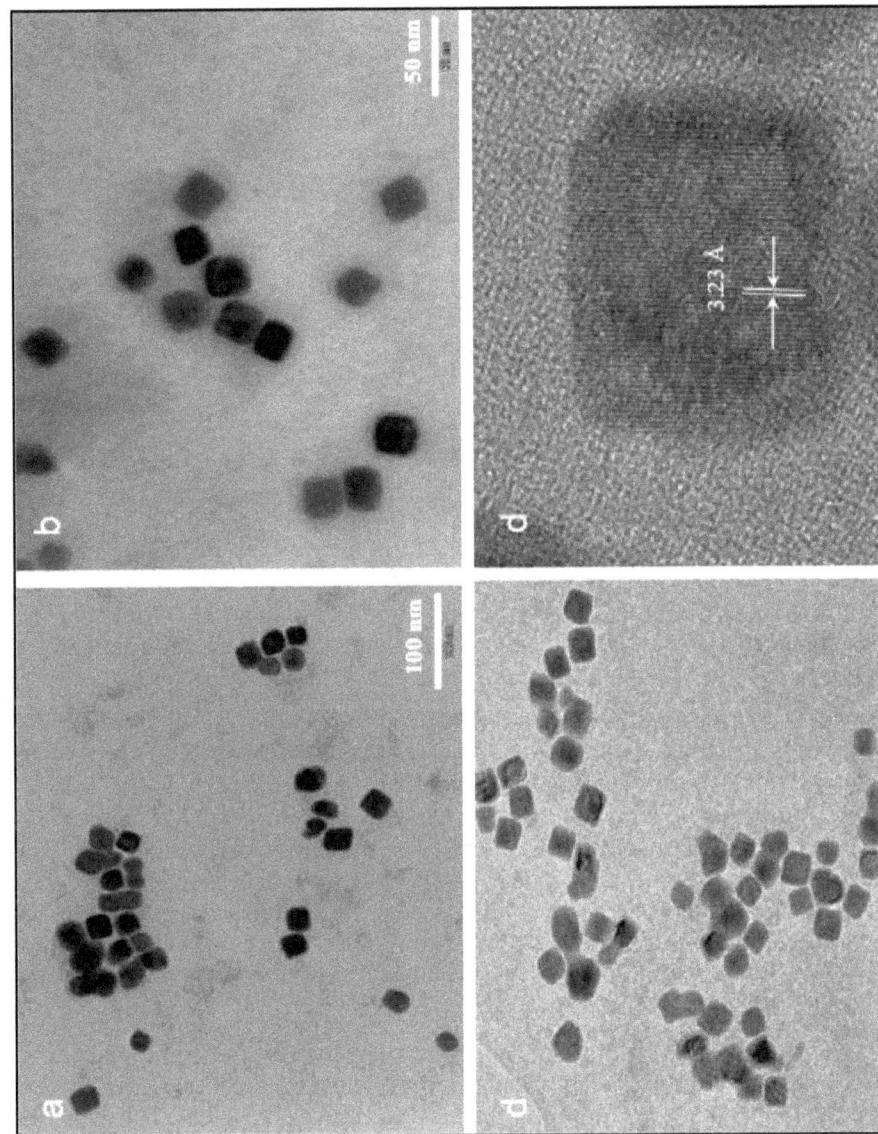

Figure 17.4: TEM and HRTEM Images of Anacardic Acid Capped PbTe Nanoparticles Synthesized at 160 °C when PbCl$_2$ was Used as Lead Source (1h)

further evidence for the fusion of particles. There are discontinuities in the lattice fringes as shown by the arrows which suggest that growth occurs via an oriented attachment mechanism. There have been previous reports of PbSe nanowires formed through the oriented attachment of nanocrystal building blocks by Cho *et al.*, 2005.

The anacardic acid capped PbTe synthesized in the same way as PbSe nanoparticles had regular cubes with an average size of 24.4 ± 4.10 nm as shown in Figure 17.4. It has been previously reported by Lee *et al.*, that lead chalcogenide nanoparticles undergo shape evolution from spherical to cubic with increasing particle size (Lee *et al.*, 2002). In a separate work by Ziqubu *et al.*, hexadecylamine(HDA) capped PbTe nanoparticles displayed shapes close to spheres and rods (Ziqubu *et al.*, 2010). The growth rate on different facets of the particles is usually dominated by the surface energy. The cubic rock salt structure of PbTe possesses different surface energies and hence allows particle growth to occur along different facets. It is apparent from this work that anacardic acid capping group allows the [111] facet to grow faster than the lower surface energy [100] face, favoring the formation of cubes (Dowty, 1976). The cubic morphology is also confirmed by the HRTEM (Figure 17.4 d) image which shows a cube shaped particle with distinct lattice fringes with lattice spacing of 3.23 Å that are assigned to the (200) cubic PbTe.

The X-ray diffraction pattern of PbS has broad peaks that are assigned to the (111), (200) and (220) planes of cubic PbS (Figure 17.5a). The X-ray diffraction pattern of PbSe show peaks corresponding to the (111), (200) and (220) reflections of cubic PbSe. For the PbTe, the (111), (200), (220) and (222) planes of cubic PbTe are visible in the X-ray diffraction pattern (Figure 17.5c). The estimated particle size from the XRD analysis using the Scherrer equation are 11.67 nm, 12.49 nm and 23.24 nm for PbS, PbSe and PbTe nanoparticles respectively. The estimated sizes are in good agreement with the TEM size measurements.

Figure 17.6 (c) shows the TEM image of the anacardic acid capped CdS nanoparticles synthesized at 140 °C. The particles are anisotropic ranging from oblate to elongated shaped particles with an average size of 13.42 ± 2.1 nm. The anacardic acid capped CdSe nanoparticles and CdTe nanoparticles also showed anisotropic morphologies. The CdTe particles (Figure 17.6b) were more oblate in shape with an average size of 15.80 ± 2.8 nm. The assembly of all anacardic acid capped CdS, CdSe and CdTe nanoparticles are well ordered, mosaic type arrangement of particles as seen in the TEM images (Figure 17.6c). There is almost an equal inter particle distance of approximately 3 nm for the CdS, CdSe and CdTe particles as observed from the TEM images.

Figure 17.7 (a) shows the powder X-ray diffraction pattern of the anacardic acid capped CdS nanoparticles. The XRD pattern indicate a hexagonal phase due to the presence of (100), (002), (101), (102), (110) and (103) reflection planes. The average crystallite size was calculated to be 12.84 nm, using the Scherrer formula (Patterson, 1939) close to the size determined by TEM.

The wide angle powder X-ray diffraction peaks (Figure 17.7 b) of the as-synthesized anacardic acid capped CdSe nanoparticles show five distinct peaks for a wurtzite crystalline structure of the bulk materials. The diffraction peaks at 2θ

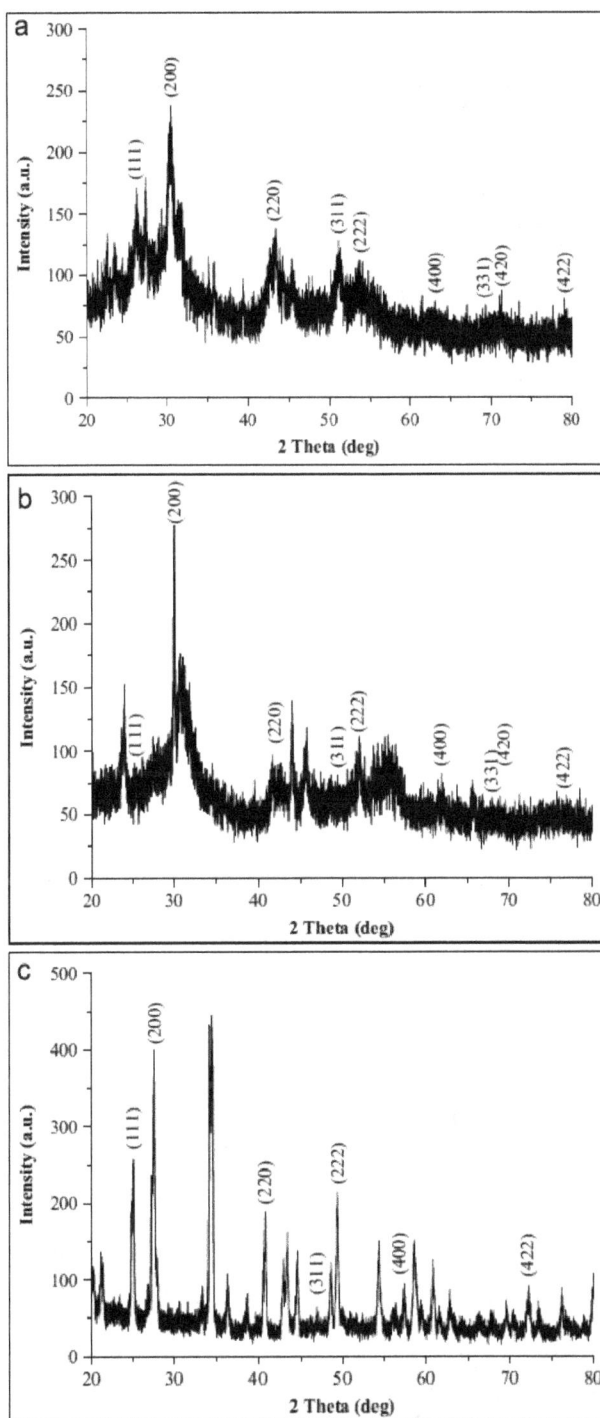

Figure 17.5: Powder X-ray Diffraction Spectra of Anacardic Acid Capped
(a) PbS, (b) PbSe and (c) PbTe Nanoparticles

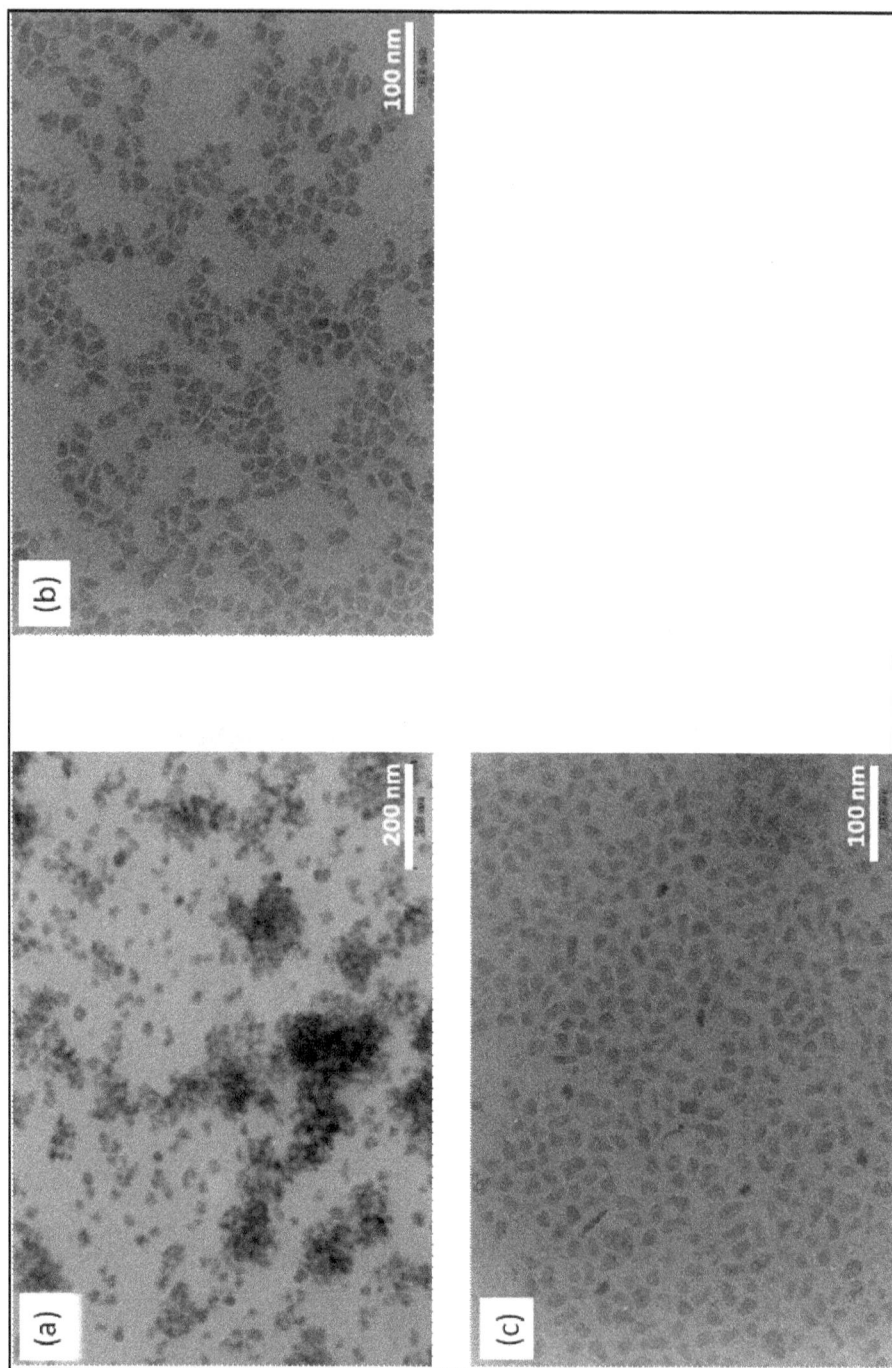

Figure 17.6: TEM (a, b, c) Images of Anacardic Acid Capped CdSe, CdTe and CdS respectively

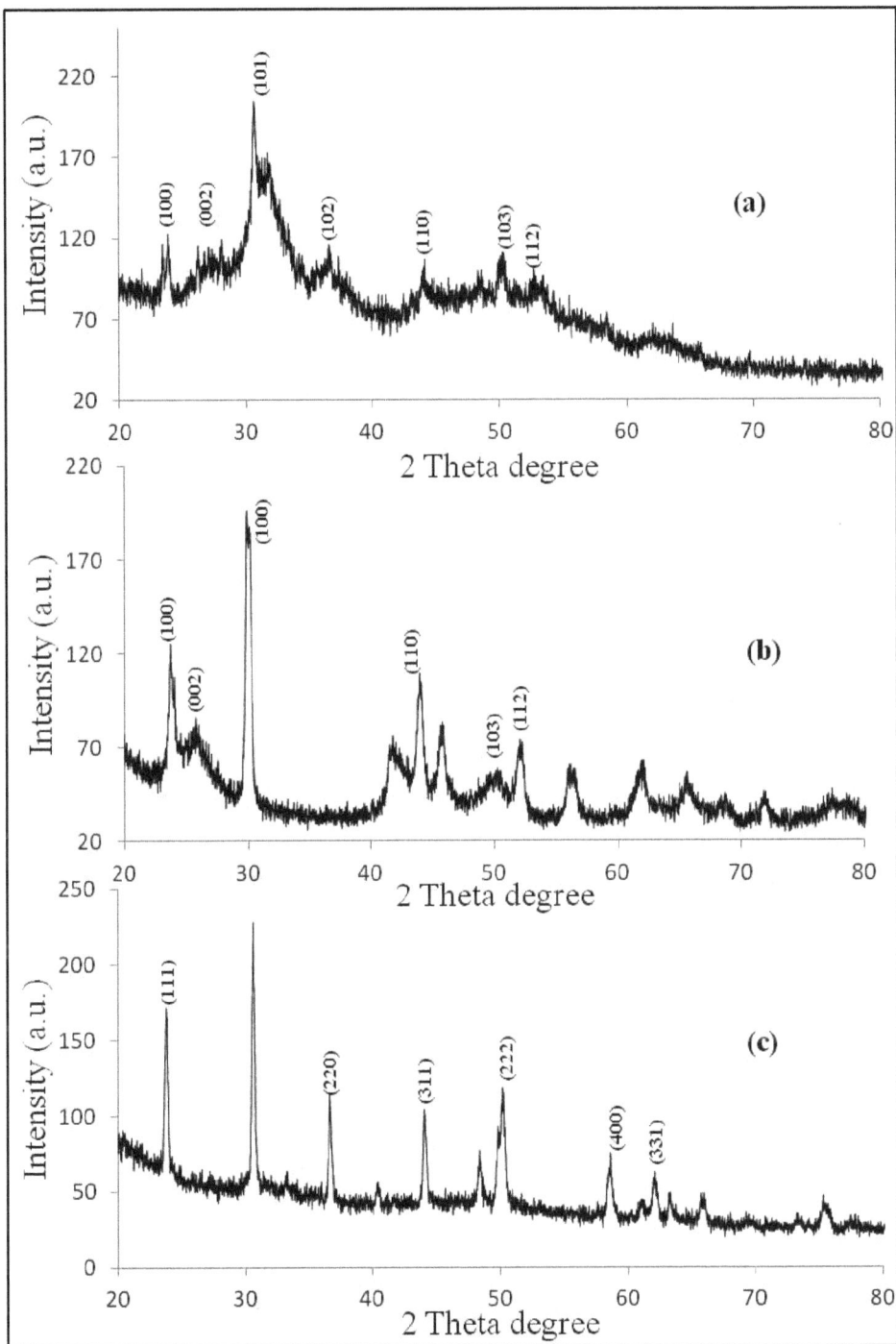

**Figure 17.7: Powder X-ray Diffraction Spectra of Anacardic Acid Capped
(a) CdS, (b) CdSe and (c) CdTe Nanoparticles**

values of 23.65°, 29.92°, 43.91°, 49.94° and 52.02° are observed corresponding, respectively to the (100), (101), (110), (103) and (112) crystalline planes of hexagonal CdSe. The high intensity of (101) peak indicates that the elongated particles have a large number of (101) planes thus making that peak the dominant reflection in the first diffraction feature (Rogath, 1999).

Figure 17.7 (c) shows XRD patterns obtained from powdered fractions of anacardic acid capped CdTe nanoparticles. The nanocrystals belong to the cubic (zinc blende) structure which is also the dominant crystal phase of bulk CdTe. The reflections could be indexed to the (111), (220), and (311) prominent planes of the cubic (zinc blende) CdTe (Ithuria, 2008). The presence of (222), (400) and (331) planes further supports the existence of cubic structure of CdTe nanoparticles. The additional peaks could be due to the unreacted cadmium carbonate used as Cd-source.

FT-IR spectroscopy was performed in order to investigate the possible chemical interactions between the semiconductor nanoparticles and the anacardic acid matrix. The surface of nanocrystals exist many metal or chalcogen defects, which may be passivated by organic ligand or inorganic materials (Shan *et al.*, 2005). The FT-IR spectrum of the isolated anacardic acid (Figure 17.8 a) showed all fingerprint peaks

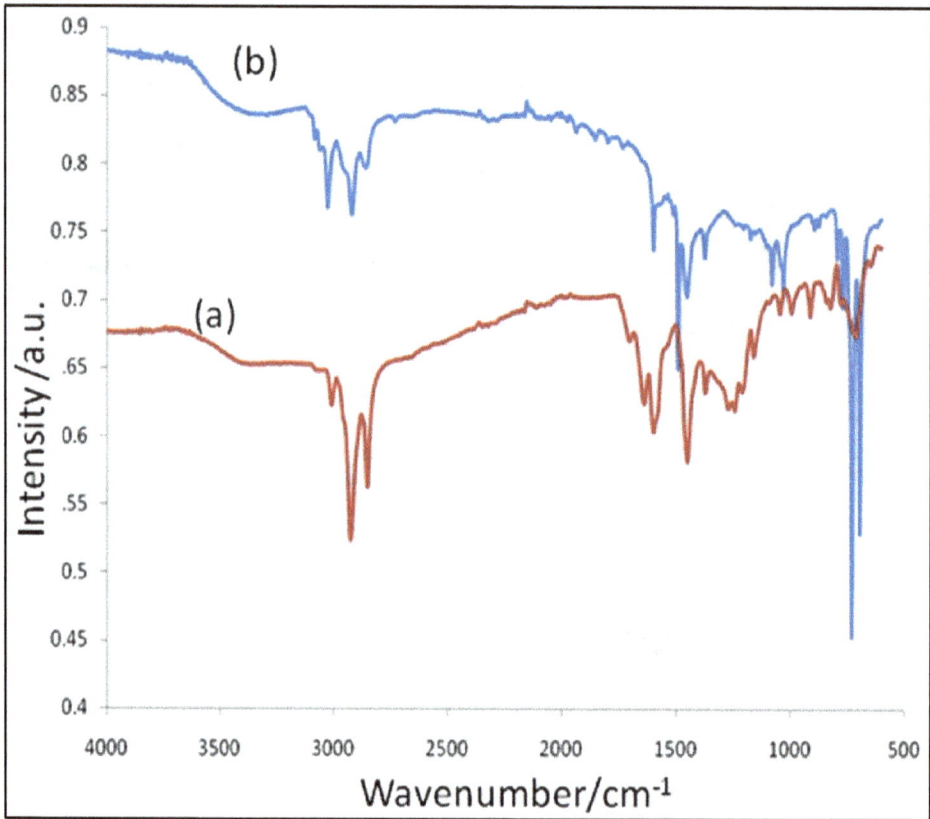

Figure 17.8: FT-IR for (a) Anacardic Acid and (b) CdTe Semiconductor Nanoparticles Capped by Anacardic Acid at 140 °C when CdCl-$_2$ was Used as Cd-Source

for anacardic acid as reported elsewhere (Phillip *et al.*, 2008). The obscured band at 3467 cm⁻¹ was attributed to the O-H stretching of the acid. The frequencies of the capped materials (Figure 17.8 b) are shifted to slightly higher wave numbers in the anacardic acid passivated CdTe nanoparticles. The shift in the COOH stretching position is probably due to a change in the dipole moment when anacardic acid binds to the metal surface that has high electron density. Strongly hidden C=O stretch on the capped nanoparticles confirm the capping of nanoparticles surface by anacardic acid, which coordinates to the CdTe via the carboxylate group.

CONCLUSIONS

Lead and cadmium chalcogenides (PbE and CdE) have successfully been synthesized using anacardic acid as a capping agent. The UV-Vis and PL results confirmed that both PbE and CdE nanoparticles undergo quantum confinement effects. The TEM and HRTEM further revealed a mosaic pattern for all three chalcogenide samples. The results suggest that anacardic acid could be an effective and potential capping agent in the synthesis of metal chalcogenide nanoparticles. The method is environmentally friendly as it uses non-toxic and inexpensive naturally occurring acid as a capping agent. The later qualities augment further that anacardic acid is a good capping agent for the preparation of nearly monodispersed and shape controlled nanoparticles.

ACKNOWLEDGEMENTS

The authors are grateful to the National Research Foundation (NRF), Department of Science and Technology (DST) South Africa and Royal Society Leverhulme Africa Award and STHEP (Tanzania) for funding. The authors also thank Dr. James Wesley-Smith from the Electron Microscopy Unit, University of Kwa-Zulu Natal for electron microscopy (TEM) measurements and CSIR, Pretoria, for HRTEM facility.

REFERENCES

1. Akhtar, J., Malik, MA., O'Brien, P., Wijayantha, KGU., Dharmadasa, R., Hardman, SJO., Graham, DM., Spencer, BF., Stubbs, SK., Flavell, WR., Binks, DJ., Sirotti, F., El Kazzi, M., and Silly, M., 2010. A greener route to photo electrochemically active PbS nanoparticles. *J. Mater. Chem.* 20: 2336-2344.

2. Bawendi, MG., Carroll, PJ., Wilson, WL., and Brus, LE., 1992. Luminescence properties of CdSe quantum crystallites: Resonance between interior and surface localized states. *J. Chem. Phys.* 96: 946-954.

3. Boatman, EM., Lisensky, GC., and Nordell, KJ., 2005. A Safer, Easier, Faster Synthesis for CdSe Quantum Dot Nanocrystals. *J. Chem. Educ*, 82 (11): 1697-1699.

4. Bruchez, M., Moronne, M., Gin, P., Weiss, S., and Alivisatos, AP., 1998. Semiconductor Nanocrystals as Fluorescent Biological Labels. *Sci.* 281: 2013-2016.

5. Chan, WCW., and Nie, SM., 1998. Quantum Dot Bioconjugates for Ultrasensitive Nonisotopic Detection. *Sci.* 281: 2016-2018

6. Cho, KS., Talapin, DV., Gaschler, W., and Murray, CB., 2005. Designing PbSe nanowires and nanorings through oriented attachment of nanoparticles. *J. Am. Chem. Soc.* 127: 7140-7147.

7. Dowty, E., 1976. Crystal structure and crystal growth: I. The influence of internal structure on morphology. *Am. Mineral.* 61: 448–459.

8. Efros, AL., Rosen, M., Kuno, M., Nirmal, M., Norris, DJ., and Bawendi, MG., 1996. Band-edge exciton in quantum dots of semiconductors with a degenerate valence band: Dark and bright exciton states. *Phys. Rev.* B. 54 (7): 4843-4856.

9. Gautam, UK., and Seshadri, R., 2004. Preparation of PbS and PbSe nanocrystals by a new solvothermal route. *Mater. Res. Bull.* **39:** 669–676.

10. Greenham, NC., Peng, X., and Alivisatos, AP., 1996. Charge separation and transport in conjugated-polymer/semiconductor-nanocrystal composites studied by photoluminescence quenching and photoconductivity. *Phys. Rev.* B. 54 (24): 17628-17637.

11. He, R., and Gu, H., 2006. Synthesis and characterization of monodisperse CdSe nanocrystals at lower temperature. Colloids and Surfaces A: *Physicochem. Eng. Aspects.* 272: 111-116.

12. Ithuria, S., and Dubertret, B., 2008. Quasi 2D Colloidal CdSe Platelets with Thicknesses Controlled at the Atomic Level. *J. Am. Chem. Soc.* 130: 16504-16505.

13. Lee, YW., Jun, SN., Cho, and Cheon, JW., 2002. Single crystalline star-shaped nanocrystals and their evolution: Programming the geometry of nano-building blocks. *J. Am. Chem. Soc.* 124: 11244-11245.

14. Lucio, PLL., Santos, CO., Romeiro, LAS., Costa, AM., Ferreira, JRO., Cavalcanti, BC., Moraes, OM., Costa-Lotufo, LV., Pessoa, C., and Santos, ML., 2010. Synthesis and cytotoxicity screening of substituted isobenzofuranones designed from Anacardic acids. *Eur. J. Med. Chem.* 45: 3480-3489.

15. Maseko, NN., Revaprasadu, N., Rajasekhar Pullabhotla, VSR., Karthik, R., and O'Brien, P., 2010. The influence of the cadmium source on the shape of CdSe nanoparticles. *Mater. Lett.* 64: 1037-1040.

16. Mlowe, S., Nejo, AA., Rajasekhar Pullabhotla, VSR., Mubofu, EB., Ngassapa, FN., O'Brien, P and Revaprasadu, N., 2013. Lead chalcogenides stabilized by anacardic acid. *Mater. Sci. Semicond. Process.* 16: 263-268.

17. Mntungwa, N., Rajasekhar Pullabhotla, VSR., and Revaprasadu, N., 2011. A facile route to shape controlled CdTe nanoparticles. *Mater. Chem. Phys.* 126: 500-506.

18. Mokari, T., Zhang, M., and Yang, P., 2007. Shape, Size, and Assembly Control of PbTe Nanocrystals. *J. Amer. Chem. Soc.* 129: 9864–9865.

19. Murray, CB., Norris, DJ., and Bawendi, MG., 1993. Synthesis and Characterization of Nearly Monodisperse CdE (E = S, Se, Te) Semiconductor Nanocrystallites. *J. Am. Chem. Soc.* 115: 8706-8715.

20. Norris, DJ., Efros, AL., Rosen, M., and Bawendi, MG., 1996. Size dependence of exciton fine structure in CdSe quantum dots. *Phys. Rev.* B. 53: 16347-16354.

21. Paramashivappa, R., Kumar, PP., Vithayathil, PJ., and Rao, AS., 2001. Novel Method for Isolation of Major Phenolic Constituents from Cashew (Anacardium occidentale L.) Nut Shell Liquid. *J. Agric. Food Chem*. 49: 2548-2551

22. Patterson, AL., 1939. The Scherrer Formula for X-Ray Particle Size Determination. *Phys. Rev.* 56: 978-982.

23. Philip, JYN., Francisco, JC., Dey, ES., Buchweishaija, J., Mkayula, LL., and Ye, L., 2008. Isolation of Anacardic Acid from Natural Cashew Nut Shell Liquid (CNSL) Using Supercritical Carbon Dioxide. *J. Agric. Food Chem.* **56**: 9350–9354.

24. Raniero, L., Fereira, CL., Cruz, LR., Pinto, AL., and Alves, RMP., 2010. Photoconductivity activation in PbS thin films grown at room temperature by chemical bath deposition. *Phy. B: Condensed Matter*. 405: 1283-1286.

25. Rogach, AL., Kornowski, A., Gao, M., Eychmuller, A., and Weller, H., 1999. Synthesis and Characterization of a Size Series of Extremely Small Thiol-Stabilized CdSe Nanocrystals. *J. Phys. Chem.* B. 103: 3065-3069.

26. Sapra, S., Rogath, AL., and Feldmann, J., 2006. Phosphine-free synthesis of monodisperse CdSe nanocrystals in olive oil. *J. Mater. Chem*. 16: 3391-3395.

27. Shan, G., Kong, X., Wang, X., and Liu, Y., 2005. The structure and character of CdSe nanocrystals capped ZnO layer for phase transfer from hexane to ethanol solution. *Surface Sci.* **582:** 61–68.

28. Thomas, PJ., Mubofu, EB., and O'Brien, P., 2013. Thin films of metals, metal chalcogenides and oxides deposited at the water–oil interface using molecular precursors. *Chem. Commun.*, **49**, 118-127

29. Wang, Y., Tang, ZY., Tan, SS., and Kotov, NA., 2005. Biological Assembly of Nanocircuit Prototypes from Protein-Modified CdTe Nanowires. *Nano Lett.* 5 (2): 243-248.

30. Xie, Y., Su, HL., Li, B., and Qian, YT., 2000. A direct solvothermal route to nanocrystalline selenides at low temperature. *Mater. Res. Bull.* 35: 459-464.

31. Zhu, JJ., Palchick, O., Chen, SG., and Gedanken, A., 2000. Microwave assisted preparation of CdSe, PbSe, and $Cu_{2-x}Se$ nanoparticles. *J Phys Chem B*. 104: 7344-7347.

32. Ziqubu, N., Ramasamy, K., Pullabhotla, VSRR., Revaprasadu, N., and O'Brien, P., 2010. Simple route to dots and rods of PbTe nanocrystals. *Chem. Mater*. 22: 3817-3819.

Chapter 18

Synthesis of Aluminum-Doped Zinc Oxide (ZnO) Nanoparticles as a Buffer Layer in Organic Solar Cells by Chemical Bath Deposition (CBD) Method

Kekeli N'konou*, Y. Lare, M. Baneto,
S.Ouro-Djobo, and K. Napo

Laboratoire sur l'Energie Solaire (LES), Département de physique,
Faculté des Sciences, Université de Lomé –TOGO
*E-mail addresses: kekelidavid@yahoo.fr

ABSTRACT

In this work, our objective was the test of the technique for obtaining nano-structured Zinc Oxide (ZnO) films by chemical bath deposition (CBD) method, then the development and characterization of aluminum doped ZnO nanoparticles while optimizing the deposition parameters, in order to obtain ZnO nanoparticles with properties ideal for organic photovoltaic applications.

The development of nanostructured films (nanorods) by CBD method involves two steps. In the rst step, spin-coating ZnO seeds on the substrate and in the second, the layers obtained were annealed at a temperature of 300°C before being immerging in a ZnO solution to ensure the growth of nanorods on layers obtained after the first step. X-ray diffraction (XRD) and Scanning Electron Microscopy (SEM) analyses were used to investigate the effect of Al doping on the crystallinity and surface morphology of the lms. Structural analysis by XRD showed that the ZnO nanostructured films of doped and undoped have a wurtzite hexagonal structure. The results obtained by the SEM showed that doping can promote the production of nanorods. At the end of this study, there was a clear difference in morphology observed in SEM images of intrinsic and aluminum-doped ZnO samples. This structural difference depends on the choice of substrates, chemical system used and the effect of doping.

Keywords: *Nanoparticles, Zinc oxide, Chemical bath deposition.*

INTRODUCTION

Now-a-days, the importance given to the development of renewable energies is ever increasing, due to the high share of energy demand still growing, the environmental problems and climate-related sources fossils. In the table of various renewable energy sources, solar photovoltaic occupies a prominent place mainly because of the abundance of the solar field. However, this sector still faces today a limited access to its operations due to the relatively high cost of cells, mostly in silicon technologies. To overcome this problem, different solutions are being explored by researchers, one of the most promising is the use of organic materials which have major benefit: first it requires less expensive and relatively simple technology, and it uses very little work material (of the order of several hundreds of nanometers). Efforts done by the scientific community in recent decades have helped make organic photovoltaic a very promising alternative for solar energy.

Recently, extensive investigation on the synthesis of 1D nanomaterials including wires, tubes, rods, and belts has attracted much attention, owing to their unique properties and prospective applications in nanometer-scale devices. So far, most of the research has focused on inorganic compounds and organic polymers. Nowadays, low molecular-weight organic nanomaterials have attracted increasing attention, because their electronic and optical properties are fundamentally different from those of inorganic ones (Uthirakumar, 2008; Firdaus, 2013; Grundmann, 2010; Dutta, 2008; Yogeswaran, 2008; Lu, 2011).

The basic idea is to adapt the solar spectrum solar cells by inserting oxide film converter photons. One solution to realize this concept is to insert a transparent oxide layer which may be doped to increase the absorption spectral range of the photovoltaic cells. Oxides such as Zinc Oxide (ZnO) or Titanium Oxide (TiO_2) are materials that are part of the family of transparent conductive oxide (TCO).

Different techniques such as sputtering (Z.L. Pei, 2006; H.K. Park, 2009; D.C. Look, 2006), spray pyrolysis (M. Jiang, 2009), chemical vapour deposition (K.H. Yoon, 1997), pulsed laser deposition (S. Major, 1984); sol–gel (A. Umar, 2005; V. Srikant,1997) and chemical bath deposition (CBD) methods (T. Tsuchiya,1994; J.H. Lee,2003) have been used to prepare ZnO nanorods.

The chemical bath deposition (CBD) method has many advantages over other deposition techniques, including simplicity, low cost, ease of chemical composition control and homogeneity of the solution. These advantages make CBD processing an attractive and appealing method for ZnO nanorods preparation because they offer an inexpensive way of producing solar cells and the possibility of large-area deposition (Ennaoui, 1998).

In this paper, we report results from chemical bath deposition (CBD) synthesis of Al-doped ZnO nanorods. ZnO nanorods are deposited on glass substrates by using a CBD technique with varying precursor and doping level. X-ray diffraction (XRD) and Scanning Electron Microscopy (SEM) analyses were used to investigate the effect of Al doping on the crystallinity and surface morphology of the ûlms.

MATERIALS AND METHODS

For deposition of undoped and Al-doped zinc oxide nanostructured lms, small sectioned coupons of soda-lime glass, 10×10 mm^2 in size, were used as substrates. The substrates were cleaned using Alcohol 95 per cent, and then washed with methanol and nally thoroughly rinsed in excess of deionized water. The solution prepared for spin coating onto substrates had the following constituents: zinc acetate dehydrate $(Zn(CH_3COO)_2.2H_2O)$, zinc nitrate hexahydrate $(Zn (NO_3)_2.6H_2O)$, aluminium nitrate nanohydrate $(Al(NO_2)_3, 9H_2O)$, ammonia (solution), sodium hydroxide (NaOH), and methanol (CH_3OH). All the reagents used were of analytical grade purity (> 99.99 per cent).

ZnO films were grown using a simple two-step process: spin-coating ZnO seeds on the substrate and growth of films on the seeded substrate.

In the first step, ZnO seed was prepared by a modified spin-coating method. Basically, 0,09g $Zn(CH_3COO)_2$ and 0,12g NaOH were dissolved into 50ml methanol, respectively. They were mixed rapidly and stirring at 60°C for 5 minutes, then cooled to room temperature. The resultant solution was transparent with ZnO nanoparticles. The solution was then spin-coated on the substrate at 500 rpm for 5s and 3000 rpm for 30s. After processing, the substrate was heated at 60°C for 10 minutes to remove the solvent.

In the second step, ZnO growth was carried out by suspending the substrate in a 40 ml beaker filled with an aqueous solution of zinc nitrate hydrate and ammonia at 90°C for 1 hour. Subsequently, the substrate was removed from the solution, rinsed with deionized water and dried in air at 60°C, $([Zn^{2+}] =0.1M)$. For nanostructured Al doped ZnO layers (ZnO: Al), we added the following doping levels, a weighted amount of aluminum nitrate nanohydrate$(Al(NO_2)_3.9H_2O)$ in the solution previously prepared.The concentration of zinc acetate was 0.1M and Al/Zn ratio in the solution varied between 2 and 4 at per cent.

After deposition and drying of the layers, the samples obtained are a mixture of zinc hydroxide and zinc oxide. Finally the samples were annealed at temperature of 300 °C. This annealing allowed us to obtain the conversion of Zn $(OH)_2$ in ZnO (M.Baneto,2011).

The phase composition of the samples was characterized by X-ray diffraction (XRD, Siemens D5000, diffrac tometer with CuKα radiation λ =1.5406 Å). The morphologies of the samples were observed by scanning electron microscopy (SEM; JSM-6400F, JEOL,).

RESULTS AND DISCUSSION

Structural Properties

The XRD patterns recorded for undoped ZnO film (Figure 18.1) are comparable with the standard JCPDS data card no. 36-1451 and confirmed that ZnO films are polycrystalline in nature and belong to the hexagonal wurtzite structure. It is noticed that doping influences the orientation of the obtained films. This is probably associated to the nucleation process. Figure 18.1 shows that the (100) direction is the preferential growing orientation for the undoped films. However, one can see in Figures 18.2 and 18.3 for aluminum doped ZnO films that the preferential orientation is (101). In addition, the ratio of lattice constants c/a was found to be around 1.60 for all doped and undoped layers. This is in good accord with values of the bulk wurtzite ZnO. Similar results were also obtained by Alver *et al.* (2007) The lattice constants (Table 18.1) were calculated using the following formula (Fang, 2003):

$$\frac{1}{d_{hkl}^2} = \frac{4}{3a^2}(h^2 + hk + k^2) + \frac{l^2}{c^2}$$

and

$$2d_{hkl}\sin\theta = n\lambda$$

where,

a and c are the lattice constants and d_{hkl} is the crystalline surface distance for *hkl* indices

Furthermore we noticed that for samples doped with aluminum, no secondary phases (*i.e.* no aluminum compound) were detected from XRD patterns. This may due to either the replacement of Zn^{2+} (considering that the ionic radius of aluminum (0.56 Å) is smaller than that of zinc 0.74Å) or occupation of Al^{3+} at the interstitial site in the hexagonal lattice structure and thus shows the absence of Al_2O_3 or zinc spinel ($ZnAl_2O_4$) phase formation. The crystalline quality of film is found to be deteriorated with the increase of Al doping. A similar behavior has been also reported (D. Goyal, 1992) and found that interstitial inclusion of dopant atoms deteriorate the film structure and lead to the amorphization of films. However, we noticed that the lattice parameters of ZnO (Table 18.1) decrease with the increase of Al doping. This indicates that Al^{3+} substitutes to Zn^{2+} more than occupying the interstitial sites in the ZnO hexagonal structure. An estimation of the average crystallite size applied to (100) peak (Table 18.1) has been done using Scherrer formula:

$$D = \frac{0.9\lambda}{\beta\cos\theta}$$

where,

β is the observed angular width at half maximum intensity (FWHM) of the peak, λ is the X-ray wavelength (1.5406 Å for CuKα1) and θ is the Bragg's angle. It can be

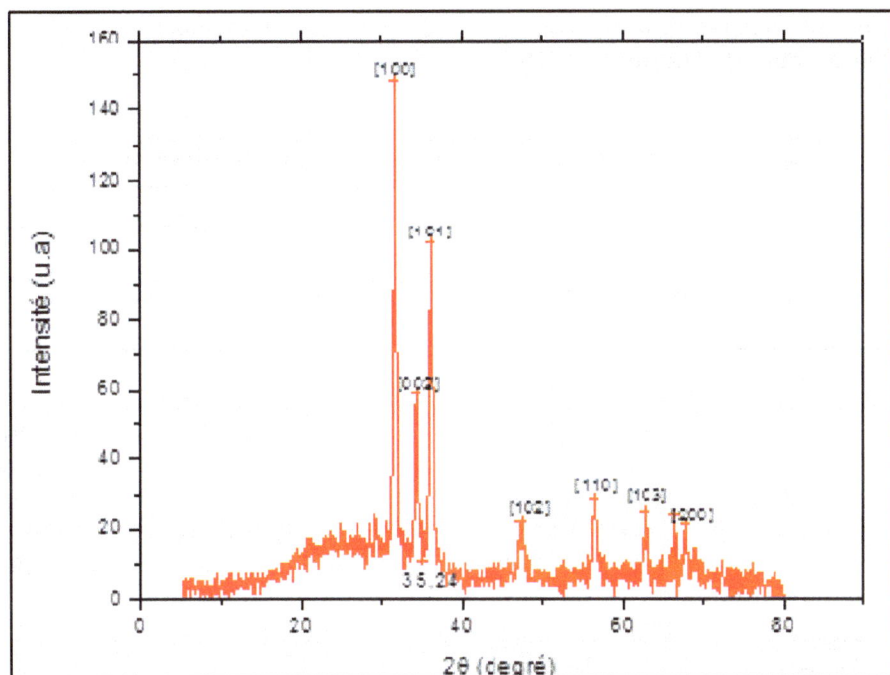

Figure 18.1: XRD Pattern of Intrinsic ZnO Nanorods

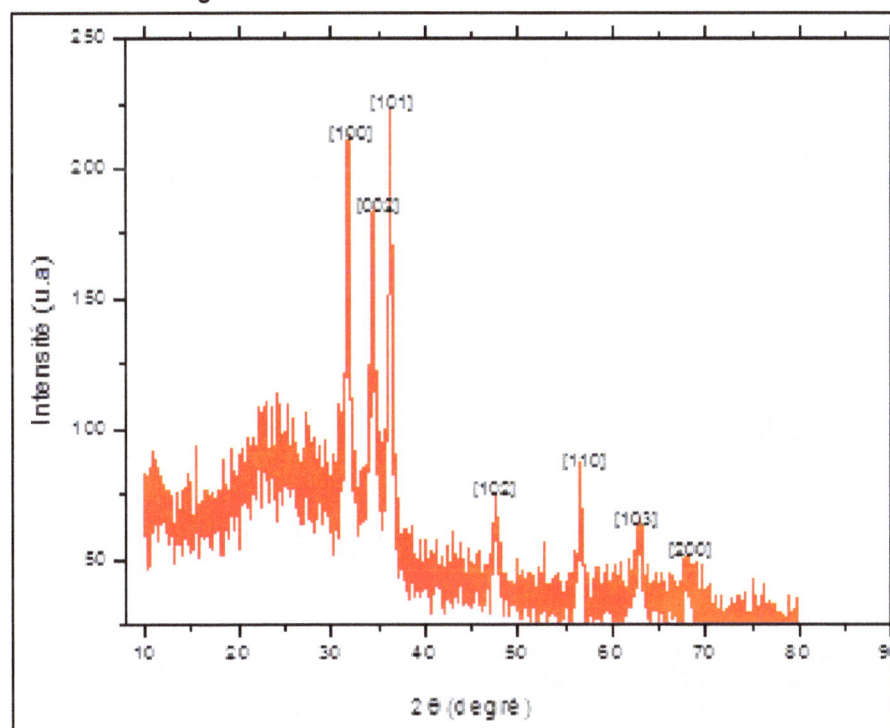

Figure 18.2: XRD Pattern of 2 at per cent ZnO:Al Nanorods

seen that, crystallite size decreases with increase of doping level. This can be explained by the fact that Al^{3+} substitutes to Zn^{2+} in ZnO hexagonal structure.

Table 18.1

Samples	Crystallite Size (nm)	Lattice Parameters (Å)	
		A	c
ZnO	40.32	3.234	5.352
ZnO:Al (2at. per cent)	35.60	3.231	5.349
ZnO:Al (4at. per cent)	32.45	3.229	5.348

The ionic radius of aluminum (0.56 Å) is smaller than that of zinc (0.74Å) and excess Al may also occupy interstitial positions in ZnO lattice resulting in distorted crystal structure, thus decreasing the carrier mobility (Dewei Chu,2009). The absence of any peak characteristic of Al_2O_3 or zinc spinel ($ZnAl_2O_4$) phases indicates interstitial substitution of Zn^{2+} by Al^{3+} to be the predominant effect of Al doping and Al segregation to grain boundary region as another possibility especially for 2 at per cent Al-doped ZnO lms.

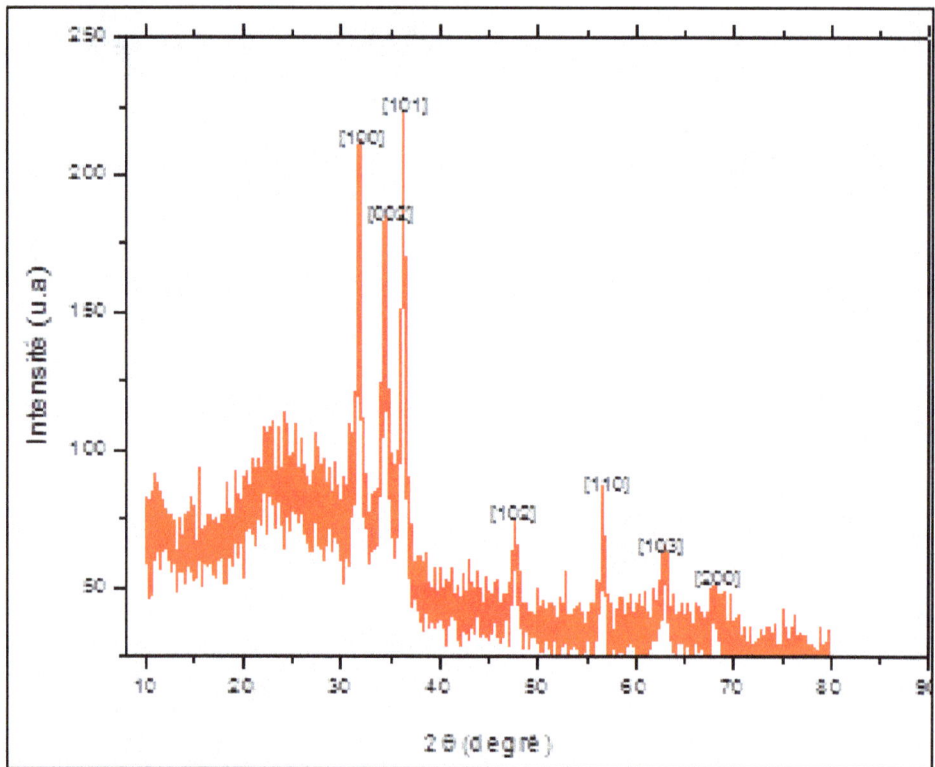

Figure 18.3: XRD Pattern of 4 at per cent ZnO:Al Nanorod Microstructural Analysis

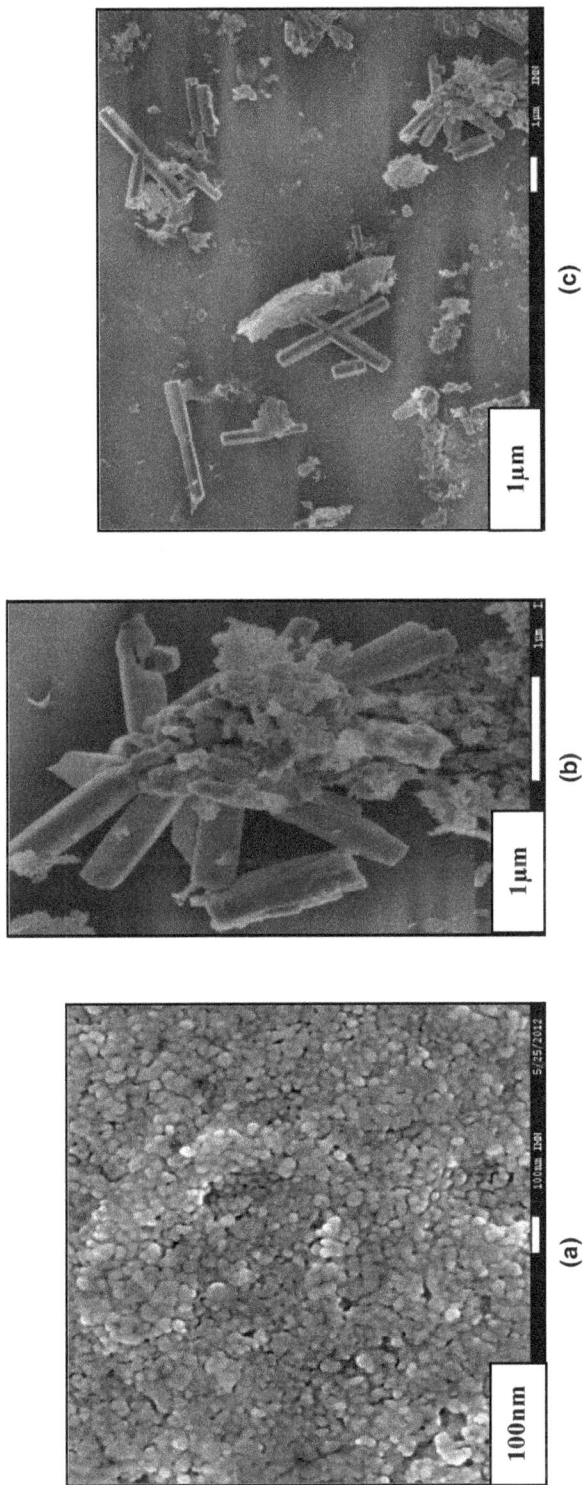

Figure 18.4: SEM Images of ZnO Nanorods
(A) Undoped, (B) 2 at per cent Al-doped, and (C) 4 at per cent Al-doped

Figures 18.4 (a, b and c) shows the SEM images of undoped and aluminum (2 at per cent and 4 at per cent) doped ZnO films. The undoped ZnO film surface (Figure 18.4a) is rough and is composed of fine particles of several tens of nanometers. We remarked that, after doping ZnO films the SEM images (Figures 18.4(a) and (b)) indicate a drastic change in the surface morphology. It can be clearly seen that aluminum doping leads to the formation of nanorods. Figure 18.4b shows for sample obtained with 2 at. per cent aluminum doped ZnO, nanorods are well exhibited. Meanwhile, by increasing the aluminum dopant level, the formation of nanorods is inhibited due to the saturation of aluminum in the precursor solution. Hence, by increasing the aluminum dopant level, the diameter of nanorods decreased. A similar result was obtained by Zhiguang Wang *et al.* (Zhiguang Wang, 2009) by studying the effect of the substrate on the growth and interconversion of nanostructured ZnO films. It can be conclude in this work that aluminum act as a catalyst in the formation of nanorods. However, many other factors can lead to the formation of ZnO nanorods. Many groups have reported the growth of highly oriented ZnO nanorods and other nanostructures from aqueous solution. Andrés-Vergés *et al.* (Andrés Vergés, 1990) reported the aqueous solution growth method for the first time in 1990. More than 10 years later, Vayssieres *et al.*(Vayssieres, L., 2001) used this method to grow nanorods on conducting glass and Si substrates. For this type of growth, a ZnO seed layer is needed to initialize the uniform growth of oriented nanorods. In our case, the ZnO seed layer was obtained from zinc acetate precursor and the ZnO nanorods were grown using zinc chloride precursor.

CONCLUSIONS

ZnO nanorods have been successfully grown by chemical bath deposition method on glass substrates using two steps deposition. Structural analysis by X-ray diffraction showed that all the ZnO films are polycrystalline with hexagonal structure. We remarked that crystallites size decreases with increase of aluminum dopant. The undoped ZnO film surface is rough and composed of fine particles of several tens of nanometers while aluminum doped ZnO films exhibited nanorods. The diameter of nanorods decreases with increase of aluminum dopant indicating the effect of aluminum on the formation of ZnO nanorods.

ACKNOWLEDGMENTS

The work has been funded by the Solar Energy Laboratory, Department of Physics, Faculty of Science at University of Lomé-TOGO.

REFERENCES

1. Alver.U, T. K1ll1nc, E. Bacaks1z, S. Nezir, *Materials Chemistry and Physics* 106 (2007). 227–230.

2. Andrés Vergés, M., *et al., J. Chem. Soc., Faraday Trans.* (1990) **86**, 959

3. Baneto.M, 2011. PhD Thesis, September 2011, Université de Lomé, Togo

4. Dewei Chu, 2009. *Phys.Status Solidi* A 206,No.4,718-723

5. Dutta.M, 2008, *Appl. Surf. Sci.* 254 (2008) 2743.

6. Ennaoui,1998. *Solar Energy Materials and Solar Cells* 54 (1998) 277-286

7. Fang.G, D. Li, Bao-Lun Yao, *Journal of Crystal Growth* 247 (2003) 393–400.

8. Grundmann.M, 2010, *Phys. Status Solidi* A 207 (6) (2010) 1437.

9. http://www.heliatek.com

10. Jiang.M, 2009.*Surf. Coat.Technol*. 203 (2009) 3750.

11. Lee J.H., 2003. *J. Cryst. Growth* 247 (2003) 119.

12. Look D.C. 2006. Doping and Defects in ZnO, in Zinc oxide: Bulk, thin lms, and nanostructures, Elsevier Ltd., 2006, p. 23.

13. Lu W.-L.,2011. *Mater. Chem. Phys*. 130(2011) 619.

14. Major.S, 1983. *Thin Solid Films* 108 (1983) 333.

15. Mohd Firdaus, 2013. *Thin Solid Films* 527 (2013) 102 –109

16. Park H.K., 2009.*Sol. Energy Mater. Sol. Cells* 93(2009) 1994.

17. Pei Z.L., 2006. *Thin Solid Films* 497 (1 –2) (2006) 20.

18. Periyayya Uthirakumar, 2008. *Journal of Luminescence* 128 (2008) 1629 – 1634

19. Srikant.V, 1997. *J. Appl. Phys*. 81 (1997) 6357.

20. Tsuchiya.T, 1994. *J. Non-Cryst. Solids* 178 (1994) 327.

21. Umar.A,2005. *Nanotechnology* 16 (2005) 2462.

22. Vayssieres, L., *et al., J. Phys. Chem. B* (2001) **105**, 3350

23. Yogeswaran.U, 2008, Sensors 8 (2008) 290.

24. Yoon.K.H, 1997. *Thin Solid Films* 302 (1997) 116.

25. Zhang.H.Z, 2004. *Journal of Crystal Growth* 269 (2004) 464–471

26. Zhiguang Wang, 2009. *Applied Surface Science* 255(2009) 4705-4710.

Chapter 19

Current Status of Nanoscience and Nanotechnology in Venezuela

M.S. López[1], C. Trocel[1], A. Hasmy[2] and H. Vessuri[1]

[1]*Venezuelan Institute for Scientific Research (IVIC),*
Caracas 1020-A, Venezuela
[2]*Department of Physics, Simon Bolivar University (USB),*
Valle de Sartenejas Baruta, Estado Miranda, Venezuela

ABSTRACT

Through the manipulation of nanosized materials to create new products and processes, Nanotechnology is an industry leading driver technology that can help in socio-economic development in emerging countries. Venezuela starts to promote the training of students, to disseminate this field in Venezuelan society as well as to design and implement national strategies in order to lever up the industrialization and competitiveness of the manufacturing sectors. In this study, nanoscale activity in Venezuela is briefly reviewed, with emphasis on research groups, research lines, and institutions involved. The work summarizes and highlights the behavior reflected in bibliometric indexes as well the activities organized in the last years by the Nanotechnology Venezuelan Network in strength collaboration with many institutions. A summary exploration is made of international cooperation through scientific co-authorship, as well of the efforts to build nano capacities, available infrastructure, public policies and relationships to the productive sector. The study also analyses the national capacities for managing risks, regulations and control of nanomaterials in Venezuela. Finally, the prospects of all these efforts will be discussed.

Keywords: *Nanotechnology, Nanoscience, Public policies, Building capacities, International cooperation, Venezuela.*

INTRODUCTION

New technologies can produce socio-economic benefits to developing countries. Few decades ago, by implementing relevant policies, some Eastern Asian countries benefited economically from the emergence of Information Technology industry. Most recently, Nanotechnology, in convergence with other New Technologies (Biotechnology, Materials and Information Technology), is introducing a new technological paradigm in the productive sector, referred also as the next global technology revolution (Silberglitt *et al.*, 2005). Central countries have taken full concern over the development of Nanotechnology and its socio-economic implications, by implementing national strategic plans and high investments.

By identifying national capacities and opportunities and by designing relevant policies, peripheral countries could get a variety of benefits from Nanotechnology which includes water remediation, clean energy, new health therapies, among other applications (Juma *et al.*, 2005). Argentina, Brazil, Iran, Malaysia, South Africa, are examples of emerging countries that have implemented specific policies for Nanoscience and Nanotechnology development. This work revises the current status of Venezuela in such knowledge and analyses Venezuelan conditions for launching a National Nanotechnology Initiative in the near future.

To identify human and infrastructure capacities, this study analyses the different Nanoscience and Nanotechnology activities where academy, industry and/or government have been involved. Regarding research activities, a previous study revealed that they are concentrated in four institutions responsible of more than 80 per cent per cent of scientific publications: the Venezuelan Institute of Scientific Research (IVIC), Central University of Venezuela (UCV), Simon Bolívar University (USB) and Los Andes University (ULA). The areas of expertise are focused on heterogeneous catalysis, electronics, health therapies, coating, and new materials, among others. The study also revealed that Venezuela ranks in the 7th position in Latin America and the Caribbean in number of published scientific articles, and the country ranks 6th (with Colombia) in *per capita* publications (approximately 4 times less than Argentina, Chile or Brazil and 40 times less than South Korea) and occupies the 4th place in citation average per paper (behind Argentina, Brazil and Mexico) (López *et al.*, 2011). This work updates these indicators and the inventory of special schools, workshops, courses and other building capacities. International cooperation and activities in the productive sector is also discussed.

Since Venezuela supports national and international policies for sustainable development and in view of probable risks on the use of some nanomaterials, this study also analyses national capacities for managing risks, regulations and control, and social awareness activities. The methodology used includes surveys and interviews. Finally, the article shows some conclusions and perspectives of Nanotechnology development in Venezuela.

Nanoscale Research in Venezuela

As part of the analysis of research capacities, we implemented a similar bibliometric technique as used before (López *et al.*, 2011), in particular, the analysis based on Porter *et al.* (2008)'s methodology, in order to identify the Venezuelan publications in Nanoscience and Nanotechnology from the *Web of Science* (WOS) databases. This analysis reflects the trend followed by the development of the field at the national level, in spite of the fact that it tends to give greater coverage to journals publishing basic research and excludes monographs or technical reports produced in industry, as well as most national and regional scientific journals. The analysed period covers from year 1997 to 2012 (Figure 19.1).

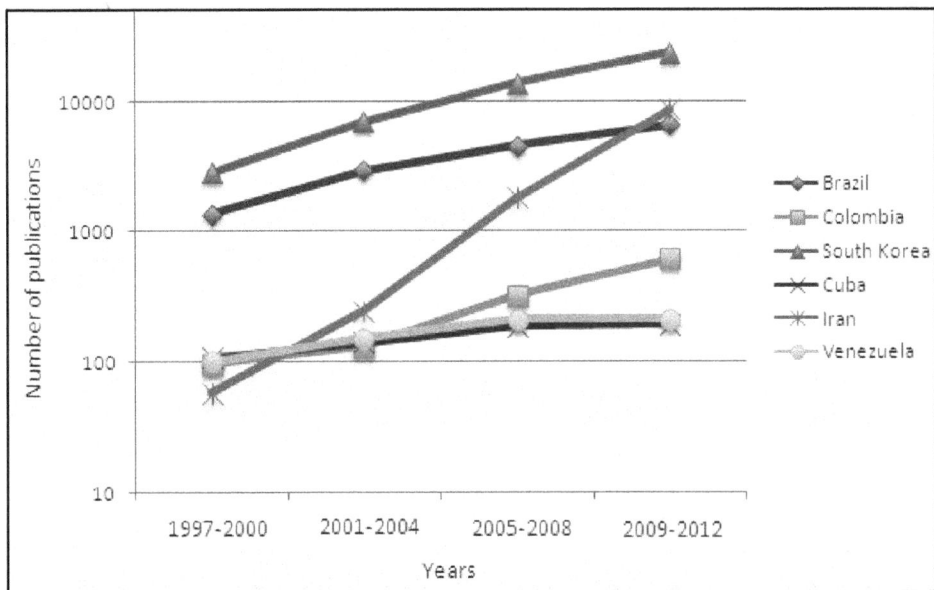

Figure 19.1: Evolution in the Number of Scientific Papers from Venezuela, Iran, Brazil, Colombia, Cuba, South Korea

Source: Authors' Elaboration on the Base of SCI Data

As observed previously, Venezuela occupies the 7th position in number of publications in Latin America and the Caribbean, and shares the 6th position with Colombia in per capita articles with 679 papers between 1997 and 2012. Figure 19.1 compares the number of publications in Venezuela with other Latin American countries, as well as with Iran and South Korea. In general the trend leads to the increase of publications in the countries analysed. However, it is evident that the production of publications in Brazil, Iran and South Korea is stronger. The figure also shows that the production of papers from Cuba and Venezuela is quite similar; then it is observed that Colombia presented a similar trend to these two countries until 2005-2008; however, in the following period it shows an important rise in its paper production, essentially due to the increase of researchers and funding in that country.

According to these trends, it may be concluded that the high rise in publications of Iran, Brazil and South Korea is linked to the strategies implemented by these countries through the implementation of specific public policies aimed to the development of Nanoscience and Nanotechnology.

The distribution trend of publications in Venezuela by knowledge field linked to Nanoscience and Nanotechnology is shown in Figure 19.2. Most publications are related to disciplines like physics, chemistry and materials science, 22 per cent, 20 per cent and 16 per cent respectively. Then, in lesser proportion, are health, polymer science, engineering and metallurgy, among others. This marked amount of publications linked to physics, chemistry and materials science, is due to the fact that in Venezuela most research related to Nanotechnology is carried out by researchers that were trained or had pursued graduate studies in these disciplines.

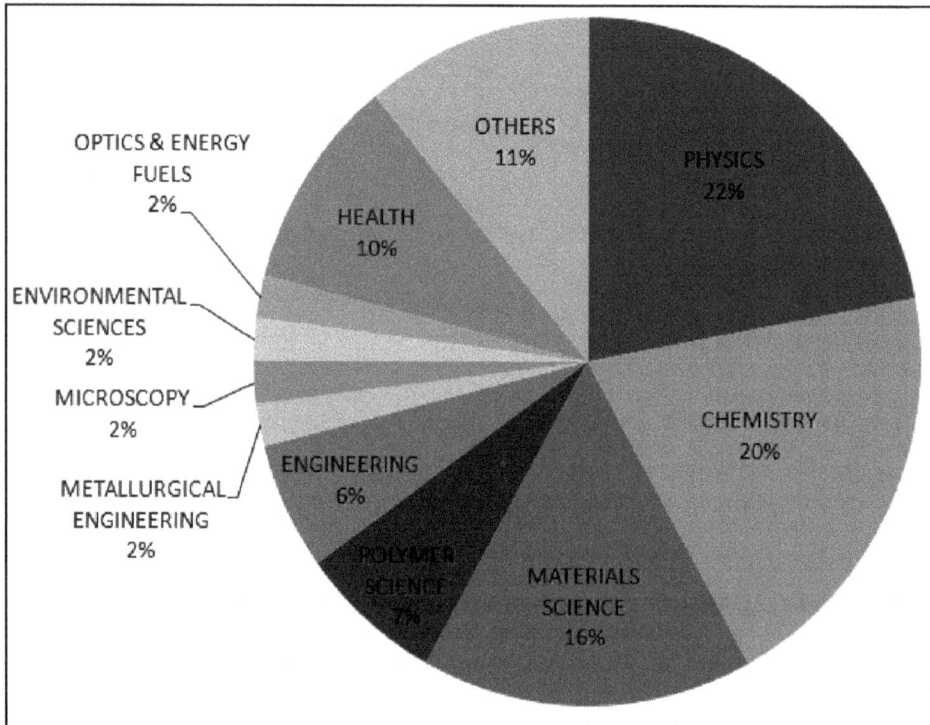

Figure 19.2: Distribution of Nanoscience and Nanotechnology Articles by Field
Source: **Authors' Elaboration on the Base of SCI Data**

The top four institutions that represent the largest number of publications are the Venezuelan Institute of Scientific Research (IVIC) (27 per cent), the Central University from Venezuela (UCV) (22 per cent), Simon Bolivar University (USB) (21 per cent) and Los Andes University (ULA) (16 per cent) (Figure 19.3), which in general confirms previous results (Lopez *et al.*, 2011). This is due to the fact that these institutions host the largest proportion of researchers and graduate students in the country, as well as the largest infrastructure adequate for research in Nanoscience and Nanotechnology. Other institutions with a lower article production are Zulia University (LUZ) with 5 per cent, the technological research institute of the national oil industry (PDVSA-INTEVEP) with 2 per cent, Eastern University (UDO) with 2 per cent, among others.

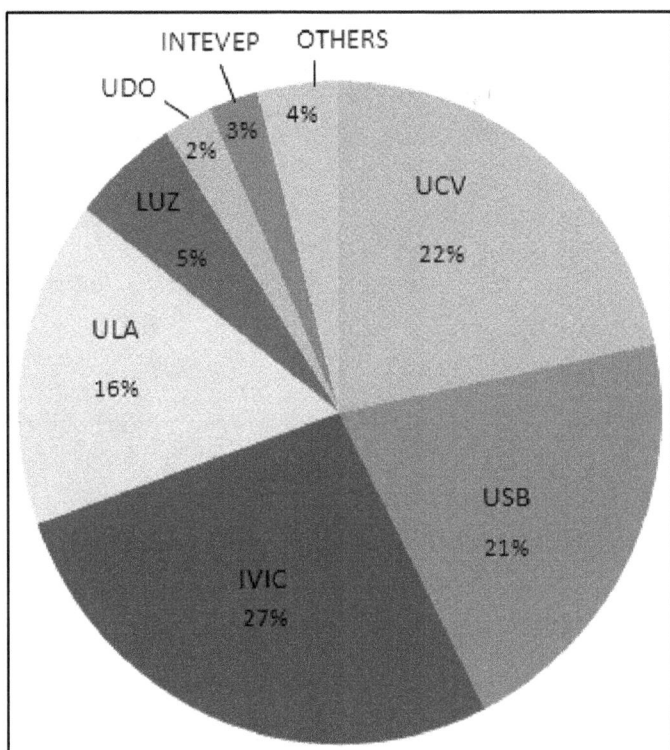

Figure 19.3: Published Article Distribution by Institution
Source: **Authors' Elaboration on the Base of SCI Data**

According to the database of the Venezuelan Nanotechnology Network (473 members), the field expertise its members is distributed as shown in Figure 19.4 (a single member may have expertise in more than one field). The largest quantity of expertise is connected to synthesis of nanomaterials (180 members), specifically concentrated in the production of metallic oxides, semiconductor, polymeric and carbonaceous nanoparticles as well as also nanostructured porous materials, among others. Then with a similar distribution prevails the expertise related to modelling and simulation of nanomaterials techniques (105 members), and analysis, control and measurement techniques (118 members), as well as nanomanufacturing, manipulation and integration (125 members). This analysis also reveals the available expertise in other fields of transversal interest to Nanotechnology such as the norms and regulations (67 members) and to the social study of Nanotechnology (79 members). Indeed it shows that in Venezuela there is a base of human capacity for the development of public policies geared to improving the conditions for the adequate use of the nano field.

International Cooperation

According to bibliometric analysis, the main partners of Venezuelan international collaboration are from the U.S.A. (22 per cent), Spain (18 per cent), France (11 per

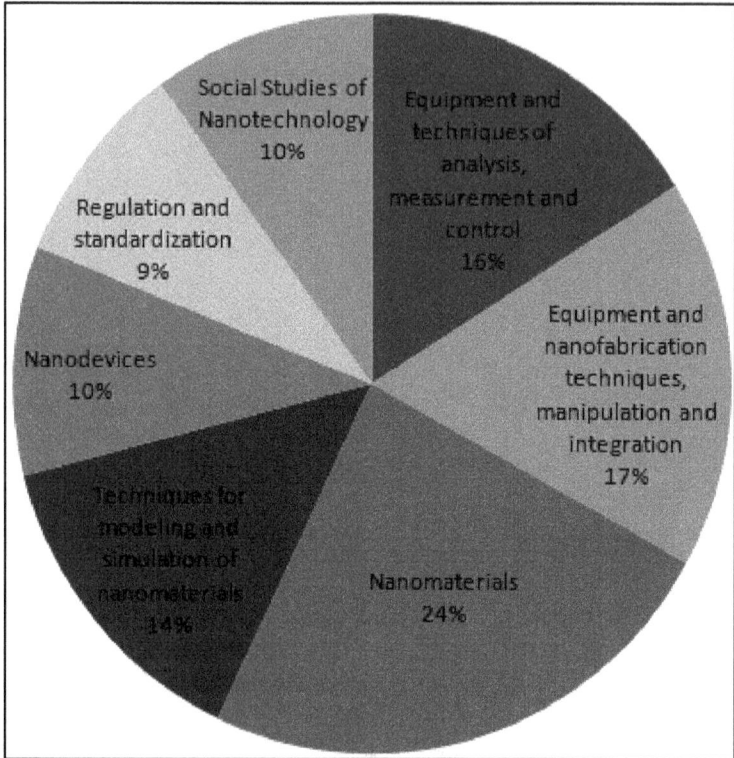

Figure 19.4: Nanoscience and Nanotechnology Expertise of Members of the Venezuelan Nanotechnology Network
Source: Authors' Elaboration on the Base of RedVnano Data

cent). Then come other countries with which it keeps a lesser cooperation percentage, as is the case with England (5 per cent), Germany (5 per cent), Argentina (4 per cent), Mexico (3 per cent), Italy (3 per cent), Canada (2 per cent), Belgium (2 per cent) and Japan (2 per cent) (Figure 19.5). Additionally in this period Venezuela has also collaborated with other 33 countries among which can be mentioned Cuba, China, India, Iran, the Netherlands, Portugal, Russia, Sweden, Turkey and Uruguay.

Although in the last four years referred to in this study (2009-2012) some institutions have acquired fundamental equipment for research, the view of researchers in the field is that Venezuela depends mostly on foreign collaboration to develop projects in Nanoscience and Nanotechnology, because the country lacks some basic instruments for nano manipulation and nano characterization, tying research lines to the agendas of collaborators from outside the country.

In connection with international cooperation two phases can be identified. A first one can be considered to last until 2011, primarily focused in the training of human resources at the fourth level. Among the most important ones we may mention the PCP Programme, which co-funded the mobility of Nanotechnology students and researchers between Venezuela and France and the PREFALC NANO$_2$ programme,

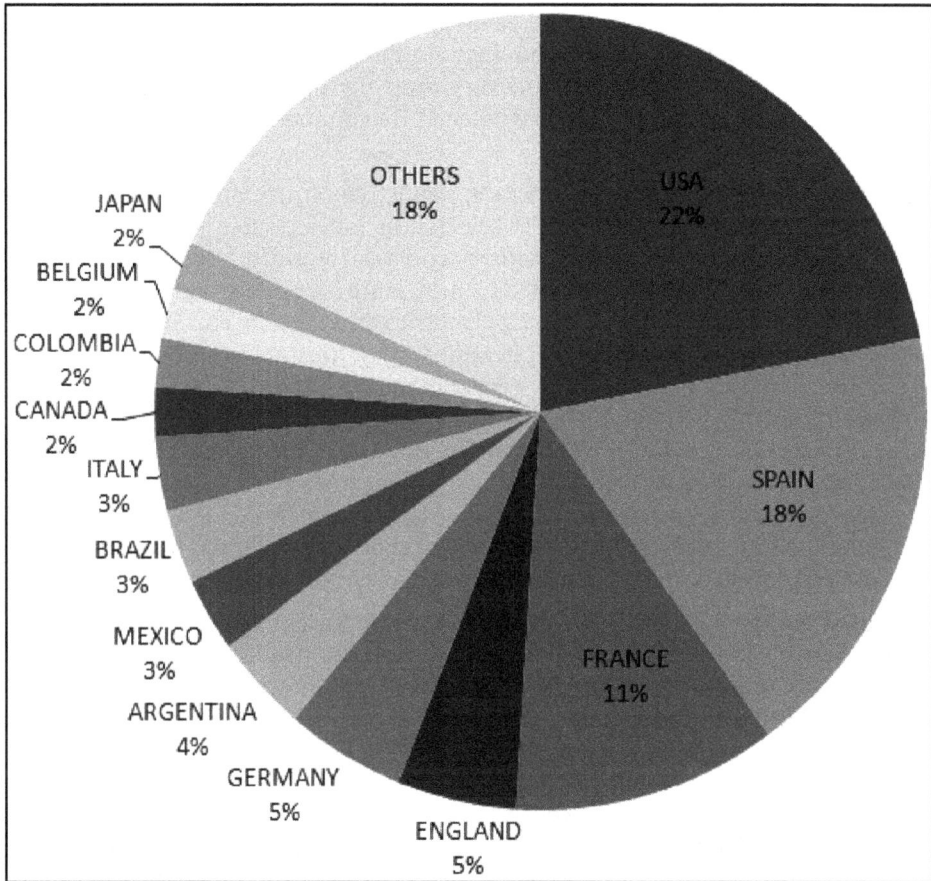

Figure 19.5: International Cooperation in Scientific Papers
Source: Authors' Elaboration on the Base of SCI Data

which co-funded mobility of teachers at master level between Argentina, Brazil, France and Venezuela. The inter-governmental agreement between Cuba and Venezuela, in a project for training of Human Resources in Nanoscience and Nanotechnology in both countries, and extended to students from the Bolivarian Alternative for the Peoples of Our America (ALBA) countries has helped to improve human capacities in Venezuela.

A second phase that was recently started adds a more integral view of scientific cooperation, in which new agreements stand out with countries such as Iran, with which in 2012 a Memorandum of Understanding was signed between the Venezuelan Ministry of the Popular Power for Science, Technology and Innovation, and the Centre for Innovation and Technological Cooperation of the Islamic Presidency of Iran, aimed to carry out joint programs of education and training, as well as research and development in Nanoscience and Nanotechnology in association with other ALBA countries. The subject of Nanotechnology was also included in the follow-up bilateral meeting held in June 2013 of the agreements signed between 2011 and 2012 with Ecuador related to science and technology. In the field of standards, regulations, metrology and nanotoxicology, a Working Group of experts will be formed between Cuba and Venezuela early in 2014, and other ALBA countries as Ecuador and Bolivia have been invited to participate.

Other cooperation activities include the active participation of Venezuelan researchers in NANOANDES, a network that includes participants of almost all South American and other world countries, and most recently, Venezuela started to participate in nano activities promoted by the Centre for Science and Technology of the Non-Aligned and Other Developing Countries (NAM S&T Centre). Furthermore, as far as topics such as social implications, Nanotechnology governance and knowledge socialization in the field, Venezuela also collaborates mostly with Ibero-American countries through the Latin American Network of Nanotechnology and Society (ReLANS) and the CYTED "José Roberto Leite" Network of Diffusion and Education in Nanotechnology. Additionally, Venezuela participates in the forum Strategic Approach to International Chemical Management (SAICM), which is a policy framework to foster the sound management of chemicals (includes nanomaterials). All these points will be developed further on.

For strengthening regional cooperation, an important step forward has been undertaken by Venezuelan government by recently proposing the creation of NANOSUR Community in the 50th Specialized Meeting of S&T (L RECyT) of MERCOSUR (a trade market union that includes Argentina, Brazil, Paraguay, Uruguay and Venezuela, and have associated other South American countries). The initiative will be open to extra regional institutions as Collaborator Member institutions. The main objective of NANOSUR is to constitute an inter-institutional cooperation platform for the strengthening of human, material and organizational capabilities of the region, and its linking to Industry and Society. The Project establishes a series of activities that will allow attacking structural problems that block a greater development of Nanotechnology in South America. The proposal includes the creation of a call program for the mobility of graduate students and teachers in Nanoscience and Nanotechnology, the creation and strengthening of work groups and knowledge networks in topics of interest to academia, industry and government in specific topics of social interest, in norms and regulations, exchange of curricular experiences, the organization of courses and workshops of regional interest, and the promotion of activities of socialization of knowledge in the field.

Training Capacities

In Venezuela, the majority of domestic nanotechnologists got their training locally thanks to existing third and fourth level studies in physics, chemistry, engineering, materials science, among other disciplines. Besides the IDB-CONICIT Program of New Technologies agreement (1991-1999), had an important component for training of researchers, mainly through student fellowships for PhD studies in Europe and the U.S.A. Others got their Ph.D. degrees writing theses co-directed by researchers from France and Venezuela, within the framework of FONACIT-French Graduate Cooperation Program (PCP). Projects included non linear optics, nanoparticles employed as catalysts, nanostructured coatings, nanoemulsions, nanostructured porous media, nanocosmetics, carbon nanotubes, nanoelectronics, among others (FONACIT, 2004, cited by Vessuri and Sanchez, 2007).

Additionally, some training initiatives emerged to promote Nanoscience and Nanotechnology through the organization of a series of national and international events on the field. These activities started in the 90s with organization of schools, workshops and conferences on topics of interest to Nanoscience and Nanotechnology as electronic microscopy, catalysis, electronic transport and other nanomaterial properties. The earliest training activities that used the prefix "nano" were organized in 2005, 2006 and 2008, in Mérida, Venezuela by ULA's Science Faculty, IVIC and INTEVEP. Other two schools were organized in 2009 and 2013 at IVIC, Venezuela, within the framework of an inter-governmental agreement between Cuba and Venezuela, in a project for training of Human Resources in Nanoscience and Nanotechnology in both countries, and extended to students from the Bolivarian Alternative for the Peoples of Our America (ALBA) countries.

In 2009 started the series of Schools of Nanoscience and Nanotechnology, ENANO, organized mainly by the Venezuelan Nanotechnology Network, RedVnano, with the support of different academic institutions (UCV, IVIC, USB, ULA, among other institutions) and the support of the Ministry of Science and Technology in Venezuela. The first edition was organized in strong cooperation with French scientific institutions (20 French researchers were invited) and covered different topics of Nanotechnology (López *et al.*, 2011). The activity also served as the scenario for the foundational assembly of the Venezuelan Nanotechnology Network, RedVnano, which at the beginning of 2010 was formally established with 127 founder members (and has today 473 members). The main goal of the Network is to help reinforce national capacities on Nanotechnology, by promoting cohesion and synergies among actors of the national science and technology system, and improve social awareness about risks and opportunities of Nanotechnology. Network Members represent institutions from the productive domain (PDVSA, SIDOR-CVG, VENALUM-CVG, etc.), higher education (UCV, UC, UDO, ULA, UNEXPO, USB, LUZ, etc.) and/or R&D (IVIC, Institute of Advanced Studies –IDEA, Engineering Institute Foundation - FII, Zulian Institute of Technological Research -INZIT) and some State organs.

From 2009 in RedVnano converged different initiatives for the promotion of schools, workshops, conferences on Nanoscience and Nanotechnology. Very important, there was also a series of converging initiatives promoting an Interinstitutional Master's Program on Nanotechnology, for which this network has signed cooperation agreements with most of the higher education institutions having Nanotechnology capacities. This Master's programme has been already approved at IVIC and USB (these institutions are waiting for the final approval of the Ministry for Higher Education), and other institutions are assessing it (LUZ, ULA, among others). The study *pensa* were elaborated by an interinstitutional commission organized by RedVnano, turning out to be quite similar in all these institutions, which agreed that the main scope of the Nanotechnology programme is to provide professionals with skills and competences for the deep and systematic study of Nanoscience and Nanotecnology. Scientific concepts, methods and techniques of the field are to be managed aiming at solving complex problems of social interest, with an interdisciplinary vision and high ethical sense (Hasmy, 2011).

RedVnano has also managed to obtain the support of the PREFALC Program of the French Foundation Maison des Sciences de l'Homme, for co-funding the mobility of Nanotechnology teachers at the master level among several countries of the South American region and France. The project helped to organize the ENANO 2011 school, which aimed to implement a pilot experience for tuning future plans for the inter-institutional Nanotechnology Master Programme. The school included a nine-week program of courses, in nine different topics, which included synthesis and characterization techniques for nanostructured materials, physical and chemical properties of nanostructured materials, Nanotechnology applications to human health and oil industry, social implications, among other topics. Approximately 300 course-hours were taught by invited teachers (21 international and 34 national). Most of the courses were transmitted in 5 universities located in different Venezuelan cities (Caracas, Cumaná, Maracaibo, Mérida and Puerto Ordaz) by using videoconferencing. The number of registered students was 91 and they had the option to ask for evaluation at the end of each course, but only 16 students asked for evaluation and validated the course in their respective postgraduate study program.

The latest edition of ENANO was organized in January 2013. The format was similar to the first experience. The program included a week of courses focused on nanocomposites, coating and nanostructured porous materials. Most of the international invited (ten) are collaborators of two Nanotechnology FONACIT-PCP projects in progress.

Other events on Nanotechnology organized in Venezuela include the International Conference in Nanoscience (ICON 2006). Since many years ago UCV's Engineering Faculty as well as the Science Faculty include in their Research Days a program of activities focused on Nanotechnology. Most recently, June 2013, RedVnano organized the Regional Days of the Venezuelan Nanotechnology Network, which included a program of seminars from project and laboratory leaders of Nanoscience and Nanotechnology. The Days were held in three different Venezuelan cities: Caracas, Maracaibo and Mérida. In all these events international and national invited researchers have participated as well students from different Venezuelan institutions and in some cases from the Latin American region.

Infrastructure

According to the RedVnano, the distribution of the main equipment of technological interest in Venezuela corresponds to Caracas, Mérida, Maracaibo, Cumaná and Puerto Ordaz (Figure 19.6). Most equipment is found among the main academic institutions and some in industry.

The available infrastructure for nanocharacterization and nanomanufacturing includes equipment for chemical analysis, particle size and nanostructured coatings, scanning probe microscopes, SEM, TEM, XRD, NMR, among others. In Caracas the largest concentration of equipment and varied laboratories is to be found. In Maracaibo and Mérida prevail techniques such as FTIR, CVD, BET and XPS, and in Cumaná

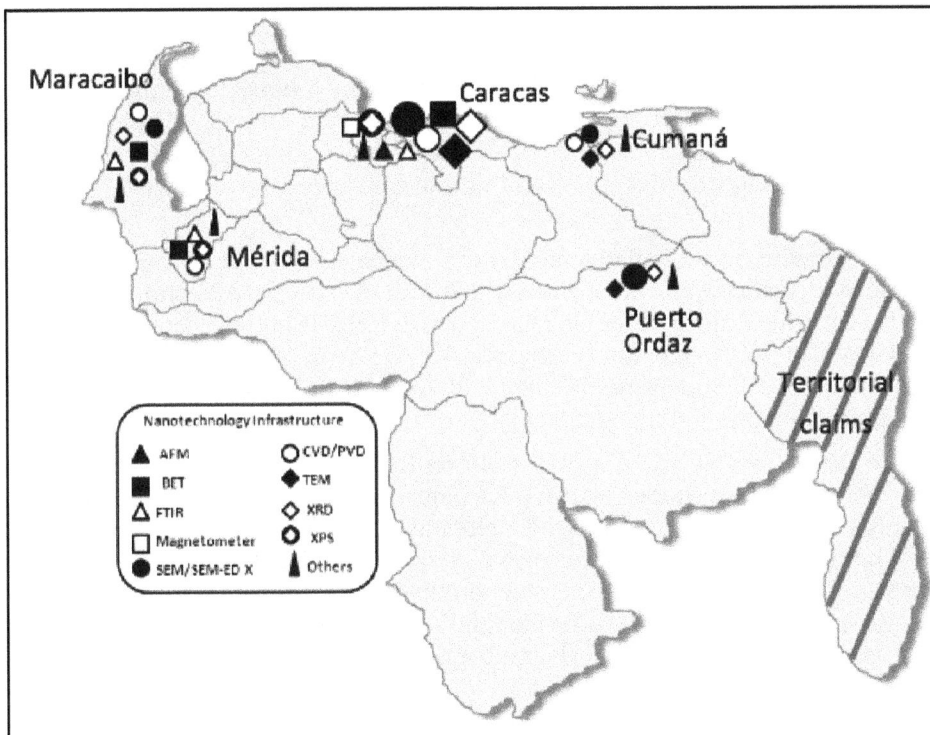

Figure 19.6: Venezuelan Map with Distribution of Nanotechnological Infrastructure (Largest symbols indicate more than one equipment)

***Source*: Authors' Elaboration on the Base of RedVnano Data**

and Puerto Ordaz, although presenting a lesser proportion of equipment, they have techniques such as DRX, SEM and TEM. A specific mention merits the recent acquisition of many nano characterization equipment by the National Institute of Hygiene "Rafael Rangel", organism responsible for pharmaceutical protocols and regulations located in Caracas, Venezuela.

Some of the equipment present in the different regions of the country is not fully functioning, due to different reasons related to repair and maintenance. The establishment of specific public policies, which among their aims include the formation of a national laboratory network to guarantee the full operation of the Nanotechnology infrastructure (as has happened in Brazil, the U.S.A. and Iran, among other nations), continues to be an overdue task.

Nanotechnology and the Productive Sector

As mentioned in a previous work (Lopez *et al.*, 2011), one of the challenges still pending that the Nanotechnology development poses to Venezuela is to aim R&D towards the production of goods and services. The country has little tradition in intellectual property instruments, as evidenced by different studies (Goncalves, 2006, De la Vega, *et al.*, 2007 and OICTS, 2008), which show that the majority of patent applications to Autonomous Service of Intellectual Property (SAPI) belonged to foreign institutions, most of them from the U.S.A., while the major part of the patents made by Venezuelan institutions originate from the national oil industry, PDVSA. The main applications exploited by the oil industry are associated to oil refining through heterogeneous catalysis, but developments also include fields for oil production sector, as is the use of nanoadditives in cementing and control of sand in oil wells (PDVSA, 2009).

Other public sector initiatives to develop Nanotechnology at the industrial level are the construction of a Chitosan Plant with the use of waste from the shrimp industry by the Zulia Institute of Technological Research (INZIT) and the construction of a pilot Plant of Hidroxiapatita on the basis of the association between IVIC and QUIMBIOTEC, all organisms affiliated with the Ministry of the Popular Power for Science Technology and Innovation.

In the private sector, important efforts have been done by some national pharmaceutical laboratories, which have embarked in initiatives of staff training, including some nanopharmacology development and innovation activities. Besides, the Clinical Nanomedicine Venezuelan Association (ASOVENAC) was constituted this year and since a few years ago a Nanotechnology session is usually included in the Venezuelan General Medicine Congress. The interest in Nanotechnology has also been present in other *fora* such as those of the food and information technology industry.

Social Implications and Awareness

A key challenge in the development of a normative framework for Nanotechnology is to overcome the current information deficits, which include the lack of scientific information and understanding of the potential risks of nanoparticles upon human health and environmental safety, the limited understanding of the different socio-technical trajectories that the technology can follow in the short, medium and long term, and the ethical and social implications of developing certain nanotechnological applications.

In the case of Venezuela, as we will see in Table 19.1, some of guidelines of the second Simon Bolivar National Development Plan (PNSB II) related to health, food safety, energy, housing, ICTs, etc., might be reached by reinforcing the use and development of nanodevices and nanostructured materials, but it is also important to take care of the risks that the development of applications with Nanotechnology in those fields might represent for the country, in terms of adverse effects to health and the environment through the contact with new materials; social upheavals due to the deep transformations of activities such as work and leisure; displacement of nature by an artificial environment, among others.

One of the current challenges faced by science and technology lies on the expectation that the design and technological practice become more democratic; this is a demand strongly associated to the current debate and questioning about the capacity of international scientific-technical systems to give answers on the possible risks derived from the new techno-scientific developments. In their practice,

Table 19.1: Correlation between Nanotechnology Applications and the Guidelines of the Venezuelan II National Simón Bolívar Plan (2013-2019)

PNSB II Guideline (2013-2019)	Sector/Nanotechnological applications
2.2.2.22 *"...Increase the proportion of essential medicines produced in the country..., required inputs by the National Public Health System"*	**Health/** ➢ Controlled liberation of pharmaceuticals ➢ Regenerative nanomedicine ➢ Lab-on-a-chip ➢ Nanotechnologies for medical imaging
1.4.10.1. *To promote innovation and the production of technological inputs for small agriculture, increasing the indexes of efficacy and productivity*	**Agrifoods/** ➢ Early detection of pathogens ➢ Water and nutrients nanodosifiers for self-sustainable crops ➢ Nanocomposite materials for food packaging and preservation
3.4.1.9 *To preserve hydric basins and watercourses.* And 3.4.12.8 *"...sanitation of wastewater"* 5.4.2. *"..., National Mitigation Plan, that covers the productive sectors issuing greenhouse gases, ..."*.	**Environment/** ➢ Nanocatalysts for water treatment and remediation ➢ Green chemistry ➢ Nanostructured porous materials for encapsulating atmospheric and other contaminants
1.2.5.2. *To consolidate the effective control of key activities in the oil and gas chain value* 3.1.7.1. *To develop petrochemical projects for processing natural gas, naphtha and refining currents, transforming them in products of higher added value*	**Hydrocarbon energy /** ➢ Nanostructured porous materials and nanoparticles for hydrocarbon refining Nanomaterials for sweetening natural gas and recovery of contaminants for the production of nanoparticles of interest to hydrocarbon refining ➢ Nanoadditves for cementing oil wells
3.1.12.2. *To diversify the matrix of primary energy and adequate energetic consumption to the best efficiency standards, incorporating coke, coal and other alternative energies.*	**Renewable energies /** ➢ Flexible solar cells based on nanomaterials ➢ Lithium batteries based on nanoparticled systems ➢ Fuel cells ➢ Nanocomposite materials for the production of eolic energy
1.5.1.3. *To guarantee the opportune access and adequate use of telecommunications and information technologies, through the development of the necessary infrastructure...*	**ICT's/** ➢ LCD, LED monitors and intelligent phones ➢ Devices based on silicium or carbon nanostructures ➢ Nanosensors for satellite technology ➢ Nanodevices for modulators and optical switches
3.1.7.*... To secure, accelerate and develop project of adding value associated to the following industrial entries: 3.2.5.1Iron and steel, 3.2.5.4-5-6. Aluminium, 3.2.5.13 Construction materials*	**Housing** ➢ Lighter, more resistant and durable metallic and polymeric nanocomposite materials for the house construction ➢ Paints with additives that are more resistant to water, corrosion and aging ➢ Antibacterial and self-cleaning ceramics based on nanomaterials

Source: Authors' Elaboration on the Base of RedVnano Data.

contemporary scientific researchers face the need to think in the ethical implications of their research activity, incorporating concepts such as risks, public perceptions, precautionary principles, responsibility, morality and ethics.

In this sense RedVnano has made important efforts to effectively include the discussion about risks and social implications. Among them the Workshop Opportunities and Risks of Nanotechnology, carried out in May 2012 stands out. In it relevant actors for the development of Nanotechnology at the national level were called in (staff from the Ministry of the Popular Power for Environment, the Ministry of the Popular Power for Health, Ministry of the Popular Power for Science, Technology and Innovation, IVIC, UCV, USB, the Rafael Rangel National Institute of Hygiene, PDVSA and basic industries), and 16 hours of introductory modules were delivered about concepts and themes transversal to the development of Nanotechnology at the national, regional and world levels, that would allow to strengthen its capabilities in decision-making in its domains of influence related to Nanotechnology. This workshop was structured to generate debate from the perspectives of the academic, governmental and productive sectors.

Other initiatives have been the recent elaboration of surveys and semi-structrured interviews to members of the Venezuelan nano community to explore and analyse the perceptions of risk associated to Nanotechnology in topics related to the ethics of

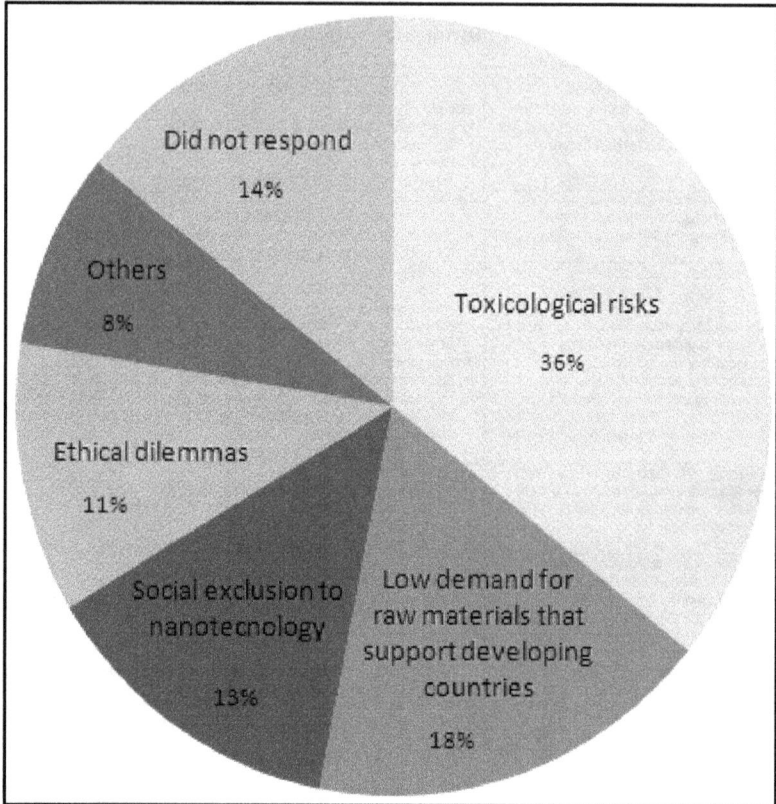

Figure 19.7: Perception of the Venezuelan Nano Community about the Potential Risks of Nanotechnology

Source: Authors' Elaboration on the Base of RedVnano Online Survey

science; the role of the scientific community in the debate about risks and opportunities posed by Nanotechnology for Venezuela and the role of states and society in governing the risks associated with this emerging technology. In what follows we present some results that gather the impressions of 74 interviewees and 21 in-depth interviews to the question: Can you identify potential environmental, health, social or economic risks in the applications you seek to develop with your research?

For the nano community in Venezuela, the toxicological risks of nanomaterials occupy the first place, followed by socio-economic risks such as the substitution of raw materials that support the economies of developing countries and the social exclusion by access to the application of Nanotechnology; these data indicate that although the perception of risk is mostly defined by risks related to the physical-chemical applications of nanomaterials, the Venezuelan nano community understands the risks of this technology in an integral manner and not only linked to scientific-technical factors. This undoubtedly represents a positive aspect of the development of the national agenda about social implications of Nanotechnology for it facilitates social mobilization around this problematic as well as the formulation of a public policy in regulatory concerns incorporating more easily the national research and development community.

Confronted with the question whether it is considered that there must be special regulations for developments in Nanoscience and Nanotechnology, 95 per cent of persons surveyed responded positively, while 3 per cent preferred not to answer, and only 2 per cent considered that there should not be special regulations; in parallel with this 58 surveyed individuals would be ready to participate in work group about norms and regulations. This coincides with the results obtained to the question about the disposition to participate in studies about nano risks and toxicology, which 53 persons out of the 74 so far surveyed asserted to be ready to participate in researches of this sort.

The qualitative analysis of the interviews reflects that for the development of research on risks and nanotoxicology, among the topics of greatest interest are biomedical applications, applications for the food sector and for environmental treatment, this due to the fact that most interviewees associated the risks to the dual use of scientific knowledge and admit the ethical dimensions of science, especially in sectors such as health, food and environment, claiming that the ethical implications of research in these fields are indifferent to the scale in which one works. In this sense they recognize as valid the concerns about the possible military use of nanotechnological applications, but they identify this problematic as being beyond the reach of their particular practice, for they conceive of the use of the technology as being separate from the process of knowledge production upon which it is based.

Venezuela is taking a step forward to establish norms and regulations for Nanotechnology in order to promote a sustainable development of this new technology. The plan to form a Working Group of experts from Cuba and Venezuela on these themes and the active participation of the country in the SAICM *fora*, through its Ministry of the Popular Power for Environment, also reflects the interest of the country to collaborate in an international Action Plan for nanomaterial management.

Diffusion of Nanotechnology in Venezuela

Since its early days RedVnano set for itself –as space of articulation between researchers, productive sector and policy decision-makers- specific aims addressed to the domain of popularization, through the promotion of social debate around the opportunities and challenges Nanotechnology poses to society and the need of developing at the national level norms, regulations and controls of goods and services generated by this technology.

In the activities of education, diffusion and popularization of Nanotechnology carried out in Venezuela two phases can be distinguished. A first phase (2004-2011) began in the context of the Happy Hour with Science in the Café Mediterráneo in Caracas. This event organized since 2004 by the Venezuelan Association for the Advancement of Science (Caracas Chapter) served as platform for several talks intended to diffuse topics of interest for Nanotechnology, among other fields of scientific knowledge. Later these activities were transferred to universities, research institutes and public and private industries. The talks dealt with basic notions of

Nanoscience and Nanotechnology, the situation of scientific and technological capabilities in this field in Venezuela and the presentation of RedVnano. The second phase, from 2011 to the present, supposes a broadening of these activities by addition of new actors such as the Students Nano Network of Los Andes University (RedNano.Est.ULA), which makes use of social networks and web spaces to diffuse Nanotechnology. They have carried out Diffusion Days in primary and secondary schools and held dialogues in universities, although with a limited scope to the western part of the country.

The "Nanotechnology Opportunities and Risks" workshop mentioned above was the basis for establishing the need of bringing the discussion about Nanotecnology to a broader space than university labs, research institutes, state apparatus and firms. Thus RedVnano aims to formulate a much more integral strategy that allows to build spaces of public debate around Nanotechnology, starting with the strengthening of ongoing activities at several levels of the domestic educational system but including new initiatives as well. These new initiatives share the assumption that science and technology communication is an integral and multidisciplinary process that must be compatible with the social and political dynamics in which it takes place. In this sense, science communication is conceived as being both an internal process inherent to the scientific community, through the publication and participation in events, and also an external and multidirectional process, from and towards the scientific community.

In this second phase the display of activities as the propagation of programs in the national circuit of radio and TV geared to Nanotechnology, in particular the Nano Universe program, made and transmitted by the Conciencia public TV channel, stands out. Other popularization spaces are accessible on the Internet through micros carried out by public organs and universities, as well as through photographical exhibitions.

Public Policies

Due to the opportunities and risks of Nanotechnology, central and emerging countries have taken full concern over the development of Nanotechnology and its implications, with national strategic plans and high investments. Venezuela does not have specific public policy for Nanotechnology, but the country has been involved in some initiatives that helped to create likely conditions. The first experience was the agreement signed between the Interamerican Development Bank (IDB) and the National Science and Technology Council of Venezuela (CONICIT) (today National Fund of Science and Technology, FONACIT) to fund a New Technologies Program (1991-1999).

In 1999, the new Venezuelan constitution established among priorities the science and technology sector. As a consequence two years later the Organic Law of Science and Technology and Innovation (LOCTI) came into being. The LOCTI established an obligation for the productive sector to support science and technology development. However, due to some changes done to the law, the LOCTI was implemented in 2006. Besides, the National Plan of Science, Technology and Innovation (2005–2030) (MCT, 2005) was launched focusing interests in transdisciplinary knowledge. The plan recognizes explicitly the importance of Nanotechnology, but in the agenda of priorities only emphasis in biotechnology and information technologies is made. However, in 2008 the Ministry of S&T started a foresight study in converging technologies (Nanotechnology, biotechnology, material and information technologies), and that same year the Engineering Institute Foundation (an organ ascribed to that ministry) published a foresight study in the field of nanomaterials (FII 2008).

While the term Nanotechnology does not yet appear explicitly in public financial calls, most of the projects developed on Nanoscience and Nanotechnology were funded by the Funding Agency FONACIT of the Ministry of S&T, financed through the LOCTI organic law. Support focused on some thematic priorities such as energy, new materials, and health among others, all of them of transversal interest to Nanotechnology. All these projects resulted in the improvement of some equipment and of the human resource training.

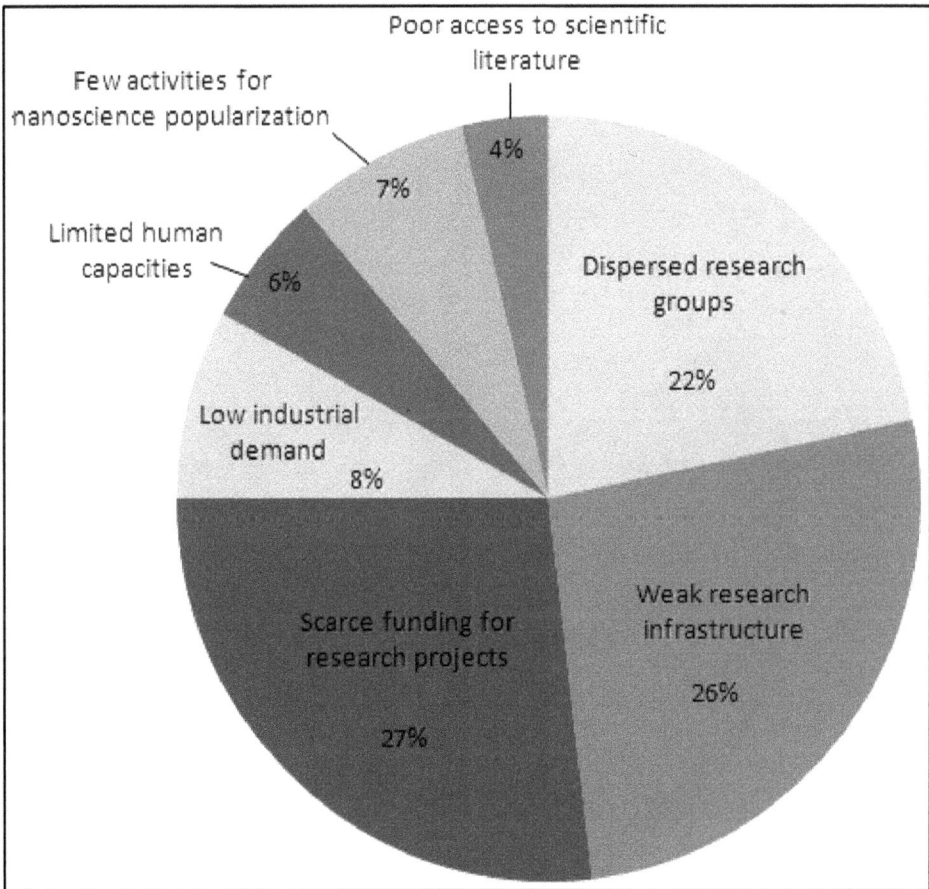

Figure 19.8: Perception of the Venezuelan Nano Community on Problems that Hinder the Nanoscience and Nanotechnology Development in Venezuela

Source: Authors' Elaboration on the Base of RedVnano Online Survey

Similarly, all schools, workshops and conferences on Nanoscience and Nanotechnology organized in Venezuela got support from the Ministry of S&T. Activities included round tables and meetings addressed to social implications of Nanotechnology. Particular mention merit two activities, one organized in 2007 by the Center of Science Studies at IVIC on an assessment of the elements for a public policy of Nanotechnology in Venezuela, and the second one mentioned above, organized in 2012 and addressed to risks and opportunities of Nanotechnology, aimed to promote a debate on elements of interest for elaborating public policies.

The cooperation agreement between Cuba and Venezuela for training nanotechnologists (2009-2013), and a new one to be started in 2014, are expected to conform a Work Group on norms and regulations, among other objectives, and to include other ALBA countries. The NANOSUR proposal led by Venezuela at MERCOSUR, the Memorandum of Understanding with Iran, are some of the public policies advanced by the Venezuelan government for international cooperation in Nanotechnology.

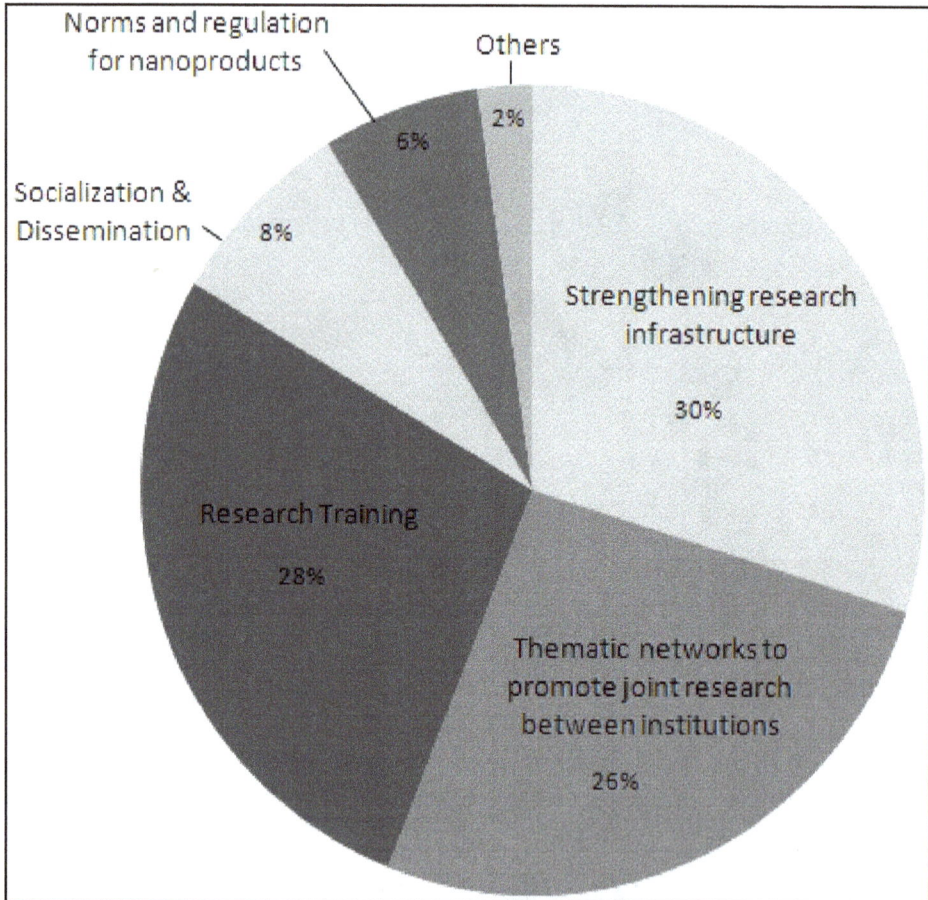

Figure 19.9: Issues that Should be Included in a Nanotechnology National Plan
Source: Authors' Elaboration on the Base of RedVnano Online Survey

In order to identify relevant issues for a national policy on Nanotechnology, the Venezuelan Nanotechnology Network, RedVnano, elaborated and distributed a survey among the Venezuelan nano community (74 persons answered the questionnaire). The results are shown in Figure 19.8. Three main difficulties for Nanotechnology development in Venezuela were identified: Scarce funding to support research projects, weak research infrastructure and dispersed research group.

Besides, persons were consulted about possible strategies to overcome difficulties. In particular, people considered that a national initiative for Nanotechnology development should include policies for strengthening research infrastructure (30 per cent of consulted persons), improving research training capacities (28 per cent) and supporting thematic research networks (or nodes) to promote joint projects among institutions on issues of national interest (26 per cent) (Figure 19.9). These results confirm previous conclusions (López *et al.*, 2011) where problems related to human and infrastructure capacity were identified as priority issues to be solved.

Nanotechnological applications could help to four of the five objectives of the Venezuelan second National Simón Bolívar Plan of Economic and Social Development (PNSB II, 2013-2019): National independence (objective 1), 21st century Bolivarian socialism (objective 2), Venezuela a powerful country (objective 3) and life preservation on our Planet (objective 5). Table 19.1 correlates many nanotechnological applications to different guidelines of the PNSB II.

CONCLUSIONS AND PERSPECTIVES

Venezuela has not yet implemented a National Initiative on Nanotechnology, but in recent years the country has created likely conditions. To profit form nanotechnology opportunities, and to generate a virtuous circle in research, development and innovation, a Venezuelan Nanotechnology Initiative could focus on implementing programs and funding instruments for the massive training of talents, toward joint projects between institutions and industry, and promoting mechanisms to protect intellectual property and to enable the incubation of technology-based firms geared to national needs. Besides, to minimize nano risks, the initiative should promote norms and regulations and knowledge socialization programs. Available evidence of funds through the organic law for S&T, LOCTI, building capacities based, school experiences organization like the ENANO schools, different master and PhD programs in basic sciences and engineering, including the inter-institutional Nanotechnology master program whose implementation is in progress, among other considerations are relevant elements that could help the country to aspire for a better position in the world in profiting Nanotechnology benefits. Energy, coating, pharmaceutical, new materials, electronic, environmental and human health are some of the sectors that can directly get benefits by using Nanotechnology. Some social awareness experiences on Nanoscience and Nanotechnology have been undertaken and the status of regional and international cooperation could help to improve conditions for a Nanotechnology plan development in Venezuela. NANOANDES networks and the Latin American Network for Nanotechnology and Society meeting will be held in Venezuela in 2014, as satellite activities of the first Venezuelan Nanotechnology Conference, and the International Workshop on

Nanotechnology, IWoN, of Non-Aligned and Other Developing Countries will be held also in Caracas in 2015. All these activities may provide a good scenario for launching a national initiative hopefully in 2014.

REFERENCES

1. De la Vega I, Suárez M, Blanco F, Troconis A, Aponte G (2007) Las tecnologías nanoscópicas en los centros y las periferias. El caso de los nanomateriales en Venezuela. Red Latinoamericana de Nanotecnología y Sociedad (ReLANS). http://estudiosdeldesarrollo.net/relans/documentos/VENEZUELA.pdf.

2. FII (2008), Fundación Instituto de Ingeniería, MCTI, *Estudio prospectivo de nanomateriales en Venezuela*, Caracas, Venezuela.

3. Goncalves E (2006) "Estudio exploratorio acerca de los recursos existentes en las tecnologías convergentes en Venezuela. Caso: Nanotecnologías." Trabajo de grado para optar al Magíster Scientiarum. IVIC. Caracas.

4. Hasmy, A (2011) Formación y Divulgación de la Nanotecnología en Venezuela: Situación y Perspectiva. Mundo Nano 4: 72-82

5. Juma, C. and Yee-Cheong, L. (Coords.) (2005) Innovation: Applying Knowledge in Development. UN Millennium Project: Task Force on Science, Technology, and Innovation. London: Millennium Project and Earth Scan

    http://www.unmillenniumproject.org/reports/index.htm

6. López M.S., Hasmy A. and Vessuri H. (2011) Nanoscience and Nanotechnology in Venezuela. J. Nanopart. Res. 13: 3101-3106

7. MCT Ministerio de Ciencia y Tecnología (2005). Plan Nacional de Ciencia, Tecnología e Innovación: Construyendo un futuro sustentable. Venezuela

    http://www.fonacit.gov.ve/documentos/MCT.pdf

8. OICTS (2008) Observatorio Iberoamericano de Ciencia, Tecnología y Sociedad. La Nanotecnología en Iberoamérica. Situación actual y tendencia.

    http://www.oei.es/salactsi/nano.pdf

9. PDVSA (2009) Intevep avanza en estudios para la aplicación de nanotecnología en pozos. May 14th. http://www.pdvsa.com/index.php?tpl=interface.sp/design/readsearch.tpl.html and newsid_obj_id=7557 and newsid_temas=0

10. Porter A, Youtie J, Shapira F, Schoeneck D (2008) Refining search terms for Nanotechnology. *J Nanopart. Res*. 10: 715-728

11. Silberglitt R, Antón PS, Howell DR, Wong A. *et al.* (2005) The Global Technology Revolution 2020, In-depth analyses:Bio/Nano/Materials/Information trends, drivers, barriers, and social implications. Rand Corporation Technical Report Series

    http://www.rand.org/pubs/technical_reports/2006/RAND_TR303.pdf

12. Vessuri H, Sanchez I (2007) Estudio Nacional Venezuela. InRoKS/IDRC 2003 – 2004 (2007) Comprendiendo las Dimensiones Sociales y de Política Pública de Tecnologías Transformativas en el Sur. Proyecto: Tecnologías Convergentes: ¿Qué está siendo hecho y qué debería hacerse sobre ellas en los Países Andinos? Informe Final de Investigación. La Paz, Bolivia.

http://www.redvnano.org/documentos/proyecto.pdf

Chapter 20

From Laboratory to Market: The Challenges of Transferring Nanotechnology Concepts Towards Business Perspectives in Africa

Trust Saidi

Department of Technology and Society Studies,
P.O. Box 616, 6200MD Maastricht University, The Netherlands
E-mail: t.saidi@student.maastrichtuniversity.nl

ABSTRACT

Throughout the history of mankind, materials have defined the technology of the age. We refer to the Stone Age and Iron Age because of the types of materials that were used or developed during those eras to make the technologies for everyday life. Materials are the essence of nanotechnology as at the nanoscale, materials exhibit properties that are different from the raw materials. At the nanoscale, materials configure themselves in different atomic arrangements not seen in the bulk form of the same materials. The laws of physics that operate on objects at the nanoscale combine classical mechanics, which govern the operations of everyday life with the fundamental laws of nature. Nanotechnology typifies revolutionary technologies which have the potential for broad applications and provide opportunities for entrepreneurship, not just in the specific technology, but also in its uses and support. Nanotechnology presents prospects for commercial applications leading to the creation of new businesses. Without useful applications, nanotechnology will remain an abstract curiosity, largely unknown except to a few interested people. However, when applications begin to appear, there is need for a business, or its equivalent, to fully exploit the technology. In order for nano-products to be made commercially viable, they must have characteristics that make them profitable for those who make them. On a very basic level, the products must be made with a process adaptable to a production environment and the production process must be able to be monitored to ensure that the products function properly without posing risks to the people and environment. The novelty and pervasiveness of nanotechnology, the established interests of stakeholders and the challenges that scientists have in communicating the value proposition of nanotechnology applications to the industry makes the process of transferring nanotechnology concepts into business perspectives complex.

Keywords: *Nanotechnology, Business, Applications, Laboratory, Market.*

INTRODUCTION

Nanotechnology is the manipulation of materials at the molecular level between 1 and 100 nanometres resulting in nanoscale particles which are different from the raw materials in terms of physical and chemical properties (Mantovani and Porcari, 2009; Salamanca-Buentello *et al.*, 2008). The development of nanotechnology is driven by the exploitation of the unique characteristics of the resultant superior materials, which occur in the transitional area between atoms and microscopic scale. The scale of nanotechnology, according to Selin (2007) is the most significant delineator of what kinds of activities, artifacts, tools, knowledge and structures embrace the technological realm. At the nanoscale, the materials possess extraordinary and enabling properties, which are capable of transforming both the industrial and social facets of human life (Parr, 2005). In this regard, the size dependent technology is expected to bring a technological paradigm in the form of a revolutionary wave of innovation, which is expected to surpass previous technologies such as Biotechnology and Information and Communication Technologies (ICT).

The ability to manipulate atoms and molecules at nanoscale in order to fabricate new materials and devices that possess remarkable properties has spurred the establishment of nanotechnology research and development centres at universities and government laboratories all over the world. The expectations are that the various inventions and discoveries associated with nanotechnology will spawn many new businesses in an endeavour to exploit the discoveries (Booker and Boysen, 2005). This comes in the wake of the fact that business is one of the vehicles through which new technology is made available to the consumers via manufactured products. However, with nanotechnology, the entry barriers are much higher than those for previous technologies. Despite this, many countries around the globe are investing significantly in the development of nanotechnology within their borders (Meridian Institute, 2005; Einsiedel and McMullen, 2004). The countries are driven by the recognition that nanotechnology has the potential to transform the business sector in every country of the world, hence they do not want to be left behind. The drive is towards harnessing innovation and tapping business opportunities with the ultimate goal of bringing nano-products to the market.

Applications of Nanotechnology

There is an incredibly broad range of prospective uses of nanotechnology, as the technology has the potential to affect virtually every industry. In South Africa, nanotechnology is being applied in adding value to minerals at DST/Mintek Nanotechnology Innovation Centre through the exploitation of gold nanoparticles. For example, the Biolabels group at Mintek has developed point of care diagnostic kits for rapid qualitative determination of antigens in human blood or serum while the Sensors group is developing electrochemical sensors for monitoring and surveillance of communicable diseases or virus outbreaks (Mintek, 2012). At the Centre for Scientific and Industrial Research (CSIR), the Nanomedicine Research Platform is developing a nano-enabled drug that facilitates targeted delivery for treating tuberculosis (CSIR, 2012). At the University of Johannesburg, a group of researchers are working in collaboration with the Water Research Platform at Mintek in applying nanotechnology for water purification. At University of Witwatersrand, the Centre of Excellence in Strong Materials is exploiting the unique properties of carbon nanotubes for catalysis (SAASTA, 2010).

In Kenya, a group of researchers at University of Nairobi are working on the application of nanotechnology in dye-sensitised solar cells with the aim of enhancing the efficiency. The Institute of Primate Research, which is located in Kenya, is a participating partner in the EU-FP7 funded Nano-Trypanosomiasis Project, which is aimed at assessing the applicability of nanotechnology in the diagnosis and treatment of human African trypanosomiasis. The researchers are developing new simple to use diagnostic tests as well as new, nanobody based treatment methods for trypanosomiasis (Institute of Primate Research, 2011). In Zimbabwe, researchers at National University of Science and Technology (NUST) successfully patented a smart nano filter for water treatment, while at the University of Zimbabwe, scientists are working towards developing nano-enabled medicine. While there has been remarkable progress in basic research, the process of transferring nanotechnology concepts towards business perspectives is proving to be a challenging not only for developing countries but also developed countries.

While governments and industries around the world are investing large sums of money towards research on nanoscience, it appears too easy to overestimate the impact of nanotechnology as most of the more spectacular expected products are far from being rolled to the market. Though nanotechnology is commonly referred to as a major upcoming business opportunity, the process of transferring nanotechnology concepts towards business perspectives is proving to be neither linear nor automatic. There is a strong consensus in industry, academia and government that the future competitiveness of nanotechnology and all that it underpins will be determined, in large part by research, innovation and how quickly firms and industries apply and incorporate new technologies into high-value-added products and high-efficiency processes (Rothrock, 2008). There are barriers that adversely affect the exploitation of nanotechnology and these relate to the complexity of nanotechnology research, bottlenecks in human resources and funding as well as poor process of transition from basic research to pilot and industrial scale production (OECD, 2010).

The challenges in the exploitation of nanotechnology have resulted in the technology being limited primarily to basic research with huge and partly hyped commercial expectations. The confinement of the technology to the laboratory is an inhibiting factor for business development and the subsequent exploitation of commercial opportunities (Boaccorsi and Piccaluga, 1994). As such, nanotechnology is still in an early and uncertain phase of development with various directions of commercialisation pending. This immaturity and uncertainty interferes with the transfer of the technology from the laboratory to the market (Valentin, 2000). One fundamental issue in transforming nanotechnology concepts into business perspectives is how the scientific knowledge base residing at universities can be applied in the commercial sphere (Bozeman, 2000). In the African countries like Kenya and Zimbabwe, few early adopters, fragmented markets, lack of infrastructure and few efficient manufacturing methods hinder the exploitation of the technology. This delay the time over which nano-enabled products are expected on the market.

Time is a critical factor in the development of nanotechnology and is more pronounced when it comes to converting basic research into products of economic value. In Zimbabwe, most of the work on nanotechnology is primarily basic research in which scientists are tinkering with nanotechnology ideas and concepts. It is not known when the research that is confined to the laboratory will reach the market. The ideal scenario is when nanotechnology concepts closely follow business perspectives to ensure that companies transform innovation into products. While it has been emphasised that the development of technology follows a predictable and traceable path as per the linear model of innovation from invention to diffusion (Rogers, 2003), the case of nanotechnology reveals that converting nanotechnology concepts into business perspectives is not an easy task as the rapid advancement of the technology is yet to be achieved as shown in Figure 20.1.

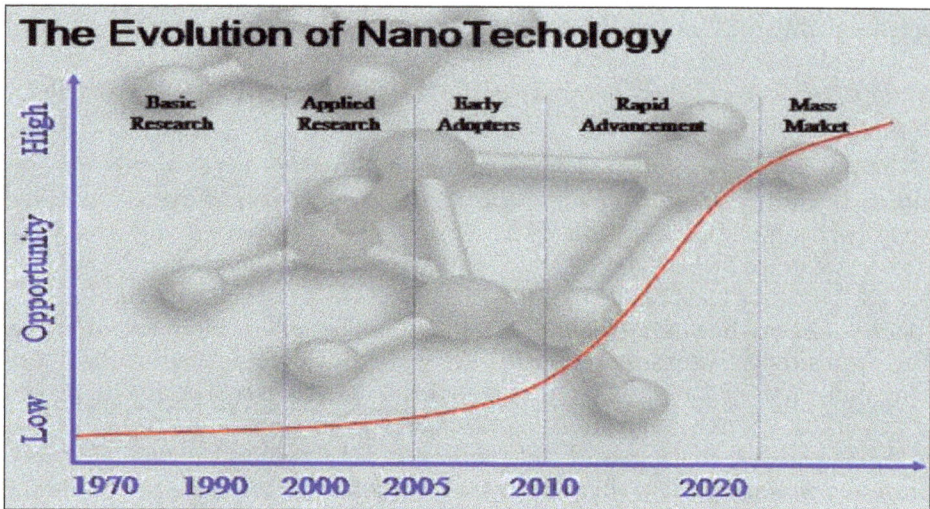

Figure 20.1: Linear Development of Nanotechnology
(Kurniawan and Sillanpaa, 2009)

Figure 20.1 shows that the period between 2010 and 2020 is the phase when nanotechnology is projected to reach rapid advancement. However, an analysis of the situation on the ground reveals that countries such as Zimbabwe and Kenya are still preoccupied with the first stage of basic research, which means that the countries are lagging behind in the adoption of the technology by approximately 20 years. This is an indication that there are challenges in converting nanotechnology concepts into viable products for the benefit of society. In this regard, the business opportunities associated with nanotechnology are yet to be fully harnessed.

Challenges in Transforming Nanotechnology Concepts into Business Perspectives

Much of the research which is done on nanotechnology resides at universities. With regard to Zimbabwe, institutions of higher learning, namely University of Zimbabwe, National University of Science and Technology and Chinhoyi University of Technology are actively engaged with nanoscience. On the other hand, there is reluctance by the companies which are expected to exploit the technology to come up with commercially viable products. What is becoming more explicit with the emergence of nanotechnology is that universities and companies are driven by different mandates and motives. The interactive models of innovation suggest that the main objective of companies is to carry out applied research for realising innovations (OECD, 2010). In contrast, universities by their nature are focused on basic research for the general advancement of knowledge and academic degrees.

Since research on nanotechnology in Kenya and Zimbabwe is still basic, companies most of which are foreign owned and directed, are reluctant to invest in nanotechnology research because of its high entry costs. As such, companies are not yet visible in the exploitation of nanotechnology. There is a missing link between basic research conducted at universities and applied research by manufacturing companies. This is a challenge in the sense that companies possess production technologies and their absence in the exploitation of nanotechnology results in little prospects of applied research. This is an issue of primary concern towards the development of nanotechnology as it makes it difficult to cross the so-called "valley of death" between basic and applied research. As such, university researchers are more focused on activities further upstream almost by default and companies are expected to take over from there to satisfy the market.

Although, Zimbabwe is endowed with minerals such as gold, platinum and diamonds, the country suffers from imbalance of payments. This is attributed to the export of minerals in their raw state. Through the application of nanotechnology, value can be added to the minerals so that they fetch better prices on the market. However, several companies in the mining sector are adopting a wait-and-see attitude and the potential opportunities brought by nanotechnologies are left unexplored. Little is being done to apply nanotechnology in mineral beneficiation. This results in an innovation chasm which depicts a missing link between basic research at universities and applied research at companies as shown in Figure 20.2.

The innovation chasm shown in Figure 20.2 is more pronounced when there is no interaction and meaningful engagement between universities and industries. The lack of tighter modes of interactions, where companies fund research and development at universities results in challenges in transforming nanotechnology concepts into business ideas. Ideally, the government and industry should be instrumental in

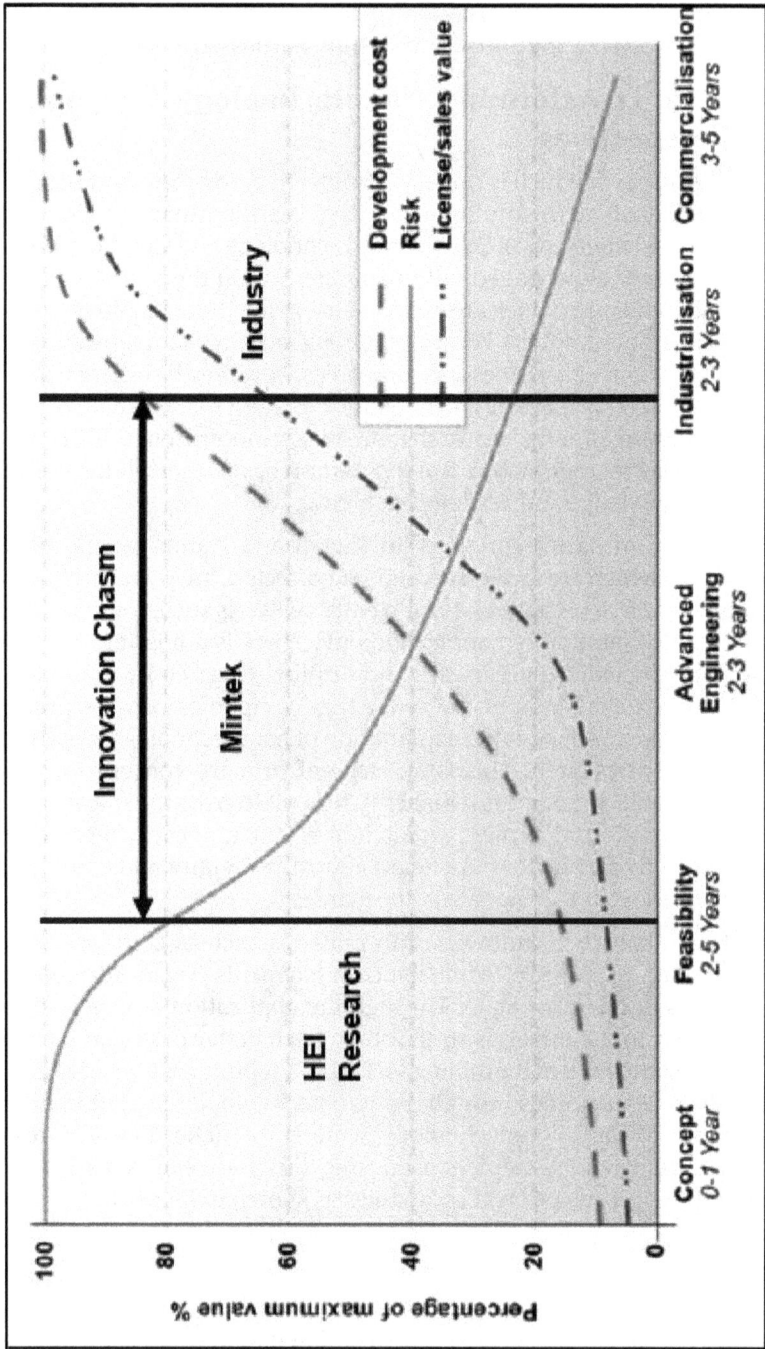

Figure 20.2: The Innovation Chasm (Mintek, 2011)

financing research and development, but in most developing countries, it is more of a vision than reality. Although the National Partnership for Africa's Development (NEPAD) set a target for African countries of spending 1 per cent of GDP on Research and Development as endorsed by the Executive Council of the African Union (AU-NEPAD, 2010), only a very few countries have reached the recommended level.

Intellectual Property Rights are a formidable barrier in the development of nanotechnology. As nanotechnology is an emerging technology driven by research and development, it gives rise to innovative manufacturing processes and products which need to be protected by intellectual property rights. There is an emerging nano race among the developed countries as indicated by the number of nanotechnology patents as shown Figure 20.3.

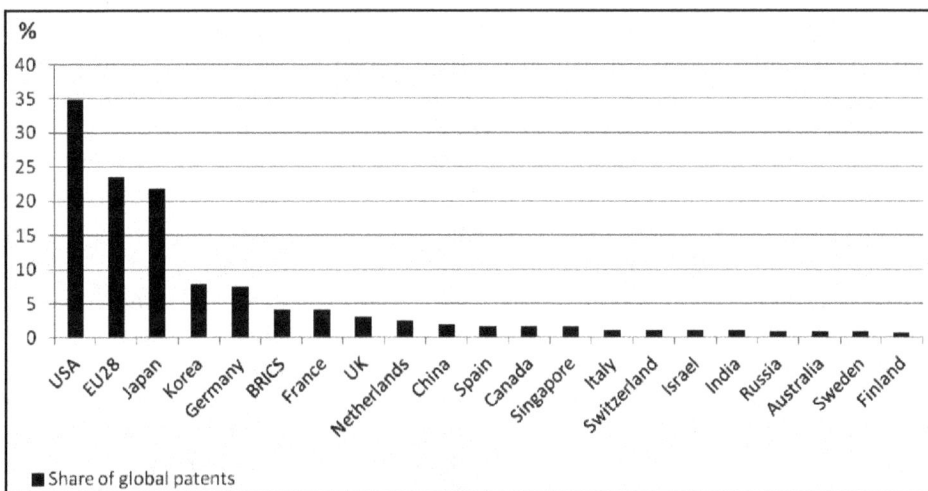

Figure 20.3: Share of Countries in Nanotechnology Patents 2008-2010 (OECD, 2013)

What is explicit from Figure 20.3 is that most nanotechnology patents are filed by the leading players from the developed countries, which are making heavy financial commitments in research and development of the technology (Battelle, 2008). In sub-Saharan Africa, South Africa, which is part of the BRICS, is the only country with notable nanotechnology patents.

While the expectations of nanotechnology applications, such as nanomedicine seem imminent, the challenge lies on the extent to which the technology will be able to diffuse to the poor, particularly in developing countries (Parr, 2005). For example, there is hardly any patent registered on nanotechnology in Zimbabwe and Kenya and there are no prospects of registering one in the near future as the two countries are lagging behind in the exploitation of the technology. This raises questions about whether African countries will ever benefit from nanotechnology because these countries will have to rely on patents from developed countries. This comes at a cost and the challenge is pronounced in poor countries where the financial resources to secure the necessary licenses to exploit patents are scarce. The paradox is that nanotechnology promises cheap solutions, which make it a pro-poor technology, but intellectual property rights make the technology beyond the reach of many intended beneficiaries. This illustrates how patents interfere with the transformation of nanotechnology concepts into practical benefits for human development.

Moreover, the exploitation of intellectual property rights on nanotechnology is complicated by the wide range of patent claims and the formation of patent thickets. These mount a significant barrier in the sense that the costs of navigating patent thickets are high and can outweigh some of the commercial gains (OECD, 2010). For example, carbon nanotubes have resulted in a frenzy of patenting leading to overly broad patent claims, which create a dense thicket of interlocking and overlapping patents. Still on patents, Bleeker and Uhlir (2007) argue that the emerging nature of nanotechnology makes it difficult to identify the prior art in order to determine whether patent applications should be granted. As African countries are lagging behind in terms of registering patents on nanotechnology, the situation paints a gloomy picture towards transferring nanotechnology concepts into business perspectives because patents filed by other countries serve as monopolistic guarantees of earnings for a period of twenty years. The skewed ownership of patents works against the rapid diffusion of the potential benefits of nanotechnology in developing countries.

Knowledge translation, including communication challenges interfere with transferring nanotechnology concepts into business perspectives. Scholars such as D'Este and Patel (2005), Zucker *et al.* (2002) and Schartinger *et al.* (2001) have analysed how the degree of codification of knowledge and different modes of interaction relates to the challenges and outcomes of technology transfer. According to their assessment, the transfer of knowledge of more tacit nature as the case with nanotechnology tends to require human mobility across organisational boundaries or other more intense and direct modes of interactions with companies. In Zimbabwe, companies used to collaborate particularly with the University of Zimbabwe in conducting research, but of late the level of interaction has decreased since the country started experiencing economic problems. Several manufacturing companies are closing down, citing viability problems. Instead, the gap between universities and industries is widening and this is not ideal in the commercialisation of technologies. While Valentin (2000) highlights a general lack of interest on companies as a challenge with universities being perceived as taking a passive role towards companies at the outset, the situation in Zimbabwe indicates that the collapse of the industrial sector is the major drawback. This is happening within a context of the inherent socio-economic and political challenges in which externally driven industries in the form of transnational companies and multinational companies are adversely affected by the indigenisation policy. The indigenisation policy of Zimbabwe requires all foreign owned companies to shed 51 per cent ownership to locals, a situation which makes the country less attractive for investment.

Cultural issues interfere with the commercialisation of nanotechnology. Universities and companies operate according to different ethical codes. The former prioritises common ownership of scientific knowledge, freedom to publish research results, professional prestige and independency. In contrast, companies tend to protect the secrecy and privacy of research that feeds into new technologies, products or processes and they invest in research to obtain short-term and commercial benefits for their shareholders, although they sometimes do so to enhance their absorptive capability vis-à-vis university research (Palmberg, 2007). Universities are almost by default more bureaucratic in their organisational set-up and less flexible to rapid shifts in research needs than companies (Valentin, 2000). This reflects the fundamental differences that universities and companies have concerning their incentives to interact with each other and engage in technology transfer (Schartinger *et al.,* 2001; Stephan, 1996). There tends to be a continuum of looser and tighter forms of interactions, ranging from conferences or seminars, supervision and joint publications to joint research facilities between universities and companies. In Kenya and Zimbabwe, the level of interaction between universities and companies is minimal. South Africa provides an interesting case in which universities and companies complement each other despite their cultural differences. The notable examples are companies such as Sasol, Element 6, Johannesburg Water and NECSA, which work in liaison with the University of the Witwatersrand, University of Johannesburg and Tshwane University of Technology among others.

Nanotechnology poses risks, some of which are known while others are not known. Some of the unknown risks are anticipated to have disastrous effects to the environment and human health in the end. The process of investigating the potential risks of nanotechnology, especially the toxicity of nanomaterials is a challenge towards transforming nanotechnology concepts into business perspectives. The complexity in the regulation of nanotechnology as a result of unknown environmental and health risks poses challenges in the development of the technology. (Swiss National Science Foundation, 2009). The lack of a sound framework on the risk governance of nanotechnology creates uncertainty on the fate of nanoproducts on the market. According to OCED (2010), the lack of regulatory protection means that producers of nano-enabled products are left without any immunity from false claims. In such an environment, companies are hesitant to bring important and useful nanotechnology products to market, because of fear of potential liability, even if the harm is not real. For example, in South Africa, a local manufacturing company once flighted an advertisement in the electronic media of the nano-enabled washing machine, only to remove it after concerns were raised on the safety of nanoparticles. Thus, the potential for overreaction to both actual and perceived risks, combined with regulatory fears complicates the business environment for companies. Due to fear of a possible lawsuit, some companies prefer to use nanotechnology in their products without making it explicit by labelling the nano component(s) used. This results in many nanoproducts entering the market without the knowledge of the consumers.

From a historical perspective, public perceptions of technologies shape the trajectory taken in generating innovation and its subsequent diffusion to the market. Lessons learnt from the development of ICT and Biotechnology (in particular GMOs in food crops) offer some perspectives worthy of urgent and serious consideration by governments in African countries. There is a possibility that nanotechnology may typify other technological advancements, which were once predicted to be relevant to the problems of the poor in developing countries, but failed to deliver the expected results (Invernizzi *et al.,* 2008; Invernizzi *et al.,* 2007). For example, the benefits of genetically modified organisms that were regarded as a solution to the challenge of hunger in the African countries were accrued in the developed world, which had the resources to adopt the new technology. Freeman (2003) argues that the slow industrial uptake and societal use of Biotechnology in some African countries was due to problems of social and political appreciation, understanding and eventual acceptance. The development of nanotechnology may follow the same path as a result of perceived health and environmental impacts, which are a source of controversy in the exploitation of the technology.

The absence of clear, concise and compelling business plans, including translation of emerging technologies into the market create formidable barriers in transforming nanotechnology concepts into business perspectives (Waitz and Bokhari, 2003). This comes in the wake of the fact that a good business plan shows that the investors have thought through all the major issues that they are likely to encounter in building their business, both at home and abroad. The critical components of a business plan focus on the issues that enable companies to bring their products to the market (Battelle, 2008). A good plan allows for efficient communication of the business and it is comprehensive to cover more than just the technology. Some researchers in science and technology do not consider thoroughly key business issues such as manufacturing and sales channel strategies and this present bottlenecks when it comes to transforming nanotechnology concepts into business perspectives. As such, a general lack of business orientation towards research results in blue-sky research, which is more of academic interest than problem solving of real life challenges. Waitz and Bokhari (2003) cite the lack of business and market skills by the university researchers as one of the biggest challenges. This adversely affects the development of nanotechnology as the lack of essential business and entrepreneurial skills makes it difficult to establish a value proposition of research to potential investors.

The absence of dedicated and coordinated teams in nanotechnology at all levels, be they national, sub-regional and global militates against effective transformation of nanotechnology concepts into business perspectives. As noted by Waitz and Bokhari (2003), one of the success factors in the exploitation of nanotechnology is a well balanced team of researchers. The teams need to have the multi-disciplinary skill sets to facilitate the exploitation of the technology. If members of the nanotechnology research teams are from the same academic discipline, yet the technology demands multi-disciplinary skills, challenges are bound to arise in the exploitation and development of the product. The lack of alignment and collaboration results in many researchers working in 'proverbial silos'. At University of the Witwatersrand, the research on carbon nanotubes has resulted in the fusion of disciplinary boundaries with chemists, physicists, engineers and toxicologists working together as a unit. However, the situation is quite different in Kenya and Zimbabwe, where disciplinary boundaries in institutions of higher learning are conspicuous. With the establishment of National Nanotechnology Programme by government of Zimbabwe, there is a drive towards multidisciplinary approaches in the development of nanotechnology.

It is common for researchers in the academia to underestimate the difficulties in commercialising new technologies. Blakely (2005) argues that it is much more difficult to make products in high quantities at a certain level of quality and consistence than to demonstrate something in a laboratory With reference to nanotechnology, the poor scalability of outputs from the technology research raises costs and prolongs new product development (OECD, 2010). This makes nanotechnology less attractive to investors. For example, the production of carbon nanotubes by chemists at University of the Witwatersrand has proven that the process of scaling up to meet growing demand is difficult. This result in demand outstripping supply, hence the application of the carbon nanotubes is limited to research at laboratory scale. This is an impediment towards commercialisation of nanotechnology as it confines the application of the technology to experimentation. There are several companies in need of large quantities of carbon nanotubes, but meeting the demand is difficult. Various methods of making carbon nanotubes have been explored at the University of the Witwatersrand, but the yield has remained relatively low. The irreproducible performance and complex properties of some nanomaterials present formidable challenges in the transition of nanotechnology from laboratory scale to pilot and prototype manufacturing. In Zimbabwe, researchers at National University of Science and Technology developed a water filter that works well at laboratory scale. However, the process of scaling up the filter to provide water at community level has proven to be a mammoth task.

By virtue of being a platform technology, nanotechnology underlies many other new technologies, thereby deriving revenue streams from many different application domains. This makes the technology a de-facto standard of the emerging technology revolution. Palmberg (2007) describes the potential economic impacts of nanotechnology by making reference to the concept of general purpose technology. It refers to a technology with a range of characteristics that makes it particularly well placed to generate longer-term productivity and economic growth across a broad spectrum of industries. Nanotechnology already bears some of the hallmarks of a general purpose technology, the remarkable one being its potential applicability in a wide range of industries as well as its multi-purpose nature (Youtie, *et al.*, 2008; Lipsey *et al.*, 2005). However, the challenge with platform technologies is that they result in the lack of focus, particularly among start-up companies. The danger of not focusing on a particular application can often be detrimental for new companies, especially if venture capitalists are not interested in multiple divergent products. South Africa is an example of a country that is geared towards making specific applications of nanotechnology in the water, health and energy sector. Also, Zimbabwe has clearly delineated its focus areas in nanotechnology research as University of Zimbabwe is focusing on applications in drug discovery, Chinhoyi University of Technology focuses on energy and National University for Science and Technology on water purification. Plans are underway for Scientific and Industrial Research and Development Centre to focus on applied research, while Africa University will work on intellectual property rights issues.

Nanotechnology falls under the category of disruptive technologies which are known for displacing established technologies through new ways of doing things. They overturn the traditional business methods and practices. This is a challenge when the technology destabilises already existing markets and fails to create new ones (Christensen, 1997). Many nanotechnology based products are targeted at existing markets. To be successful, these new products may displace the incumbents based on price and/or performance. Beyond this, the nano-based products will need to be proven to have the same quality and reliability as the existing solutions. In conservative industries such as ICT and medicine, gaining the record of accomplishment on reliability tend to take more time than expected (Waitz and Bokhari, 2003). As such, many nano-based companies enter the industry with the expectation that they would ramp the volume significantly within the first year after the introduction of their first commercial product, only to be disappointed. The disruptive character of the technology is a setback, which makes nanotechnology based companies bound to fall in the growth phase. While nano enabled products such as skin lotions and paints have superior qualities that give them an upper hand in the market, their disruptive character comes with a host of challenges.

Nanotechnology is a capital-intensive industry. The companies working on converting nanotechnology concepts into business perspectives in the developing countries are hindered from reaching their potential due to the lack of infrastructure and capital. Since nanotechnology is typically a cutting edge technology, companies suffer from lack of an existing well developed infrastructure (Maclurcan, 2005). What other companies can take for granted, such as abundant technically trained workforce, manufacturing equipment, support services and design software are crucial for nanotechnology applications. The companies, which lack research instrumentation, work force and institutional support encounter problems in exploiting nanotechnology. On the other hand, larger companies might also be reluctant to invest, especially when technologies are in their early and uncertain phase of development. In this regard, nanotechnology startups are forced to create more of their own infrastructure as they develop and this is not an easy task. As a result, many companies backtrack along the way as they find the costs involved to be unbearable to break even. Nanotechnology, unlike Biotechnology and other emerging technologies depends more on physical infrastructure in the form of state of art electron microscopes and clean room facilities. In Kenya and Zimbabwe, the lack of facilities for research on nanotechnology presents insurmountable challenges towards the exploitation of the technology. For example, electron microscopes, which facilitate manipulation of nano materials are expensive for companies in developing countries (Invernizzi *et al.*, 2007). In this context, the development of nanotechnology tends to favour larger established companies more than start-ups, as they possess well furnished laboratories as well as complementary assets and infrastructure.

The development of nanotechnology demands a critical mass of skilled personnel. The threshold of entry into nanotechnology sector is difficult in terms of skill requirements for most developing countries (Alemayehu, 2000). For the period stretching from early 2000, Zimbabwe lost experienced scientists through brain drain when the country went through a period of political and economic instability. This remains a challenge considering that a country's ability to foster and support the development of nanotechnology requires a ready supply of the staff necessary to work in the interdisciplinary field. Advances in nanotechnology depend on research scientists who have the expertise necessary to work at nanoscale. The research on nanotechnology requires a basic understanding of concepts of nanotechnology, such as properties of materials at nanoscale and quantum effects. This demands the collaboration of researchers from different scientific disciplines. As a result, individuals working on nanotechnology should have a basic knowledge of other scientific disciplines and be able to communicate effectively with other scientists.

The Way Forward

In order to transform nanotechnology concepts into business perspectives, African countries should adopt aggressive technology policies and devise broad based strategies that promote partnerships and cooperation between both north-south and south-south. This requires government funding and support within a framework of clearly defined goal-oriented nanotechnology strategies. South Africa is a good example of a country that has nanotechnology strategy, which consists of both the national research framework and an integrated manufacturing strategy as shown in Figure 20.4.

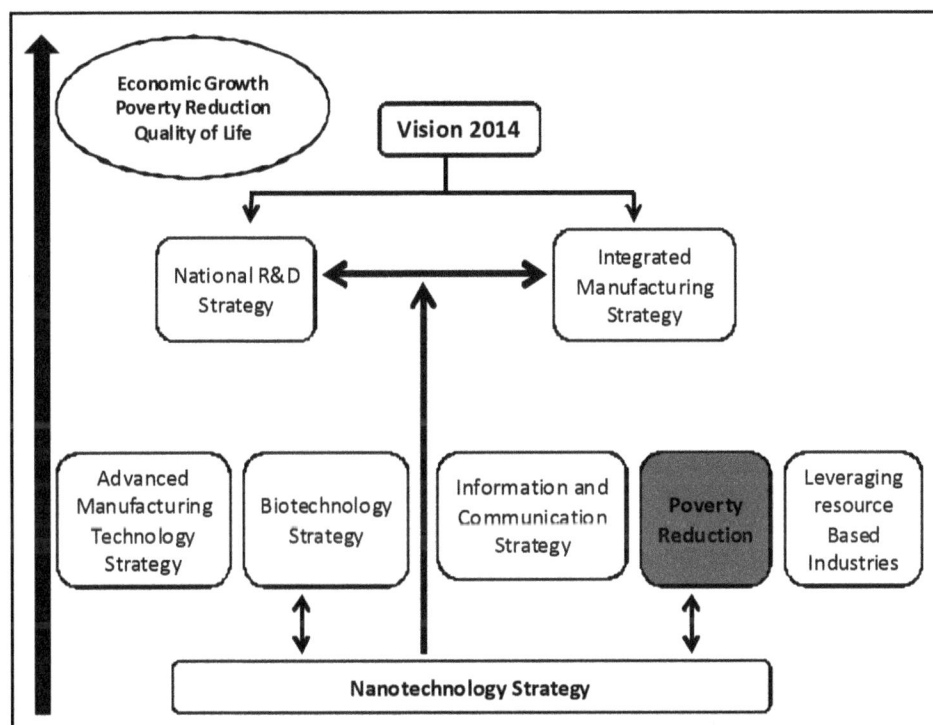

Figure 20.4: South Africa Nanotechnology Strategy (DST, 2006)

There is need for African countries to engage in nanotechnology research early to avoid the dependency syndrome which comes with late entry. Further delays in exploiting nanotechnology may result in the technology putting down its roots in the mainstream hegemonic socio-economic structure characterised by global inequality. The starting point is for the African countries to identify key areas where nanotechnology research needs to be prioritised to solve developmental challenges.

It is important that the technology is applied in areas that are crucial for the improvement of human livelihoods.

Most countries in Africa have constrained physical, human and financial resources to spearhead the development of nanotechnology. Under such a background, it is important that the few resources are pulled together for the exploitation of the technology. This can be achieved through the establishment of centres of excellence which brings together universities, colleges, not-for-profit research organisations, firms and other interested non-government organisations. The goal of the centres of excellence is to share knowledge, expertise and resources in an endeavour to bring nanotechnologies to the market faster. The centres of excellence serve as cost-shared resource centres, which stimulate research and commercialisation activities that would likely have never taken place without them.

As nanotechnology is very broad, it is imperative that African countries should prioritise domestic innovation and technological advancement which contextualise the technology to the social and economic imperatives of their citizens. On this basis, it is recommended that developing countries should not mimic the research and development programmes from the developed countries. Instead, they should align nanotechnology applications with the needs and priorities of their citizens. For example, the priorities in the development of nanotechnology in Africa should be informed by the Millenium Development Goals. By making reference to Millenium Development Goals, the idea is to focus on nanotechnology applications, namely water, health and energy that contribute to the improvement of livelihoods of the masses in developing countries. This helps to guard against being carried away by the applications of nanotechnology in "lifestyle accessories" that make the headlines in glossies. It is important that the research on nanotechnology is oriented towards solving problems that pose threats to survival of the poor in Africa.

Nanotechnology requires cooperation from both the public and private sector to accelerate the development of the technology. With limited financial resources to spearhead the development of the technology in African countries, there is need to foster public and private partnerships to pull together the limited resources. International collaboration is necessary as the case with South Africa, which works with other developing countries namely Brazil, China and India in the development of nanotechnology. These countries share expertise and other resources in the exploitation of nanotechnology.

There is need for governments in African countries to put in place intermediating structures to support technology transfer. This can be done through the setting up a range of supportive institutional infrastructures such as technology transfer offices to promote an entrepreneurial stance towards technological development. For example, University of Johannesburg has a technology transfer office, while University of the Witwatersrand has Wits Enterprises, which assist in the commercialisation of promising technologies. Still in South Africa, the government established the Technology Innovation Agency (TIA) in 2008. The objective of TIA is to stimulate and intensify technological innovation in order to improve economic growth and the quality of life of all South Africans.

It is important that African countries prioritise the process of filing patents to protect their innovation. There is a need to raise awareness and provide training on intellectual property rights in order to develop a culture among the researchers of protecting their inventions from exploitation. Though African countries have few patents on nanotechnology, it is important that they secure intellectual property rights to create incentives for investment in the costly research on nanotechnology. Universities and research institutions conducting basic research on nanotechnology should work in liaison with companies by licensing their patents to promote entrepreneurship and job creation. Without effective and high quality intellectual property protection, incentives for innovation will be greatly reduced and the technical advancement in the burgeoning nanotechnology field will suffer. The World Intellectual Property Organisation working in collaboration with African Regional Intellectual Property Organisation is working towards creating a critical mass of experts in intellectual property rights by sponsoring a Masters programme in Intellectual Property at Africa University in Zimbabwe.

There is need to develop and foster transparency and public trust in the development of nanotechnology by informing the public about both the potential risks and benefits of nanotechnology. A symmetrical analysis of both potential risks and benefits is important to raise awareness of the technology so that the consumers can make informed decisions. In South Africa, the government established the Nanotechnology Public Engagement Programme. The Nanotechnology Public Engagement programme is an initiative funded by the Department of Science and Technology and implemented by the South African Agency for Science and Technology Advancement. The programme is aimed at promoting credible, fact-based understanding of nanotechnology through awareness, dialogue and education to enable informed decision making on nanotechnology innovations.

CONCLUSIONS

The chapter has presented both the opportunities and challenges in the development of nanotechnology in Africa. What is explicit is that the opportunities which are associated with the applications of nanotechnology can be realised when the challenges in the exploitation of the technology are addressed. The opportunities include the provision of clean water, effective medicine and reliable energy. On the other hand, the challenges that militate against the exploitation of nanotechnology revolve on the novelty of the technology coupled by the innovation chasm, the difficulties that researchers have in communicating the value proposition of applications to companies and the interplay of intellectual property rights issues. There is need to put in place contingency measures to ensure that the research on nanotechnology yields products that reach the market for use by the consumers. Much of the research on nanotechnology remains in the form of promises and expectations. In some cases, the hype that was generated by the technology as a potential solution to developmental challenges is slowly diminishing. With several challenges affecting the developing countries and with nanotechnology being linked to the solutions, the impact of the technology is dependent upon capitalising the opportunities available. By drawing lessons from the general societal acceptance of

ICTs and the resistance to entry of GMOs in Biotechnology, the perceived challenges of nanotechnology in travelling to the market can be overcome. This requires a supportive environment in the form of appropriate governance structures and legal frameworks.

ACKNOWLEDGEMENTS

I acknowledge the Ministry of Science and Technology Development in Zimbabwe for nominating me to represent the country at the International Workshop on Nanotechnology in Indonesia (IWON) 2013 where I presented this paper. I am indebted to Ms. Rungano Karimanzira, Director in the Ministry of Science and Technology Development and National Focal Person for NAM S&T Centre and Professor Charles Maponga, the technical director of National Nanotechnology Programme for the valuable comments they made on this paper.

REFERENCES

1. Alemayehu, M. 2000. Industrialising Africa: Development Options and Challenges for 21st Century. Africa World Press, New Jersey, United States of America.

2. AU-NEPAD. (2010). African Innovation Outlook 2010. African Union–New Partnership for Africa's Development, Pretoria, South Africa.

3. Battelle. 2008. Global Research and Development Funding Forecast, The Business of Innovation. Research and Development Magazine.

4. Blakely, K. 2005. Engineering Breakthrough in Nanotech and MEMS.

5. Bleeker, R., and Uhlir, N. 2007. A Small Charge of Infringement: Strategic Alternatives for Nanotech Patent Defenders, Nanotechnology Law and Business, Volume. 4.

6. Bonaccorsi, A. and Piccaluga, A. 1994. A Theoretical Framework for the Evaluation of University-Industry Relationships, Research and Development Management, Volume 24 Number 3.

7. Booker, R., and Boysen, E. 2005. Nanotechnology for Dummies. Wiley Publishers, Toronto, Canada.

8. Bozeman, B. 2000. Technology Transfer and Public Policy: A Review of Research and Theory. *Research Policy*, Volume 29, Number 4-5, pp. 627-655.

9. Christensen, C.M. 1997. The Innovator's Dilemma. Harvard Business School Press, Boston MA, United States of America.

10. CSIR. 2012. The Pan African Centre of Excellence in Nanomedicine for Infectious Diseases of Poverty. Council for Scientific and Industrial Research, Pretoria.

11. D'Este, P. and Patel, P. 2005. University-Industry Linkages in the UK: What are the Factors Determining the Variety of Interactions with Industry?

12. DST. 2006. The National Nanotechnology Strategy. Department of Science and Technology, Pretoria, Republic of South Africa.

13. Einsiedel, E. F. and McMullen, G. 2004. Stakeholders and Technology: Challenges for Nanotechnology. *Health Law Review*, Volume 12, Number 3, pp.1-5.

14. Freeman, C. 2003. Policies for Developing New Technologies, SPRU Electronic Working Paper Series, Number 98.

15. Institute of Primate Research. 2011. A Research Directorate of the National Museum of Kenya, Nyani Bulletin, Volume 6, Number 1, pp. 1-4.

16. Invernizzi, N., Foladori, G., and Maclurcan, D. 2007. The Role of Nanotechnology in Development and Poverty Alleviation: A Matter of Controversy. *AZojono - Journal of Nanotechnology* Online, Volume 13, pp. 123-148.

17. Invernizzi, N., Foladori, G., and Maclurcan, D. 2008. Nanotechnology's Controversial Role for the South, *Science, Technology and Society*, Volume 13, Issue 1, pp. 123–148.

18. Kurniawan, T. A., and Sillanpaa, M. 2009. Nanomaterials: Really Small Things that can Make Things Different.

19. Lipsey, R. G., Carlaw, K.I and C. T. Bekar. 2005. Economic Transformations: General Purpose Technologies and Long-Term Economic Growth. Oxford University Press, Oxford, United Kingdom.

20. Palmberg, C. 2007. Modes, Challenges and Outcomes of Nanotechnology Transfer-A Comparative Analysis of University and Company Researchers, Paper presented at the DRUID Summer Conference 2007 on Appropriability, Proximity, Routines And Innovation, Copenhagen, CBS, Denmark, June 18 - 20, 2007.

21. Maclurcan, D. C. 2005. Nanotechnology and Developing Countries-Part 2: What Realities? *AZojono - Journal of Nanotechnology* Online, pp.1-19.

22. Mantovani, E., and Porcari, A. 2009. Mapping Study on Regulation and Governance of Nanotechnology: AIRI/Nanotech IT, The Innovation Society.

23. Meridian Institute. 2005. Nanotechnology and the Poor: Opportunities and Risks, Closing the Gaps Within and Between Sectors of Society. Meridian Institute, Washington DC, United States of America.

24. Mintek. 2011. Advanced Metal Nanoparticle Systems for Diagnostic Application. Mintek, Johannesburg.

25. Mintek. 2012. DST/Mintek Nanotechnology Innovation Centre: Biolabels Development Unit, Mintek, Johannesburg.

26. OECD. 2010. The Impacts of Nanotechnology on Companies: Policy Insights from Case Studies. OECD Publishing, Paris, France.

27. OECD. 2013. Organization for Economic Cooperation and Development-Patent Database October 2013. OECD Publishing, Paris, France.

28. Palmberg, C. 2007. Appropriability, Proximity, Routines and Innovation, DRUID Summer Conference: Appropriability, Proximity, Routines And Innovation, Copenhagen, CBS, Denmark, June 18 - 20, 2007

29. Parr, D. 2005. Will Nanotechnology Make the World a Better Place? *Trends in Biotechnology*, Volume 23, Number 8, pp. 395-398.

30. Rogers, E. M. 2003. Diffusion of Innovations. Free Press, New York, United States of America.

31. Rothrock, G. 2008. Nanomanufacturing: The Missing Link Between Discovery and Products. Liquidia Technologies, Durham, United Kingdom.

32. SAASTA. 2010. Nanotechnology, The Science of the Very Small. Department of Science and Technology, Pretoria, Republic of South Africa.

33. Salamanca-Buentello, F., Deepa, L. P., Court, E. B., Martin, D. K., Daar, A. S., and Singer, P. 2008. Nanotechnology and the Developing World. *PLoS Medicine*, Volume 2 Number 5, pp.1-14.

34. Schartinger, D., A. Schibany and H. Gassler. 2001. Interactive Relations between Universities and Firms: Empirical Evidence for Austria. *The Journal of Technology Transfer*, Volume 26 Number 3, pp. 303-328.

35. Selin, C. 2007. Expectations and the Emergence of Nanotechnology. Science, Technology and Human Values, Volume 32 Number 2, pp. 196-218.

36. Stephan, P. 1996. The Economics of Science', *Journal of Economic Literature*, XXXIV, pp.1199-1235.

37. Swiss National Science Foundation. 2009. Opportunities and Risks of Nanomaterials Implementation Plan of the National Research Programme NRP 64 Berne, 6 October 2009.

38. Valentin, E. 2000. University – Industry Cooperation: A framework of Benefits and Obstacles, Industry and Higher Education.

39. Waitz, A. and Bokhari, W. 2003. Nanotechnology Best Practices, Quantum Insight.

40. Youtie, J., Iacopetta, M and Graham, S. 2008. Assessing the Nature of Nanotechnology: Can We Uncover an Emerging General Purpose Technology? *Journal of Technology Transfer*, Volume 33, Number 3.

41. Zucker, L., Darby, M and Torero, M. (2002). Labor Mobility from Academia to Commerce, *Journal of Labour Economics*, Volume 20, Number 3, pp. 629-660.

Annexure–
Serpong Recommendations on
"Transferring Nanotechnology Concept Towards Business Perspectives"

WHILE EXPRESSING gratitude to the Ministry of Research and Technology (RISTEK), Government of Indonesia, Indonesian Institute of Sciences (LIPI) and Indonesian Society for Nano, as well as to the Centre for Science and Technology of the Non-Aligned and Other Developing Countries (NAM S&T Centre) for organizing the International Workshop on Nanotechnology (IWoN 2013): "Transferring Nanotechnology Concept Towards Business Perspectives", which was held at PUSPIPTEK, Serpong, Indonesia during 2-5 October 2013,

HAVING BEEN CONVINCED that the future technical and economic prosperity of the countries liesamong others, in the promotion of Nanoscience and Nanotechnology and their applications for industrial use to enrich and strengthen the socio-economic status of the Non Aligned Member States and other developing countries,

BY SHARING the experiences in Non Aligned and other developing countries through the presentation of their country case studies on the current status of research and development in the field,

RECOGNIZING that nanotechnology cuts across multiple disciplines such as agriculture and food, biotechnology, medicine, health, new materials, water and air purification, environmental sensing and protection, energy generation, among others, and that by exploiting the same the developing countries can create wealth to enhance the quality of life of their people,

HAVING CONSIDERED the present status and future prospects on nanotechnology in developing countries with particular focus on Materials and

Processes; and potentials of industrial applications of Nanotechnology for Health, Food and Agriculture, ElectronicDevices, Energy and Environment, notwithstanding the human capital development;

THE PARTICIPANTS FROM CAMBODIA, EGYPT, THE GAMBIA, INDIA, INDONESIA, IRAN, IRAQ, KENYA, MADAGASCAR, MALAWI, MALAYSIA, MAURITIUS, MYANMAR, NEPAL, NIGERIA, PAKISTAN, SINGAPORE, SOUTH AFRICA, SRI LANKA, SUDAN, TOGO, TANZANIA, UGANDA, VENEZUELA, VIETNAM, ZAMBIA AND ZIMBABWE EXPRESSED that the deliberations of the IWoN 2013 were a resounding success in sharing of knowledge and at the end of which the following recommendations and actions were made for adoption by the participating countries in formulating their policies and action plans for the development of Nanoscience and Nanotechnology for industrial applications, and

UNANIMOUSLY RESOLVED THAT:

☆ Emphasis should be laid on commercialization of nanoproducts to achieve socio-economic progress.

☆ The implementation, regulatory, ethical, standardization and Intellectual Property Rights (IPR) issues of nanoscience and nanotechnology should be properly addressed.

☆ Developing countries should promote need-based R&D activities and encourage entrepreneurship.

☆ Develop innovative strategies in bringing academia and R&D Institutions together with industries for mutual understanding in promoting business perspectives to tune R&D activities to the requirements of the industry which primarily aims at marketing and profit making.

☆ Create awareness among the masses regarding nanotechnology through electronic and print-media.

☆ A database of nanoscientists and nanotechnologists among the NAM and other developing countries be createdand asociety be formed under the umbrella of the NAM S&T Centre. The Indonesian Society for Nano has the mandate to spearhead this cause.The Society will further encourage the bilateral, regional and multilateral collaborations to enhance global partnerships and networking of international linkages.

The participant from Bolivarian Republic of Venezuela proposed to organize an International workshop related to nanotechnology with participation of the member countries of the NAM S&T Centre and other developing countries jointly with the NAM S&T Centre, subject to necessary approvals of the competent authorities, with date, venue, etc., to be mutually decided.

The participant from the Republic of Mauritius made a similar proposal.

The participants of the workshop heartily welcomed the above proposals.

THUS RESOLVED AND ADOPTED ON THE 3rd OCTOBER 2013 ATPUSPIPTEK, SERPONG, INDONESIA.

www.ingramcontent.com/pod-product-compliance
Lightning Source LLC
Chambersburg PA
CBHW050513190326
41458CB00005B/1522